Contents

Contributors

Dr Vishu Bhadravathi Consultant Child and Adolescent Psychiatrist, Coventry CAMHS, UK

Dr Rajan Chawla Consultant Psychiatrist (General Adult), Derbyshire Healthcare NHS Foundation Trust, Derby, UK

Dr David Clarke Consultant Psychiatrist (Learning Disability), Worcestershire Health and Care Trust, UK

Dr Jennifer Crisp (retired) formerly Consultant Psychiatrist, Psychotherapist and Safeguarding Named Doctor in North Staffordshire, UK

Mrs Dawn Crowther LLM, Mental Health Legislation Manager, South Staffordshire and Shropshire Healthcare NHS Foundation Trust, UK

Dr Martin P. Deahl Consultant Psychiatrist, South Staffordshire and Shropshire Partnership NHS Trust and Consultant Advisor in Psychiatry, Royal Air Force, UK.

Mr Roland Dix Consultant Nurse (PICU), 2gether NHS Foundation Trust, UK

Dr Stephen Dye Consultant Psychiatrist (PICU), Norfolk and Suffolk NHS Foundation Trust, UK

Dr Manjit Gahir Lead Consultant Forensic Psychiatrist, National High Secure Deaf Service, Rampton Hospital, Nottinghamshire, UK

Dr Simon Gibbon Consultant Forensic Psychiatrist, East Midlands Centre for Forensic Mental Health, Arnold Lodge, Leicester, UK

Dr Carol Henshaw Consultant in Perinatal Mental Health, Liverpool Women's NHS Foundation Trust, and Honorary Senior Lecturer, University of Liverpool, UK

Dr Richard Hodgson Consultant Psychiatrist, Lyne Brook Centre, Stoke-on-Trent, UK

Dr Christian Hosker Consultant Liaison Psychiatrist and Lead Clinician, Leeds Liaison Psychiatry Service, UK

Professor Peter Lepping Consultant Psychiatrist, Betsi Cadwaladr University Health Board, North Wales, UK, and Honorary Professor, Centre for Mental Health and Society, Bangor University, UK, and Mysore Medical College and Research Institute, Mysore, India

Dr Ken Ma Consultant Child and Adolescent Psychiatrist, Coventry CAMHS, UK

Dr Santhusi Mendis Locum Consultant Psychiatrist, Birmingham and Solihull Mental Health Foundation Trust, UK

Dr Brendon Monteiro Medical Director, St George Healthcare Group, UK

Dr Ejaz Nazir Consultant in Old Age Psychiatry, South Staffordshire and Shropshire Healthcare NHS Fundation Trust, Visiting Lecturer at the University of Staffordshire, and Visiting Senior Lecturer at the Centre of Ageing and Mental Health at Chester University, UK

Dr Kevin Nicholls Consultant Psychiatrist, Combat Stress, Shropshire, UK

Professor Rob Poole Professor of Social Psychiatry, Bangor University, Wales, UK

Dr Faisil Sethi Consultant Psychiatrist (PICU) and Associate Clinical Director, Maudsley Hospital, South London and Maudsley NHS Foundation Trust, UK

Dr Nicholas Swift Associate Specialist in Adult Psychiatry, South Staffordshire and Shropshire NHS Foundation Trust, UK

Dr Roji Thomas Consultant in Neuropsychiatry, National Centre for Mental Health, Birmingham, UK

Dr Derrett Watts Consultant Psychiatist and Clinical Director for Substance Misuse, North Staffordshire Combined Healthcare Trust, and Training Programme Director for Higher Specialist Training, General Adult Psychiatry, Health Education West Midlands, UK

Acknowledgements

Professor Peter Lepping thanks Rebecca Hoofe for her secretarial support with his chapter, the members of the European Violence in Psychiatry Research Group and the Working Group for the Prevention of Coercion in Psychiatry for their kind support in gathering the necessary scientific information for the included table as well as their comments, discussions and their continuous research to improve psychiatric care, Doctors H Firmino, M Huber, M Krishna, G Onchev, BN Raveesh, J Rodriguez and A Salmoiraghi for information about the use of medication internationally, and Professor Vimal K Sharma from Chester University and Professor Rob Poole from Glyndwr University Wrexham for their continued mentorship.

Dr Ken Ma and Dr Vishu Bhadravathi thank the library services of the Coventry and Warwickshire NHS Partnership Trust for their assistance in searching the literature and accessing appropriate articles in the preparation of their chapter.

Dr Kevin Nicholls thanks Professor Chris Freeman for advice on the initial drafts of his chapters on electroconvulsive therapy and self-poisoning, respectively, and reserves full responsibility for any errors and omissions. He also thanks Dave Jago, Publications Director at the Royal College of Psychiatrists, without whose sponsorship, guidance and encouragement this text would not exist, Katherine Sole, Staff Editor at the College, for her expert diligence in co-ordinating the drafting and editing of the text and forging its delivery to print, and Fiona Jones of the Bryntirion Resource Centre, Welshpool for her erstwhile encouragement and secretarial support.

Dr Nicholas Swift thanks Dr Jasmeet Soar, the Resuscitation Council (UK) and Professor Richard Williams for helping to include elements of the first Resuscitation Council (UK) standards for resuscitation in mental health in-patient units.

Preface

This book originated in 2011 when I was asked to raise, coordinate and edit a book on emergencies in psychiatry by the Publications Director at the Royal College of Psychiatrists. Writing this at the end of 2014, I'm unsure whether I should not have sought expert authorship of a chapter advising on suitable treatment for editors of psychiatry books!

Recruiting authoritative contributors in the current climate of relentless and insidiously cumulative financial squeeze was difficult. On the basis of occasional comment by eminent peer reviewers, I wonder whether some much-esteemed and yet only recently retired academic colleagues fully realise the extent to which the research and teaching fabric has now become eroded by sustained cuts in NHS support of these endeavours. Resource levels as recently as the 1990s, when I was a trainee, seem positively halcyon compared with contemporary stringencies.

In this context, I especially applaud the contributors who filled the breach to produce this book. They range from exceptional trainees and non-consultant grade colleagues to senior consultants and professors. I am immensely proud of the team that stepped forward.

I was also particularly fortunate in being able to persuade the only non-clinician in the team, Dawn Crowther, to write on legal considerations relating to the Mental Health Act 1983 (as amended in 2007) and the Mental Capacity Act 2005. At the risk of embarrassing Dawn, I can report without fear of contradiction that she is a foremost authority in this field.

Unable to find an expert contributor able to commit to writing a chapter on electroconvulsive therapy (ECT), I wrote that chapter myself and take full responsibility for any failings. Given the broad readership that this book targets, detailed technical considerations and legal commentary regarding ECT is precluded. All matters relating to these and otherwise are most properly deferred to *The ECT Handbook*, also published by the College, the authoritative text on this subject.

I have also provided the final chapter, which is an overview of the treatment of self-poisoning, against advice from some quarters. I must emphasise that I am in no way implying that psychiatrists should be medically managing overdose patients. However, background knowledge of medical treatment of overdose is important as a 'level 1' awareness insight and is perhaps comparable in importance to, for example, anaphylaxis treatment training. It is not improbable that a front-line psychiatrist might have first contact with a patient who has overdosed (as I have more than once), and neither is it improbable that this might be more likely than encountering anaphylactic shock. If my efforts prevent one future misguided attempt to help with milk or inappropriate emetic treatment, it will have been worthwhile.

I am indebted to all contributors and other friends and colleagues who have generously given advice and guidance. The latter are too numerous to mention by name without risk of inadvertently and unforgivably omitting someone, so I do not attempt to do so but unreservedly record my gratitude to them all.

Finally, I would iterate that it is a very special privilege to be a psychiatrist. Trying to serve some of our most vulnerable and without exception valued people at times when they do not necessarily accept their need for help will always be a challenge truly worthy of our society's best endeavours. Further to this, I take this unique opportunity to record my especial thanks to my one-time trainers Dr David Myers and Dr Patrick Campbell (both formerly of Shelton Hospital, Shrewsbury) and Professor John Cox (formerly of Keele University and one-time Registrar and President of the Royal College of Psychiatrists). I can only hope that I have not fallen too far short of their teaching and example.

K.N.

CHAPTER 1

Assessment of suicide risk

Rajan Chawla

Suicide can be defined as self-inflicted death with evidence that the person intended to die (Kaplan & Sadock, 1998; Jacobs *et al*, 2003). It is a major cause of death: in fact, the tenth most common cause of death worldwide (1.5% of all deaths; Hawton & Heeringen, 2009). Suicide accounts for approximately 5000 deaths per year in the UK and, according to the National Confidential Inquiry into Suicide and Homicide by People with Mental Illness report (2011), this rate has decreased over the past decade. The most common methods of suicide in the UK are hanging, overdose (self-poisoning) and multiple injuries (caused by jumping from a height, for example, or train incidents). It also reports that suicide by hanging has increased, while suicides by carbon-monoxide poisoning, self-poisoning and firearms fatalities have decreased.

Assessing risk in patients presenting with suicidal ideation is fundamental to the practice of psychiatry. A structured and systematic approach that evaluates risk is needed to inform decisions about the patient's care. Many trained professionals report difficulty in assessing risk (Way *et al*, 1998), and assessment might be more complicated for informal in-patients (Mahal *et al*, 2009).

Half of all people who die by suicide have had previous contact with mental health services, and half of this group have had contact within the previous 12 months (Department of Health, 2001). This finding is consistent with the National Confidential Inquiry into Suicide and Homicide by People with Mental Illness report (2011), which estimated that 24% of suicides had been in contact with mental health services in the year before death. Predictors of suicide include male gender, substance misuse, increased age, previous suicide attempt, violent method of suicide attempt and history of psychiatric disorder (Nordentoft, 2007).

Key features in assessment

National Health Service trusts and other service providers have varying protocols, or in some cases no protocol at all, for assessing suicide risk. Junior doctors and other professionals fear that they are ill-equipped to assess suicide potential (Bongar & Harmatz, 1991; Boris & Fritz, 1998; Sudak *et al*, 2007). The effects of clinical experience on professional judgement have not been sufficiently evaluated; neither have the intuitive benefits of empathy and non-judgmental rapport on outcome been confirmed.

Risk factors

Predisposing factors for suicidal thinking and behaviour have been extensively researched. While assessment of risk is important, this can at best be but conscientious. Most individuals who have thoughts of or display behaviours of self-destruction will not kill themselves. Defensive practice when weighing this causes unnecessary admissions to general or mental health settings, not only adversely affecting the patient's well-being but also causing misuse of resources and diverting attention from the effective care of others.

Suicide risk factors have been categorised as baseline, acute, chronic high risk and chronic high risk with acute exacerbation (Bryan & Rudd, 2006). Others have classified these factors as static, stable, dynamic or future (Bouch & Marshall, 2003).

Static risk factors are usually historical facts, and cannot be changed. Examples of static factors are childhood trauma, a history of mental health problems, alcohol and illicit substance use and previous suicidal behaviour.

Dynamic risk factors, on the other hand, can change. For example, a coexisting psychiatric disorder might fluctuate. Future risk factors can be predictable; for example, an anniversary or any forthcoming likely stressful event. Physical illness can also be a risk factor, for instance patients with physical illness such as stroke, myocardial infarction, cancer, chronic pain and neurological disorders can present with suicidal ideation.

A list of factors that increase the risk of suicide is given below. Perhaps predictably, the higher the number of risk factors an individual has, the higher their risk of suicide (Schwartz & Rogers, 2004):

- increasing age (>45 years for men and >55 years for women)
- previous suicide attempts
- male gender
- family history of completed suicide
- isolation from family, friends or significant others
- any acute changes in health status, worsening of physical illness
- alcohol and other substance misuse, abuse or dependence
- domestic violence
- social isolation
- access to lethal means
- unemployment, financial difficulty
- severe anxiety, depression, psychotic disorder, or other mental illness

- impulsivity and hopelessness
- chronic pain
- poor prognosis of associated illness
- previous suicide attempt
- recent discharge from a hospital.

Klonsky *et al* (2012) investigated the association between hopelessness and attempted suicide in psychotic disorders. Their results suggest that even modest level of hopelessness seem to confer an increased risk of suicide in patients with psychotic disorders.

Patients under the care of drug and alcohol treatment services have higher rates of attempted and completed suicide (Ross *et al*, 2012). Having known someone who died by suicide increases the risk of subsequent suicide in vulnerable people (Crosby & Sacks, 2002). De Leo *et al* (2005) emphasise that suicidal tendency fluctuates over time. Crucially, the presence of mental illness increases risk and, in depressed mood, the probability of experiencing suicide ideation is increased by up to three times (De Leo *et al*, 2005).

Miret *et al* (2011) found that individuals are more likely to be treated in a psychiatric hospital after a suicide attempt if they have history of previous suicide attempts or past psychiatric treatment, show suicidal ideation or suicide planning, and when they lack family support.

Physical illness is linked with an increased risk of suicide, particularly in the presence of mood disorders or other psychiatric disorders (Jacobs *et al*, 2003). Evidence suggests that some diagnoses, including HIV, lung diseases, cancer and neurological conditions such as Huntington's chorea, are specifically associated with a higher risk of mental health problems and suicide (Goodwin *et al*, 2003)

Risk of suicide is increased after discharge from psychiatric in-patient care, and has been found to be 100 times higher than among the general population (see Hunt *et al*, 2009). Hunt *et al* (2009) have explored various possibilities that might account for this: poor follow-up in the community; disjointed continuity of care; self-discharge; and deterioration following reduction of care. The first 2–3 weeks after discharge are considered a period of high risk; the first week in particular is a time of increased vulnerability (Hunt *et al*, 2009). Association of suicide with mental illness, alcohol and illicit substance misuse might exacerbate risk and is discussed below.

Men are more likely to take their own life than women, but more women than men attempt suicide or self-harm (Kaplan & Sadock, 1998). Marriage seems to be a protective factor, at least for men. Divorced men have been shown to be nearly 2.4 times more likely to take their own life than their married counterparts (Kposowa, 2000). Social isolation, loneliness and lack of social support or network increase the risks of attempted and completed suicide, particularly in older adults (Waren *et al*, 2003).

Genetic vulnerability to suicidal behaviour might be a predictor of suicidal behaviour in adolescents, reflected in a family history of suicidal behaviour.

Assessment

An odd, widely held perception is that every suicide is predictable and consequently could have been prevented by healthcare professionals. In reality, identifying those most at risk of suicide is difficult. Even when concerns are highlighted, practical management will be necessarily constrained by resources, patient views and legal considerations. Bryan and Rudd (2006) argue that the clinician's role is not to predict suicide, but to identify when a patient is at increased risk of attempting suicide and respond appropriately. Comprehensive clinical assessment is paramount in identifying the intensity of suicide risk. The overall aims of assessment are as follows:

- to evaluate individual suicide drivers versus protective factors
- to understand the level of severity of suicidal intent
- to identify factors that can change the severity of risk
- to provide care and therapeutic interventions; this might include or preclude hospital admission.

Making decisions about suicide risk management is an integral part of psychiatric practice. A structured and systematic approach to assessment is beneficial in identifying those at higher risk. During the assessment, the following questions may be useful (the emphasis placed on each will depend on the circumstances of each case).

- What is the likelihood of an untoward incident?
- What are the possible consequences if it were to occur?
- Can this be prevented and, if so, how?
- Is there stated intent to employ violent and immediate means? If so, is there ready access to this means (e.g. dangerous weapons, railway line)?
- How and where can this individual be supported?
- What are the immediate and long-term plans to improve outcome?
- What is the overall level of risk?

Thorough assessment will allow the formulation of a management plan that is proportionate and as safe as possible. 'Safe' can have a different meaning for different individuals, depending on their unique circumstances. For example, one patient might have a partner who can take time off work to provide support, whereas another patient might have a partner with his or her own health problems, who is unable to provide the support needed.

Competent assessment is a complex process requiring training, knowledge and experience. Individual situations will vary and a checklist approach should be avoided.

Background information and current presentation

Distressed people might be reluctant to disclose their situation without prompting. Questions should be asked about the following factors:

- significant stress (e.g. death of a loved one)
- mental health problems (e.g. depression, psychosis)
- substance misuse
- previous suicide attempts and self-destructive behaviour
- emotional, sexual or physical abuse
- medical illness or chronic physical problems.

A close family member or a friend can provide invaluable information and insights into the person's history, recent significant factors and recent changes in their demeanour or behaviour. Contrary to myth, individuals who have repeatedly self-harmed are not at lower risk of fatal action. Indeed, a previous history of thoughts of self-harm predicts increased risk.

Suicidal intent

It is a common misconception that asking about suicide increases the likelihood of a person attempting suicide. This is untrue and an open discussion about suicidal ideation is crucial to thorough assessment (Schwartz & Roger, 2004). Gathering details of the persistence of such ideation and over what period of time, the drafting of a suicide note or putting affairs in order, the use of alcohol or other drugs, and an assessment of impulsivity informed by these factors, past actions, emotional state and subjective reporting of intent will all help to determine the level of risk. Further enquiry into detailed planning or efforts to access ligatures, exhaust hoses, lethal chemicals or weapons (for example) is crucial.

Repeated, frequent risk assessments

Suicide risk will change, as suicidal ideation is usually dynamic. Consequently, it is important that assessment is repeated regularly. Suicide has occurred on wards, in police stations and indeed on intensive care psychiatric units when the patient has been under constant observation (National Confidential Inquiry into Suicide and Homicide by People with Mental Illness, 2011). Ligature points (any environmental feature that could be used to support a strangulation device) on windows or doors are commonly employed and belts are sometimes used as a ligature.

Protective factors

Protective factors are crucially weighed in the assessment of suicide risk:

- strong psychosocial supports (e.g. a supportive partner)
- evidence of previously deployed coping mechanisms

- cultural and religious beliefs against suicide
- reasons for living (e.g. children or animals)
- worthwhile employment, whether paid or voluntary
- positive plans for the future
- insight into psychological distress and causes for this (e.g. comorbid physical illness)
- medication adherence
- engagement with a healthcare professional or wider services.

Mental state examination

Observation of behaviour by an informed assessor can reveal crucial information about a patient's unspoken feelings and lend another dimension to informing the formulation. Undergraduate texts describe the more obvious signs of mental illness, such as distraction, preoccupation, and psychomotor retardation. However, the experienced clinician will also be alert to more subtle evidence of distress, such as a fleeting tendency to tearfulness that might be contained or a person 'talking past' an enquiry about a potentially painful subject. Gently refocusing on relevant points and revisiting topics that the patient might prefer to skate over will be necessary. Whatever the patient's response, be it reassuring explanation, anger, tearfulness, or remaining mute, it will be helpful in determining what is going on and how best to assist. Open questions are most helpful in gauging how best to negotiate the interview and identify areas of concern for the patient in a non-threatening and non-directive fashion. Selective use of closed questions will be appropriate in defining matters more precisely at pertinent stages in the interview, and will be needed to concisely conclude matters that might be distressing for the patient. Sufficient time must be given to allow emotional topics to be kindly broached in a sensitive manner, with allowance for silences and gathering thoughts if necessary.

Suicide and mental illness

People with a history of mental illness or suffering from current mental health problems are at higher risk of suicide compared with those without mental health issues. Common psychiatric diagnoses associated with suicide in the UK are listed below (Hunt *et al*, 2006; National Confidential Inquiry into Suicide and Homicide by People with Mental Illness, 2011):

- affective disorders (32–47%)
- schizophrenia (15–20%)
- alcohol dependence (8–17%)
- personality disorder (8–11%)
- drug dependence (3–9%).

More than 90% of people who die by suicide are clinically depressed, and the presence of another mental health problem or substance use-related disorder is an added risk factor (Moscicki, 2001). Comorbidity of mental disorder and physical illness also increases suicide risk (Lönnqvist, 2000).

Mental disorders, especially depression, are present in more than 90% of suicides, and over 80% are untreated at the time of death (Lönnqvist *et al*, 1995; Henriksson *et al*, 2001). A lifetime suicide risk of about 6% has been calculated for all depressed patients (Inskip *et al*, 1998). However, the majority of individuals with suicidal thoughts do not attempt to kill themselves (Kessler *et al*, 1999).

Substantial evidence indicates that early detection of risk and subsequent risk management reduces the incidence of suicide (Appleby, 2012). Melle *et al* (2004) investigated the effects of preventive measures on the rate of suicidal thoughts and attempts. They concluded that such behaviour was significantly less common in individuals who received early assessment and intervention, including regular contact and repeated reviews. Worryingly, Hunt *et al* (2006) found that over 60% of individuals with schizophrenia who died by suicide had been in contact with mental health services in the week before. Effective treatment and intervention is the key to decreasing the risk of suicide in people suffering from mental illness. Risk factors for suicide with mental illness include not taking medication, non-engagement with mental health teams or services, and failure to seek help in case of relapse.

MacLean *et al* (2011) examined the association between suicidal behaviour and physical illness in individuals with a history of mood disorder. They found that physical problems such as respiratory diseases and hypertension are associated with increased suicidal behaviour, independent of any comorbid mental illness. Tidemalm *et al* (2008) investigated the impact of psychiatric illness on continuing risk after a suicide attempt, and confirmed that the severity of mental disorder at the time of a suicide attempt significantly influences future risk. A large number of suicides occur in the first year after an unsuccessful suicidal action, emphasising the importance of high-quality aftercare following discharge.

Individuals with schizophrenia or other psychotic conditions are often considered unpredictable and dangerous. Although some individuals might be vulnerable to a rapidly deteriorating mental state, this possibility should be factored into a risk management plan, with particular consideration given to how relapse can be quickly detected and action taken. Stereotyped generalisations regarding unpredictability and any consequential sense of misplaced inevitability is inappropriate and might result in a higher risk of suicide (Fialko *et al*, 2006). Individuals with improving insight might suffer low mood, hopelessness and a higher risk of suicide. This can occur in the wake of successful response to antipsychotic medication (Lysaker *et al*, 2007).

Suicide and alcohol and drug use

Alcohol and drug dependence, particularly substance misuse, are significant risk factors for suicide (Kessler *et al*, 1999; Darke *et al*, 2000; Coffin *et al*, 2003; Sher, 2006; Bohnert *et al*, 2010). Individuals recently discharged from prison or hospital are also at increased risk of death by overdose that might be accidental because of a reduced level of tolerance after a period of institution-imposed abstinence (Seymour *et al*, 2000).

Individuals commonly use alcohol and drugs to cope with suicidal ideation, and lifetime mortality due to suicide in people dependent on alcohol is approximately 18% (Sher, 2006). If dependency follows, this might further increase the risk of suicide (Murphy *et al*, 1992).

In their study on suicides among alcohol abusers, Murphy and colleagues (1992) found that more than four-fifths of those who took their own life had communicated that they had suicidal thoughts and over a third had made a previous suicide attempt. Two-thirds had little or no social support, half were unemployed and half had significant medical problems. Nearly two-fifths were living alone. Murphy and colleagues (1992) concluded that, as nine out of ten 'alcoholic' suicides assessed had at least three of the above factors, the assessment of suicidal risk in this group should consider these factors.

Risk minimisation

Suicide risk assessment is individual specific, requiring a systematic, yet flexible approach. Common methods of suicide in England include hanging, drug overdose, jumping from a height and car exhaust (carbon monoxide) poisoning. Men are more likely to use violent methods, such as hanging (Varnik et al, 2008).

Evidence for the effectiveness of psychotropic medication treatment is limited. Lithium is effective in reducing suicide risk in both bipolar affective disorder and unipolar depression (Baldessarini *et al*, 1999). Clozapine might reduce the suicide rate in individuals with schizophrenia, but this benefit is possibly offset by increased mortality related to metabolic syndrome.

Prevention

Prevention measures can be classified as primary or secondary. Primary preventive measures include educational programmes for mental health professionals and other healthcare workers. Providing public information about where to seek help in crisis is an important measure that can be focused on voluntary agencies and other providers that interact with high-risk populations. Other strategies include restriction of access to methods for suicide. Lester (1998) recommended a number of ways to do this, including strict gun laws, vehicle emissions control, restricting access to the tops of buildings, fencing bridges, limiting the packet size of medication frequently used for suicidal acts, packaging pills in plastic blisters, and seeking permission to remove high-risk items from the homes of those vulnerable to suicidal thinking (see also Mann *et al*, 2005).

Secondary prevention includes screening of at-risk individuals, providing appropriate support and treatment when indicated to reduce risk of further harm, and educating patients and carers about mental disorders. There has been a recent decrease in hospital suicide rates, probably due in part to guidelines by the Department of Health regarding removal of ligature points on wards (National Confidential Inquiry into Suicide and Homicide by People with Mental Illness, 2013).

Summary

Not all deaths by suicide are preventable. However, the high-quality assessment of vulnerable people, with the careful evaluation of risks and the formulation of robust care plans, is essential in preventing as many suicides as possible. The capacity of services to deliver appropriate treatment and sufficient support when early signs of relapse indicate a need is the challenge to be met.

References

Appleby L (2012) Suicide prevention: the evidence on safer clinical care is now good and should be adopted internationally. *International Psychiatry*, **9**: 27–29.

Baldessarini RJ, Tondo L, Hennen J (1999) Effects of lithium and its discontinuation on suicidal behavior in bipolar manic depressive disorders. *Journal of Clinical Psychiatry*, **60**: 77–84.

Bohnert SBA, Roeder K, Ilgen AM (2010) Unintentional overdose and suicide among substance users: a review of overlap and risk factors. *Drug and Alcohol Dependence*, **110**: 183–192.

Bongar B, Harmatz M (1991) Clinical psychology graduate education in the study of suicide: availability, resources, and importance. *Suicide and Life-Threatening Behaviour*, **21**: 231–244.

Boris NW, Fritz GK (1998) Pediatric residents' experiences with suicidal patients: implications for training. *Academic Psychiatry*, **22**: 21–28.

Bouch J, Marshall JJ (2003) *Suicide – Risk Assessment and Management Manual (S–RAMM). Research Edition*. Cognitive Centre Foundation.

Bryan CJ, Rudd MD (2006) Advances in the assessment of suicide risk. *Journal of Clinical Psychology*, **62**: 185–200.

Coffin PO, Galea S, Ahern J, *et al* (2003) Opiates, cocaine and alcohol combinations in accidental drug overdose deaths in New York City, 1990–98. *Addiction*, **98**: 739–747.

Crosby AE, Sacks JJ (2002) Exposure to suicide: incidence and association with suicidal ideation and behavior – United States, 1994. *Suicide and Life-Threatening Behaviour*, **32**: 321–328.

Darke S, Ross J, Zodar D, *et al* (2000). *Heroin-related deaths in New South Wales*, Australia, 1992–1996. *Drug Alcohol Depend*, **60**: 141–150.

De Leo D, Cerin E, Spathonis K, *et al* (2005) Lifetime risk of suicide ideation and attempts in an Australian community: prevalence, suicidal process, and help-seeking behaviour. *Journal of Affective Disorders*, **86**: 215–224.

Department of Health (2001) *Safety First: Five-Year Report of the National Confidential Inquiry into Suicide and Homicide by People with Mental Illness. Department of Health* (http://www.dh.gov.uk/en/Publicationsandstatistics/Publications/PublicationsPolicyAndGuidance/DH_4006679).

Fialko L, Freeman D, Bebbington PE, *et al* (2006) Understanding suicidal ideation in psychosis: findings from the psychological prevention of relapse in psychosis. *Acta Psychiatrica Scandinavica*, **114**: 177–186.

Goodwin RD, Marusic A, Hoven CW (2003) Suicide attempts in United States: the role of physical illness. *Social Science & Medicine*, **56**: 1783–1788.

Hawton K, Heeringen K (2009) Suicide. *Lancet*, **373**: 1372–1381.

Henriksson S, Bothius G, Isacsson G (2001) Suicides are seldom prescribed antidepressants: findings from a prospective prescription database in Jamtland county, Sweden, 1985–1995. *Acta Psychiatrica Scandinavica*, **103**: 301–306.

Hunt I, Kapur N, Windfuhr K, *et al* (2006) Suicide in schizophrenia: findings from a national clinical survey. *Journal of Psychiatric Practice*, **12**: 139–147.

Hunt I, Kapur N, Webb R, *et al* (2009) Suicide in recently discharged psychiatric patients: a case control study. *Psychological Medicine*, **39**: 443–449.

Inskip HM, Harris EC, Barraclough B (1998) Lifetime risk of suicide for affective disorder, alcoholism and schizophrenia. *British Journal of Psychiatry*, **172**: 35–37.

Jacobs DG, Baldessarini RJ, Conwell Y, *et al* (2003) Practice guidelines for the assessment and treatment of patients with suicidal behavior. *American Journal of Psychiatry*, **160**: 3–60.

Kaplan HI, Sadock BJ (1998) The brain and behaviour. In *Synopsis of Psychiatry* (8th edn). Lippincott.

Kessler RC, Borges G, Walters EE (1999) Prevalence of and risk factors for lifetime suicide attempts in the National Comorbidity Survey. *Archives of General Psychiatry*, **50**: 971–974.

Klonsky ED, Kotov R, Bakst S, *et al* (2012) Hopelessness as a predictor of attempted suicide among first admission patients with psychosis: a 10-year cohort study. *Suicide and Life-Threatening Behaviour*, **42**: 1–10.

Kposowa AJ (2000) Marital status and suicide in the National Longitudinal Mortality Study. *Journal of Epidemiology and Community Health*, **54**: 254–261.

Lester D (1998) Preventing suicide by restricting access to methods for suicide. *Archives of Suicide Research*, **4**: 7–24.

Lönnqvist JK (2000) Psychiatric aspects of suicidal behaviour: depression. In *The International Handbook of Suicide and Attempted Suicide* (eds K Hawton, K Heeringen). Wiley–Blackwell.

Lönnqvist JK, Henriksson MM, Isometsa ET, *et al* (1995) Mental disorders and suicide prevention. *Psychiatry and Clinical Neurosciences*, **49** (Suppl 1): S111–S116.

Lysaker PH, Roe D, Yanos PT (2007) Toward understanding the insight paradox: internalized stigma moderates the association between insight and social functioning, hope and self esteem among people with schizophrenia spectrum disorders. *Schizophrenia Bulletin*, **33**: 192–199.

MacLean J, Kinley DJ, Jacobi F, *et al* (2011) The relationship between physical conditions and suicidal behaviour among those with mood disorders. *Journal of Affective Disorders*, **130**: 245–250.

Mahal SK, Chee CB, Lee JC, *et al* (2009) Improving the quality of suicide risk assessments in the psychiatric emergency setting: physician documentation of process indicators. *Journal of the American Osteopathic Association*, **109**: 354–358.

Mann JJ, Apter A, Bertolote J, *et al* (2005) Suicide prevention strategies: a systematic review. *JAMA*, **294**: 2064–2074.

Melle I, Larsen T, Haahr U, *et al* (2004) Reducing the duration of untreated first-episode psychosis: effects on clinical presentation. *Archives of General Psychiatry*, **61**: 143–150.

Miret M, Nuevo R, Morant C, *et al* (2011) Suicide risk in psychiatric hospitalisation after suicide attempt. *Crisis*, **32**: 65–73.

Moscicki EK (2001) Epidemiology of completed and attempted suicide: toward a framework for prevention. *Clinical Neuroscience Research*, **1**: 310–323.

Murphy GE, Wetzel RD, Robins E, *et al* (1992) Multiple risk factors predict suicide in alcoholism. *Archives of General Psychiatry*, **49**: 459–463.

National Confidential Inquiry into Suicide and Homicide by People with Mental Illness (2011). *National Confidential Inquiry Annual Report: England, Wales and Scotland*. The University of Manchester (http://www.medicine.manchester.ac.uk/mentalhealth/ research/suicide/prevention/nci/inquiryannualreports/Annual_Report_July_2011.pdf).

National Confidential Inquiry into Suicide and Homicide by People with Mental Illness (2013). *Annual Report: England, Wales and Scotland*. The University of Manchester (http://www.bbmh.manchester.ac.uk/cmhr/centreforsuicideprevention/nci/reports/ NCIAnnualReport2013V2.pdf).

Nordentoft M (2007) Prevention of suicide and attempted suicide in Denmark. Epidemiological studies of suicide and intervention studies in selected risk groups. *Danish Medical Bulletin*, **54**: 306–369.

Ross J, Drake S, Kelly E, *et al* (2012) Suicide risk assessment practices: a national survey of generalist drug and alcohol residential rehabilitation services. *Drug and Alcohol Review*, **31**: 790–796.

Schwartz RC, Rogers JR (2004) Suicide assessment and evaluation strategies: A primer for counselling psychologists. *Counselling Psychology Quarterly*, **17**: 89–97.

Seymour A, Oliver JS, Black M (2000) Drug-related deaths among recently released prisoners in the Strathclyde region of Scotland. *Journal of Forensic Science*, **45**: 649–654.

Sher L (2006) Alcohol consumption and suicide. *Quarterly Journal of Medicine*, **99**: 57–61.

Sudak D, Roy A, Sudak H, *et al* (2007) Deficiencies in suicide training in primary care specialties: a survey of training directors. *Academic Psychiatry*, **31**: 345–349.

Tidemalm D, Langstrom N, Lichtenstein P, *et al* (2008) Risk of suicide after suicide attempt according to coexisting psychiatric disorder: Swedish cohort study with long term follow up. *British Medical Journal*, **337**: a2205.

Varnik A, Kolves K, van der Feltz-Cornelis CM, *et al* (2008) Suicide methods in Europe: a gender-specific analysis of countries participating in 'the European Alliance Against Depression'. *Journal of Epidemiology and Public Health*, **62**: 545–551.

Waren M, Rubenowitz E, Wilhelmson K (2003) Predictors of suicide in the older elderly. *Gerontogist*, **49**: 398–406.

Way BB, Allen MH, Mumpower JL, *et al* (1998) Interrater agreement among psychiatrists in psychiatric emergency assessments. *American Journal of Psychiatry*, **155**: 1423–1428.

CHAPTER 2

Violence and aggression

Peter Lepping

It is an uncomfortable truth that violence and aggression is a common occurrence in health settings. It has been argued that, among all occupational groups, 'healthcare workers are ranked as one of the most likely groups to experience workplace aggression' (Chappell & Di Martino, 2006). Anecdotally, there is a perception by many health workers that psychiatric-unit staff are particularly prone to experiencing violence because of a perceived link between mental health problems and aggression. However, the reality is that violence and aggression is widespread in all medical settings (Hahn *et al*, 2008; Lepping *et al* 2013), with serious consequences for staff and patients.

In the management of such violence, healthcare staff commonly employ de-escalation techniques, but occasionally there is also a need for measures of restraint, including physical restraint, enforced medication and, in psychiatric settings, seclusion. These measures are often considered with great trepidation by staff and patients. There are a number of significant ethical issues with regard to restraint. Although most healthcare workers would consider proportionate restraint to be occasionally necessary, there are many who advocate that medicine should never use any form of restraint at all. However, most guidelines employed across the European Union allow proportionate, reasonable, appropriate and considerate restraint to avoid imminent harm. It is less clear to what degree restraint can occasionally be used beyond those limited circumstances. Keski-Valkama and colleagues (2010), for example, found that although agitation and disorientation were the most frequent reasons for the use of restraint and seclusion, the duration of those measures was not determined directly by the reasons for using them. They concluded that 'clinical practice may deviate from theoretical and legal grounds established for such measures'. This exemplifies the importance of sound ethical structures and guidance around the use of restraint to manage violence and aggression (Steinert & Lepping, 2011).

Although it is obviously important to protect patients from inappropriate and unnecessarily long restraint measures, it is equally important for employers to protect their staff from workplace violence and assaults. In the UK, many initiatives of so-called 'zero tolerance' have been tried over the years, with limited success in reducing the incidence of violence. However, it is well proven that work-related violence negatively affects the psychological and physical well-being of healthcare staff (Richter & Berger, 2000; Needham *et al*, 2005). Worryingly, there is some evidence that violence towards staff can adversely affect the quality of care they subsequently provide (Needham *et al*, 2005). Workplace violence, therefore, has the potential to have a negative impact on both staff motivation and patient care.

As Professor Taylor from Cardiff University points out in her review on psychosis and violence, 'individuals with psychosis are often feared' (Taylor, 2008). She confirms the well-established, small but consistent relationship between schizophrenia and violent acts. However, she concludes that 'public fears about individuals with psychotic illnesses [regarding violence in the community] are largely unfounded, although there would be benefit in greater attention to the safety of those in their close social circle' (Taylor, 2008). It is probably in part this public fear that has fed the assumption that violence is particularly prevalent in psychiatric hospitals and among psychiatric patients. However, this is not the case, as Hahn and colleagues (2008) showed in their review of patient and visitor violence in general hospitals, which included 31 studies from around the world. Patient and visitor violence is commonplace in medical wards (Hahn *et al*, 2008; Lepping *et al* 2013), as well as in psychiatric wards. However, there seems to be a better awareness and subsequently more widespread training about violence in psychiatry compared with other medical specialities. The task for health staff and healthcare providers is to ensure a safe environment and appropriate management of violent and aggressive incidents.

Prevalence

Current research suggests that about 10% of hospitalised psychiatric patients have engaged in some form of violence prior to admission (Bjørkly, 1995). Given that this is a much higher rate of violence than in the psychiatric population as a whole (Taylor, 2008), prevalence of violence might be overestimated if we only take into account the hospitalised psychiatric population (Nijman *et al*, 2006). The prevalence of violence among psychiatric in-patients is as difficult to estimate as the prevalence of restraint used in psychiatric settings. Many of the reasons are methodological. What seems an easy enough epidemiological task actually becomes very complex in detail. The problem starts when we try to define what violence and aggression is. The World Health Organization defines violence as 'the intentional use of physical force or power, threatened or actual, against oneself, another person, or against a group or community, that either results in or has a high likelihood of resulting in injury, death, psychological harm, maldevelopment, or deprivation' (World Health Organization, 2012). This definition is commonly used in violence research and has a degree of face validity. It has somewhat superseded older definitions that focus on injury (Bandura, 1986). Even accepting the World Health Organization's definition of violence, not all studies necessarily follow this definition. Depending on their settings, they might look at verbal abuse, threats or physical assaults separately or in combination.

Another issue is the way in which violence is measured. There are problems with any type of measurement and its accuracy. In the past, people have used self-reporting, staff observational scales, and staff self-reports. All these measures rely on the accuracy of the reporter. The main problem with any attempt to collect prospective data is that staff can be too busy to report every incident. In addition, there are difficulties with the statistics of the epidemiology of violence. In many settings, it is a few patients who are responsible for the majority of violent incidents. The same is true for restraint. The question, therefore, is whether we should use the mean or the median as the preferred statistical measure, as only the use of medians would accurately manage statistical outliers. There are also problems with measuring what actually happens in individual hospitals. It is unclear whether we ought to look at incidents per admission, per patient or per hospital day. All of these can yield very different results, because some patients have long and others have short lengths of stay. Some might have only one admission, whereas others might have several admissions in the same year. It becomes even more difficult if we want to calculate incidents per 100 000 population, which is only possible to a reasonable extent if we have hospitals that cover defined catchment areas. All this makes national and international comparisons very difficult. However, Steinert and colleagues have suggested the use of the following definitions to analyse violence and restraint: separate outcome reporting for different diagnostic groups; the use of median rather than mean to avoid over-proportionate influence of outliers when restraint episodes per patient are measured; and violence/coercion measured in relation to in-patient days (Steinert et al, 2010).

Despite all of those methodological problems, it is estimated that the proportion of psychiatric in-patients who are involved in assaults is around 15–30% (Nijman et al, 2006). However, significant differences seem to exist between various European countries. Nijman et al (2005) examined the use of the Staff Observation Aggression Scale (SOAS). Its research version, SOAS-R, has been the recommended tool for logging incidents of violence for some time. In their review of 15 years of SOAS research, the number of aggressive incidents per patient per year on acute admission wards throughout Europe varied considerably, with a range of 0.4 to 33.2 incidents (mean 9.3). They concluded that, even when data were obtained in a comparable manner, substantial differences in aggression rates remain between wards and countries, with the Netherlands seeming to have a particularly high rate of incidents of aggression on acute wards

(Nijman *et al*, 2005). It has to be added that the Dutch tradition of using long times of seclusion is not at all characteristic of psychiatric settings across Europe. The other country that is a relative outlier in this respect is Switzerland, where the average length of one restraint episode is about 40 hours. However, both countries have made enormous efforts to reduce these times. Organisations such as the European Violence in Psychiatry Research Group, founded in 1997, have significantly contributed to a better understanding of violence and restraint across Europe. Understanding the international context has led the outlying countries in particular to seriously rethink policy and practice. These collaborations play an important part in gathering data and finding ways to reduce violence and restraint across healthcare settings in Europe and elsewhere.

The same geographic variation exists for the number of restraints in psychiatric units. The best available review to date shows the mean number of measures per patient ranging between 1.4 in Finland, Spain and Switzerland to 5.6 in Norway. Similarly, the mean duration of an intervention varies between 10 minutes in Wales and 1,182 hours in the Netherlands. The number of patients subjected to restraint per admission varied between <3% in Norway and Wales and 35.6% in Austria (Steinert *et al*, 2010). The problem with these data is that they only provide a snapshot of particular units: data for larger regions rarely exists.

The best available data on violence towards staff come from the National Audit of Violence, conducted in England and Wales in 2003–2005 and again in 2006–2007 (Royal College of Psychiatrists, 2005, 2007). The audits found that there were marked differences in results between non-nursing and nursing staff and between the types of psychiatric hospitals audited. The number of nursing staff who had experienced violence was consistently high, but ranged from 73% in forensic units up to 86% in short-stay learning disability units. Other, non-nursing members of the clinical teams experienced much lower levels of violence. The experiences of non-clinicians were also generally better: 36% of patients and 18% of visitors experienced violence on psychiatric wards. Interestingly, 48% of patients felt that staff sometimes threatened to use medication or other forms of restraint to control patients' behaviour, whereas only 30% of nursing staff and 24% of medical staff felt that this happens (Royal College of Psychiatrists, 2005). In the 2006–2007 audit, the proportion of nurses in adult units who had experienced upset or distress was 58%, those threatened was 72% and those assaulted was 46%, which were slighly lower than in the previous audit. The figures were much lower in other staff groups, and lower again in patients and visitors. Interestingly, in this audit, acute and intensive care units were much more likely to report any category of aggression (abuse, threats or assaults) than rehabilitation or forensic units (Royal College of Psychiatrists, 2007). The audit results from England and Wales are broadly in keeping with later findings from Finland (Keski-Valkama *et al*, 2010).

Bowers and colleagues (2011) calculated incidents in various ways to try and give a comprehensive overview. Their systematic review included 128 papers for which at least one measure of the rate of aggression or violence could be calculated. The studies came from a variety of settings, including acute and forensic wards. Well over 50% came from English-speaking countries (USA 35, UK 31, Australia 14, Canada 5). The remaining studies came from the Netherlands, Sweden, Italy, Germany, Israel and Taiwan. As other researchers have found, the definition of violence and aggression varied widely between studies, but they managed to calculate incidents using a variety of methodologies. They reported that '32.4% of patients displayed violence, there were 182.8 violent events per 100 admissions per month, and 26.2% of admissions per month displayed violence. Per 100 occupied bed days, there were 3.14 events, and they found 122.2 events per 100,000 population per year. The meta-analysis with random affects which takes into account sample sizes showed a combined rate of 30.7% of violent patients per 100 admissions. However, there was a high level of heterogeneity between the studies' (Bowers *et al*, 2011). These figures could give a skewed impression, as they are averages that include forensic units, where recorded violence is higher than in other wards. It is unclear whether this is an objective difference, or whether it is because of more stringent recording systems on forensic units. The 2006–2007 audit suggests that there might be fewer violent incidents in forensic units compared with other psychiatric wards (Royal College of Psychiatrists, 2007). However, in Bower's study, the UK mean patient-based percentage of recorded violent incidents was 52% for forensic units, whereas it was only 30% for acute and 15% for normal psychiatric wards. Similar trends could be seen in other countries too, where forensic units often have a far higher recorded incident rate than other psychiatric wards. The mean number of recorded events in the UK was over 6 times higher in forensic wards than in other psychiatric wards, and the same was true for the mean recorded events per 100 admissions per month (Bowers *et al*, 2011). The lesson here is to be very careful when interpreting combined data, because incident rates and recorded rates can vary significantly in different settings.

There is persistent evidence that violence is a problem not just for psychiatric wards. However, proper comparisons are difficult because the available data for violence on medical wards are much less sophisticated than the data for psychiatric wards. The most comprehensive systematic review to date was published in 2008 by Professor Hahn and colleagues from Bern, which analysed 31 studies of patient and visitor violence in general hospitals worldwide (Hahn *et al*, 2008). All were questionnaire-based and asked medical staff directly about their experience of violence in a given past time frame, such as the past year. The data were from countries as diverse as Ireland, England, the USA, Israel, Taiwan, Sweden, Turkey, Jamaica, Kuwait, Hong Kong, Poland, Australia and New Zealand. Most surveys were of nurses, but some were of healthcare staff generally or physicians in particular. The results showed wide differences: in terms of verbal abuse, the figures ranged from 9% in the past year in Sweden to 91% in the USA. Figures for actual physical assaults were significantly lower and ranged from 3% in Israel to 58% in the USA. Visitor violence, when recorded, was by and large less common than patient violence. For obvious reasons, percentages for patient and visitor violence remained high in those studies where nurses or physicians were asked for their experience during their whole career (35–60% for verbal abuse and 7.5–38% for physical assaults for patient and visitor violence; Hahn *et al*, 2008).

These results are in keeping with those from an emergency department in Vancouver, Canada, where 57% of staff had been physically assaulted in the year assessed. The vast majority had also witnessed verbal abuse, physical threats or assaults. More worryingly, 73% were afraid of patients as a result of violence and 74% reported reduced job satisfaction (Fernandes *et al*, 1999). A large survey from the University of Liverpool showed significant differences between departments: 42% of staff in medical departments and 36% of surgical staff had been assaulted, compared with 30% of accident and emergency staff. Nurses were much more likely to be assaulted than doctors (43% versus 14%; Winstanley & Whittington, 2004). Hahn and colleagues (2008) showed that medical staff were more likely to be assaulted than surgical staff or staff in intensive care units. Women and children's care as well as paediatric clinical settings were also high-risk areas for verbal abuse and threatening behaviour (Hahn *et al*, 2008). Interestingly, male nurses were at higher risk of patient and visitor violence than female nurses. Younger and less experienced staff also seemed to be more at risk (Whittington *et al* 1996; Hahn *et al*, 2008).

Patients at risk of being violent

There has been a lot of debate about the relationship between mental illness and violence. Although it is relatively well accepted that mental illness might cause a slight increase in the risk of lifetime violence in the community, it seems that, in reality, the risk of lifetime community violence is mostly related to substance misuse. Nevertheless, much research has gone into identifying particular risk factors within patients and patient groups that might lead to in-patient violence. Again, we find that violence is better researched in psychiatric settings than in any other setting.

Bo *et al* (2011) conducted a study in Denmark comparing patients with schizophrenia with people in the general population. They concluded that there were two different trajectories for violent behaviour in the schizophrenia group. On the one hand, there were patients with no history of violence or criminal behaviour, for whom active psychotic symptoms seemed to explain the violent behaviour. The other, much bigger group was made up of patients with personality disorder, which predicted violence regardless of other symptoms associated with their schizophrenic illness (Bo *et al*, 2011).

There is relatively persistent evidence that male gender, substance misuse and a history of physically aggressive behaviour are important risk factors for violence (Amore *et al*, 2008). In a comprehensive meta-analysis of 166 independent datasets, Douglas and colleagues (2009) showed that psychosis was significantly associated with increased odds of violence in the region of 49–68%, depending on the study. However, there was significant dispersion among the effect sizes analysed, which the authors explain by citing heterogeneity of study designs, definitions and measurements of psychosis, and comparison groups (Douglas *et al*, 2009). A large, Swedish cohort study found that patients with substance use disorders have a high risk of violence, as well as a high hazard ratio for excess mortality and a high risk of dying prematurely from suicide or an alcohol- or drug-related cause (Stenbacka *et al*, 2012).

Overall, the evidence that substance misuse, personality disorder and certain psychotic symptoms, such as paranoia and acute psychosis, increase the risk of violence is relatively consistent and increasingly undisputed (Cornaggia *et al*, 2011). Dack and colleagues (2013) conducted a large meta-analysis and found many factors associated with in-patient aggression: being younger, male gender, involuntary admission, not being married, a diagnosis of schizophrenia, a greater number of previous admissions, a history of violence, a history of self-destructive behaviour and a history of substance abuse. In a multi-level modelling study from England, the factors most strongly associated with verbal aggression were aggression towards objects and physical aggression against others as well as patients being involuntarily detained, locked-door wards, high patient turnover and patient alcohol use (Bowers *et al*, 2009). A number of authors have questioned the validity of the research focus on particular diagnoses or symptoms. They have argued that, instead, the role of environmental factors ought to be explored more (Steinert, 2002; Whittington & Richter, 2006). There is good evidence to suggest that many of the reasons for violence are the same for patients with various illnesses as they are for the general population. In-patient violence could be strongly associated with the more frustrating aspects of institutionalisation, such as boredom on wards, restricted environments and the inability to get one's demands met (Whittington & Richter, 2006).

Few studies have looked at the association between Asperger syndrome and violence. In a qualitative review on the topic, there was some indication of 'possible patterns of dynamics of violence that might prove to be typical of persons with Asperger syndrome' (Bjørkly, 2009). However, when a comparison was made between Asperger syndrome and psychopathy, it indicated the possibility of 'qualitative differences in the characteristics of violent behaviour between the two disorders' (Bjørkly, 2009).

Among medical patients, it seems that patients between 15 and 40 years of age, as well as those over 70, are found to be more aggressive (Hahn *et al*, 2008). Again, there is a male preponderance (McKenna *et al*, 2003). There is some evidence that traumatic brain injury increases the odds ratio for violent events, whereas epilepsy reduces it (Fazel *et al*, 2009). Other at-risk groups include patients with dementia, alcohol or illegal drug intoxication or withdrawal, delirium, confusion or high arousal (Brayley *et al*, 1994; Winstanley & Whittington, 2004; Hahn *et al*, 2008).

The previously mentioned 2005 audit looked at possible ways of improving the current situation and asked staff about reasons for in-patient violence. Inadequate staffing, overcrowding, substance misuse and high levels of patient boredom were commonly mentioned. It also emphasised that training in the prevention and management of violent incidents should be tailored to individual staff needs (Royal College of Psychiatrists, 2005). In a study conducted in the UK, Switzerland and Germany, Lepping and colleagues (2009) examined factors that would make psychiatric nurses feel safer on their wards. They found that the British ward managers perceived violence and aggression to be a smaller problem on their wards compared with the Swiss and German ward managers. This was associated with the availability of teams who would immediately attend violent incidents, regular training and clear protocols. To a lesser degree, risk assessments contributed to a feeling of safety but staffing levels, interestingly, did not seem to play a role (Lepping *et al*, 2009).

In keeping with the idea that environmental factors play a big role in violent behaviour, many studies have tried to examine specific behaviours that might be indicative of imminent violence. A number of such behaviours have been found, such as aggression against objects or persons, irritability, boisterousness, confusion and disorientation (Abderhalden *et al*, 2004; Almvik *et al*, 2006; Amore *et al*, 2008; Bowers *et al*, 2009). These types of behaviours occur in various illnesses but also in the general population, for instance on a Friday night in the pub when trouble starts to brew. These findings exemplify the complex interplay between environmental and individual factors and situational circumstances in the development of violence.

International comparisons and guidelines

Internationally, the best-known guideline on violence is arguably the National Institute for Health and Care Excellence (NICE) guideline 'Violence: The Short-Term Management of Disturbed/Violent Behaviour in In-Patient Psychiatric Settings and Emergency Departments' (National Institute for Health and Clinical Excellence, 2005). NICE guidelines are as evidence-based as current evidence allows. They take into account economic concerns as well as scientific evidence, and they try to give the best possible guidance considering all available evidence at the time of publication. They are regularly reviewed and updated. However, the level of evidence they incorporate is varied, ranging from well-conducted randomised, controlled trials (RCTs) to expert opinion. It is interesting that most of the recommendations put forward in the guideline are supported by a very low level of evidence, such as consensus and expert opinion rather than high-level RCTs. They suggest that the short-term management of disturbed and violent behaviour should begin with a prediction phase, which includes risk assessment. The next step is a prevention phase, when de-escalation techniques and observation come into play. Interventions for the continued management of violence after de-escalation has failed include rapid tranquillisation, seclusion and physical interventions such as restraint. The guidelines also emphasise the importance of post-incident reviews for staff and patients.

Physical restraint

In the UK, physical restraint is usually carried out by specially trained teams of four. It includes direct physical contact between persons where reasonable force is positively applied against resistance, either to restrict movement or mobility or to disengage a person from the harmful behaviour they display (Social Care, Local Government and Care Partnership Directorate, 2014).

Chemical restraint

Generally speaking, chemical restraint involves using medication to restrain. This can be oral or intramuscular (in some cases, even intravenous) medication. Physical restraint may be applied to allow the application of chemical restraint. Chemical restraint differs from therapeutic sedation in that it does not have a directly therapeutic purpose but is primarily employed to control undesirable behaviour. It can be difficult to measure the duration of chemical restraint, because the sedation will subside gradually and at a different rate in individual patients.

Mechanical restraint

Mechanical restraint involves the use of equipment. The equipment can be specially designed mittens or belts, which are widely used outside the UK. Other possible mechanical restraints include the use of everyday equipment such as heavy tables or bed supports to restrict a person's movement. Even keeping up a drip beyond medical necessity could be considered mechanical restraint.

Environmental restraint

Environmental restraint includes elements of the environment that limit people's ability to move around freely, such as locked doors, electronic keypads and locks. Seclusion would be the most typical example of environmental restraint. Seclusion is defined as the placing of a person alone in an area with the door shut in such a way as to prevent free exit from that area. Many psychiatric units use a seclusion room, but might keep the door open. In the UK and Scandinavia, the use of specific open spaces to allow an agitated patient to pace around freely while isolating him or her from other patients is common (called 'skjerming' in Norway and 'skerming' in Denmark, meaning 'shielding').

Psychological restraint

Psychological restraint includes telling the patient not to do something, or saying that doing what they want to do is not allowed or too dangerous. It also includes the restriction of life choices or possessions, such as walking aids, glasses, or outdoor clothing, with the intention of stopping them from leaving.

Restraint can be separated into circumstances that are unforeseen and unexpected and those that are planned. The former includes emergency situations where sudden violent behaviour needs to be constrained in order to prevent immediate harm or injury. Planned restraint, by contrast, might be needed to facilitate investigations in the patient's best interest (in patients who lack capacity). It also includes the removal of a patient who lacks capacity to a care home or some form of supported living, which might be against the patients' expressed wishes but is in their best interest and in accordance with mental health law or other legislation.

International differences

Restraint must always be justifiable, appropriate, reasonable and proportionate to a specific situation, and should be applied for the minimum possible duration (Social Care, Local Government and Care Partnership Directorate, 2014). It also has to be legal, and different countries have different legislation to cover the use of restraint in different circumstances. Many countries, such as the different countries within the UK, have legislation applicable to patients who lack capacity as well as mental health legislation that regulates the use of restraint. The European Convention on Human Rights also defines the limitations of restraint under Articles 3 and 5. Still, the current legal provisions, as well as clinical practice, are quite varied across Europe (Steinert & Lepping, 2009). The main reasons for this variation are different national traditions and experiences with the abuse of medicine and psychiatry over the decades. Although people in some countries, who are not familiar with other countries' traditions, might find various practices barbaric or undesirable, there is very little evidence to suggest that specific types of restraint are more harmful than others.

According to Steinert & Lepping's (2009) survey of 16 European countries, intravenous medication is only commonly used in restraint in Finland, Estonia, Germany, Luxemburg and Austria. Physical restraint is common in the UK, Sweden, Finland, Estonia, the Benelux countries and France, but much less common in Germany, Switzerland, Austria, Italy, Slovenia and Turkey. Mechanical restraint with belts is commonplace across Europe, with the exception of the UK and Ireland, but in many countries it is only allowed with one-to-one supervision. Equally, the practice of seclusion varies throughout Europe, although most countries have seclusion as an option. Net beds – hospital beds covered with a firm net over a metal frame that allows patients free movement within an area confined to his or her bed – are used in Luxemburg, Austria, the Czech Republic, Slovakia and Malta (Steinert & Lepping, 2009).

When it comes to involuntary admissions, doctors and, in many countries, judges are an integral part of such procedures across Europe, whereas the police only play a role in some of the surveyed countries. Outside emergency settings, involuntary admissions cannot be arranged by doctors in Germany and Turkey. Big differences exist with regard to transfers to specialised prisons or forensic psychiatric units: the level of patient violence required before considering such a transfer varies widely between countries (Steinert & Lepping, 2009).

Equally diverse is the type of medication that is given for the management of disturbed behaviour in various countries. The NICE guidelines (National Institute for Health and Clinical Excellence, 2005), for example, suggest the use of oral haloperidol and lorazepam, or lorazepam alone if the behavioural disturbance does not occur in a psychotic context. For intramuscular treatment they recommend a combination of haloperidol and lorazepam. In the event of moderate disturbance with psychosis, intramuscular olanzapine can be considered, but not within an hour of using lorazepam to avoid respiratory and cardiovascular complications. The NICE guidelines suggest that there is insufficient evidence for the safety of the combination of intramuscular haloperidol with promethazine or the safety of intramuscular midazolam alone, and therefore these agents are not recommended by the NICE guidelines despite being commonplace in some countries.

Zuclopenthixol acetate is not recommended for rapid tranquillisation because of its relatively slow onset and long duration of action. It should only be used if the patient a) is expected to be disturbed or violent for a long period of time, b) has a history of repeated intramuscular administration of sedating medication, or c) has a past history of timely response to zuclopenthixol. The NICE guidelines also consider the possibility that the patient might have made an advanced directive indicating that zuclopenthixol is their treatment of choice.

The guidelines do not recommend oral or intramuscular chlorpromazine because of the risk of cardiovascular complications and QT-interval prolongation. They do not recommend intramuscular diazepam or thioridazine. Olanzapine or risperidone should not be used for the management of disturbed behaviour in patients with dementia (National Institute for Health and Clinical Excellence, 2005). In the UK, most mental health services and hospitals have local guidelines that are based on the NICE guidelines and include protocols for the use of oral and intramuscular medication. On the whole, these local guidelines recommend de-escalation, followed by the offer of oral medication, followed by intramuscular (but not intravenous) medication. The emphasis is on lorazepam if there is no psychotic element to the disturbed behaviour, but the addition of an antipsychotic, usually haloperidol, is recommended in the case of psychosis.

With the help of the European Violence in Psychiatry Research Group, my colleagues and I conducted a survey looking at the practice of chemical restraint throughout Europe and other countries (see Table 2.1, overleaf).

Most guidelines agree that de-escalation should always be the first response to violent behaviour. This could include removing a patient to an environment with fewer stimuli. In some countries, it would automatically mean seclusion, but in others a removal to a quiet area. If de-escalation fails, a decision has to be made about the origin of the disturbed behaviour. If agitation is the main issue, most guidelines recommend the use of short-term benzodiazepines. If there is a psychotic element to the presentation and treatment is required on top of sedation and an anxiolytic, the use of antipsychotics is recommended. Most guidelines ask clinicians to be cautious when giving antipsychotics to patients who are already on other antipsychotic medication. Caution is also recommended with the combination of intramuscular olanzapine and lorazepam. Some guidelines recommend the cautious use of benzodiazepines in combination with clozapine. However, clozapine is advocated by some authors as useful in the medium-term treatment of aggressive behaviour (Krakowski *et al*, 2006; Citrome & Volavka, 2011) and is used for this purpose in some European countries. Although zuclopenthixol is still used in many European countries, its use is increasingly discouraged in the treatment of acutely disturbed or violent behaviour, because of its slow onset and long half-life.

In the specific situation of people with schizophrenia, a recent review confirmed the medium-term efficacy of clozapine and short-term benefits of adjunctive beta-blockers in the treatment of violence and aggression. There was little evidence supporting the use of mood stabilisers, depot medication or electroconvulsive therapy for this purpose (Topiwala & Fazel, 2011). The famous Clinical Antipsychotic Trials of Intervention Effectiveness (CATIE) project did not find any advantage of second-generation antipsychotics over perphenazine in reducing violence in people with schizophrenia, confirming most other research findings that show equal efficacy for first- and second-generation antipsychotics for the treatment of aggression in people with schizophrenia (Swanson *et al*, 2008).

Several authors have pointed out that there are fundamental difficulties with meta-analyses and evidence-based medicine when it comes to the development of guidelines (Steinert, 2009; Steinert & Lepping, 2011). Professor Steinert was responsible for the development of the German Psychiatric Association's treatment guidelines on aggressive behaviour. In contrast to the UK NICE guidelines, the German guidelines were put together using a consensus model that included the views of scientists as

Table 2.1 Chemical restraint guidelines and medications used in 21 countries

Countries	Guideline	Medications used
Austria	Local guidelines	Risperidone, chlorprothixenhydrochloride, lorazepam, quetiapine (oral), prothipendyl (intravenous), ziprasidone, aripiprazole (intramuscular), and (more rarely) zuclopenthixol
Belgium	None	Risperidone, droperidol, olanzapine, clotiapine with or without diazepam/clorazepate
Bulgaria	National guidelines	Haloperidol, chlorpromazine, zuclopenthixol first line, benzodiazepines, (aripiprazole in mania)
Czech Republic	National recommendations	Benzodiazepines, levomepromazine, haloperidol, chlorpromazine, olanzapine, risperidone, benzodiazepines with antipsychotics
Finland	None	Lorazepam, haloperidol, zuclopenthixol
Germany	National guidelines	Lorazepam, haloperidol
Iceland	None	Haloperidol, zuclopenthixol, lorazepam
India	None	Haloperidol plus promethazine, haloperidol plus lorazepam, olanzapine, zuclopenthixol, diazepam (in rural settings), midazolam nasal spray (in children)
Ireland	Local guidelines	Haloperidol plus lorazepam, olanzapine plus lorazepam (both oral), haloperidol plus midazolam (intramuscular), diazemuls
Italy	Local guidelines (some areas)	Zuclopenthixol, promazine, haloperidol, benzodiazepines (intramuscular/oral), wide variations
Netherlands	Local guidelines (some areas)	Haloperidol plus promethazine, olanzapine (zuclopenthixol also commonly used)
Norway	None	Lorazepam, olanzapine, zuclopenthixol
Portugal	None	Intramuscular haloperidol, zuclopenthixol, carbamazepine, less often aripiprazole, olanzapine
Romania	Local guidelines	Diazepam and/or haloperidol (intravenous or intramuscular), chlorpromazine (intravenous or intramuscular), olanzapine, aripiprazole (both intramuscular)
Slovenia	None	Intramuscular lorazepam, olanzapine, haloperidol, promazine, aripiprazole, midazolam, oral clonazepam, risperidone, diazepam, lorazepam
Spain	Regional guidelines	Haloperidol with or without benzodiazepines (intramuscular/oral), olanzapine, risperidone (oral)

Table 2.1 Cont.

Countries	Guideline	Medications used
Sweden	None	Haloperidol or promethazine plus lorazepam, zuclopenthixol plus diazepam
Switzerland	None	Haloperidol or zuclopenthixol and lorazepam or diazepam. Commonly high-potency antipsychotic plus benzodiazepine plus low-potency antipsychotic (levomepromazine, chlorprothixenhydrochloride or promazine)
Turkey	None	Oral second-generation antipsychotic or benzodiazepine (lorazepam, diazepam, clonazepam, alprazolam), intramuscular haloperidol, olanzapine, zuclopenthixol, ziprasidone
UK	National and local guidelines	Lorazepam with or without haloperidol, olanzapine, zuclopenthixol
USA	None	Haloperidol, lorazepam

Countries were included if we had at least two independent opinions from experts working in that country. The list of medications used might not be exhaustive but represents commonly used medication. Where the type of application is not specified, medication can be given intramuscularly or orally, but not intravenously.

Source: adapted from Lepping (2013).

well as patient representatives. Evidence-based medicine was not given priority over other considerations. He identified a number of sources of bias in evidence-based guidelines, in part related to commonly mentioned criticisms of RCTs, but also reflecting additional concerns (Steinert, 2009; Steinert & Lepping, 2011).

1   The level of evidence that is attributed to a particular study in the NICE guidelines and other evidence-based guidelines relates to the quality of the study rather than the reported effect size. This means you can get a high level of recommendation with any high-quality study, regardless of the actual observed effect size. It is possible that an effective treatment could get a lower recommendation than a less-effective treatment, if it was evaluated with a poorer-quality study than the less-effective treatment.

2   The external validity of the studies is not taken into account systematically. This is a particular problem in violence research, as the heterogeneity between settings and countries is usually enormous. Moreover, it is unclear whether the typical violent patient will ever be recruited into a study, because commonly occurring factors such as acute intoxication are usually exclusion criteria. This makes it more difficult to generalize from the existing studies to actual clinical situations.

3   Absence of evidence is not evidence of absence of effect. This is an important argument. There are a number of treatments regularly used in many countries without any particular evidence from RCTs. The main reason for the lack of evidence is not the absence of efficacy, but the fact that neither the pharmaceutical industry nor other funders are interested in examining the efficacy of these medications in the treatment of aggression. This is particularly true for older antipsychotics and older medication in general, because there is little financial gain in examining the efficacy of old, but usually very cheap, medication. There is therefore a clear bias towards newer, more expensive medication and their competitor drugs. Many combinations of low-potency antipsychotics and sedatives could prove to be efficacious, if only we could test them.

4   The ethical framework of many clinically relevant questions cannot be adequately examined in RCTs. This is most notably true for the comparison of different types of restraint, particularly when one type of restraint might be alien to the tradition of a particular country. For example, it would be very difficult to persuade British nurses to use mechanical restraint in an RCT. Equally, it is unlikely that an alien restraint method would be acceptable to patients if they are not familiar with it. However, attempts have been made to try and compare various types of restraint in RCTs and evidence is beginning to emerge. One recent trial in Germany showed that such studies are feasible (Bergk *et al*, 2011). It found little difference between seclusion and mechanical restraint with regard to patient acceptance and perceived restriction of human rights (Bergk *et al*, 2011).

5   The German guideline group concluded that a consensus achieved between professionals, patients and relatives might be key to achieving overall acceptance of the guidelines, a goal that many might find as important as scientific evidence.

Children and the elderly

Special considerations apply in the treatment of violence in children and older people, particularly older people with dementia. There has been significant debate about the off-label use of antipsychotic medication for agitation and confusion in patients with dementia. Significant concerns have been raised about the increased risk of cardiovascular events with second-generation antipsychotics. However, good alternative strategies to treat the often significant agitation and aggression seen in patients with dementia are in short supply. Maher and colleagues (2011) recently performed a systematic review and concluded that there are 'small but significant benefits' for agitation and mood for olanzapine, risperidone and aripiprazole, with effect sizes ranging from 0.12 to 0.20. However, adverse events were common in all the studies they included (Maher *et al*, 2011). Isaksson and colleagues (2011) found that in the week of their study, 32% of nursing home residents with dementia engaged in physically violent behaviour. The three factors independently associated with aggression were male gender, antipsychotic treatment and decline in orientation (Isaksson *et al*, 2011). Such results will continue to cast doubt on the efficacy of antipsychotics in the treatment of disturbed behaviour in patients with dementia. Others have suggested environmental adjustment and the treatment of pain as effective ways of reducing agitation in this patient group (Husebo *et al*, 2011).

The treatment of aggression in children and adolescents is even more rife with ethical problems. Currently, antihistamines, benzodiazepines and antipsychotics are the most commonly used medications (Barzman & Findling, 2008). Although most of these treatments seem relatively safe, few studies have assessed the long-term risks associated with pharmacological treatment. However, aggressive behaviour has its own potential harmful consequences in the short, medium and long term, and these must be weighed against any side-effects from medication used to control aggressive behaviour.

Conclusion

The treatment of violence and aggression is complicated by ethical and clinical difficulties. However, there is no doubt that violence and aggression have a seriously negative effect on victims, whether they are patients or staff. They undermine staff morale and have long-term physical and emotional consequences for victims. From an organisational point of view, violence and aggression cause short-term and long-term sickness, adverse outcomes and poor patient satisfaction. Therefore, it ought to be evident that it is in the interest of any organisation to reduce violence and aggression in medical settings as much as possible.

We have to consider that there are environmental reasons, as well as reasons related to illness, that make violence particularly likely in hospitals. Environmental reasons include the institutionalization of people in hospital settings. Illness-related reasons include acute confusion and irritability. These illness-related factors are particularly likely in acute delirium, dementia, psychosis, substance withdrawal and acute organic syndromes, which are all commonplace in acute hospital wards of the 21st century, where the focus is on the more acutely ill, short lengths of stay and early discharge. There are also consequences for the perpetrators of violence in terms of guilt, criminal prosecution and being subjected to restraint.

In an environment where risk is increasingly important, it is conceivable that violent patients might be treated differently to non-violent patients with the same underlying disorder or illness. The interactions between illness-related and environmental factors in the development of aggression and violence are complex. As many violent incidents occur in the same way as they do with people who do not show any signs of illness, reducing environmental triggers for violence is essential. However, some factors seem to increase the risk of violence; some of these are constant, whereas others are changeable. Constant factors include male gender and a history of violence, and changeable factors include irritability, thought disorder, substance misuse, disorientation and confusion.

There are two different types of situations that might make restraint or other management of aggression and violence necessary.
1   A planned intervention, such as medical investigations or a change of accommodation, that might provoke violence in the patient.
2   An emergency situation with acute aggression that might endanger the patient, staff or others (such as fellow patients or visitors).

Almost all guidelines worldwide seem to suggest risk assessment and de-escalation as a starting point of management. If the situation does not improve, oral medication should be offered. Most guidelines would suggest a sedating benzodiazepine. This can be supplemented with an antipsychotic, particularly when there is a psychotic element to the presentation. Should the situation still not be brought under control and the risk remain, intramuscular benzodiazepines and antipsychotics are recommended. Short-acting drugs are preferred to long-acting ones. A possible regime is the combination of lorazepam and haloperidol. In children and adolescents, as well as in patients with dementia, slightly different recommendations exist.

Most research into violence and aggression has focused on psychiatric hospitals and mental illness, despite the fact that they are equally common in medical and surgical settings. Despite methodological problems, the epidemiology of violence and aggression is relatively well known. There are a number of trials looking at the safety and efficacy of various medications for treating violence and aggression. However, less is known about the acceptability of different types of restraint in different settings, where the research is only just beginning. In the future, it might be possible to establish which types of restraint might be most acceptable to which patients in different countries around the world. Acceptability would include concepts such as perceived restrictions of personal liberty as well as patient preference.

References

Abderhalden C, Needham I, Miserez B, *et al* (2004) Predicting inpatient violence in acute psychiatric wards using the Brøset-Violence-Checklist: a multicentre prospective cohort study. *Journal of Psychiatric and Mental Health Nursing*, **11**: 422–427.

Almvik R, Rasmussen K, Woods P (2006) Challenging behaviour in the elderly – monitoring violent incidents. *International Journal of Geriatric Psychiatry*, **231**: 368–374.

Amore M, Menchetti M, Tonti C, *et al* (2008) Predictors of violent behaviour among acute psychiatric patients: clinical study. *Psychiatry and Clinical Neurosciences*, **62**: 247–255.

Bandura A (1986) *Social Foundations of Thought and Action: A Social Cognitive Theory*. Prentice Hall.

Barzman DH, Findling RL (2008) Pharmacological treatment of pathologic aggression in children. *International Review of Psychiatry*, **20**: 151–157.

Bergk J, Einsidler B, Flammer E, *et al* (2011) A randomised controlled comparison of seclusion and mechanical restraint in inpatient settings. *Psychiatric Services*, **62**: 1310–1317.

Bjørkly S (1995) Prediction of aggression in psychiatric patients: a review of prospective prediction studies. *Clinical Psychology Review*, **15**: 475–502.

Bjørkly S (2009) Risk and dynamics of violence in Asperger's syndrome: a systematic review of the literature. *Aggression and Violent Behavior*, **14**: 306–312.

Bo S, Abu-Akel A, Kongerslev M, *et al* (2011) Risk factors for violence among patients with schizophrenia. *Clinical Psychology Review*, **31**: 711–726.

Bowers L, Allan T, Simpson A, *et al* (2009) Identifying key factors associated with aggression on acute inpatient psychiatric wards. *Issues in Mental Health Nursing*, **30**: 260–271.

Bowers L, Stewart D, Papadopoulos C, *et al* (2011) *Inpatient Violence and Aggression: A Literature Review*. Institute of Psychiatry, Kings College London.

Brayley J, Lange R, Baggoley C, *et al* (1994) The violence management team. An approach to aggressive behaviour in a general hospital. *Medical Journal of Australia*, **15**: 254–258.

Chappell D, Di Martino V (2006) *Violence at Work (3rd edn)*. International Labour Office.

Citrome L, Volavka J (2011) Pharmacological management of acute and persistent aggression in forensic psychiatry settings. *CNS Drugs*, **25**: 1009–1021.

Cornaggia CM, Beghi M, Pavone F, *et al* (2011) Aggression in psychiatry wards: a systematic review. *Psychiatry Research*, **189**: 10–20.

Dack C, Ross J, Papadopoulos C, *et al* (2013) A review and meta-analysis of the patient factors associated with psychiatric in-patient aggression. *Acta Psychiatrica Scandinavica*, **127**: 255–268.

Douglas KS, Guy LS, Hart SD (2009) Psychosis as a risk factor for violence to others: a meta-analysis. *Psychological Bulletin*, **135**: 679–706.

Fazel S, Philipson J, Gardiner L, *et al* (2009) Neurological disorders and violence: a systematic review and meta-analysis with a focus on epilepsy and traumatic brain injury. *Journal of Neurology*, **256**: 1591–1602.

Fernandes CM, Bouthillette F, Raboud JM, *et al* (1999) Violence in the emergency department: a survey of health care workers. *Canadian Medical Association Journal*, **161**: 1245–1248.

Hahn S, Zeller A, Needham I, *et al* (2008) Patient and visitor violence in general hospitals: a systematic review of the literature. *Aggression and Violent Behaviour*, **13**: 431–441.

Husebo BS, Ballard C, Sandvik R, *et al* (2011) Efficacy of treating pain to reduce behavioural disturbances in residents of nursing homes with dementia: cluster randomised clinical trial. *BMJ*, **343**: d4065.

Isaksson U, Graneheim UH, Åström S, *et al* (2011) Physically violent behaviour in dementia care: characteristics of residents and management of violent situations. *Aging Mental Health*, **15**: 573–579.

Keski-Valkama A, Sailas E, Eronen M, *et al* (2010) The reasons for using restraint and seclusion in psychiatric inpatient care: a nationwide 15-year study. *Nordic Journal of Psychiatry*, **64**: 136–144.

Krakowski MI, Czobor P, Citrome L, *et al* (2006) Atypical antipsychotic agents in the treatment of violent patients with schizophrenia and schizoaffective disorder. *Archives of General Psychiatry*, **63**: 622–629.

Lepping P (2013) The use of emergency psychiatric medication: A survey from 21 countries. *Journal of Clinical Psychopharmacology*, **33**: 240–242.

Lepping P, Steinert T, Needham I, *et al* (2009) Ward safety perceived by ward managers in Britain, Germany and Switzerland: identifying factors that improve ability to deal with violence. *Journal of Psychiatric and Mental Health Nursing*, **16**: 629–635.

Lepping P, Lanka SVN, Turner J, *et al* (2013) Percentage prevalence of patient and visitor violence against staff in Welsh high-risk medical wards. *Clinical Medicine*, **13**: 543–546.

Maher AR, Maglione M, Bagley S, *et al* (2011) Efficacy and comparative effectiveness of atypical antipsychotic medications of off-label uses in adults: a systematic review and meta-analysis. *JAMA*, **306**: 1359–1369.

McKenna BG, Poole SJ, Smith NA, *et al* (2003) A survey of threats and violent behaviour by patients against registered nurses in their first year of practice. *International Journal of Mental Health Nursing*, **12**: 56–63.

National Institute for Health and Clinical Excellence (2005) *Violence: The Short-Term Management of Disturbed/Violent Behaviour in In-Patient Psychiatric Settings and Emergency Departments (NICE Clinical Guideline 25)*. NICE.

Needham I, Abderhalden C, Halfens RJ, *et al* (2005) Non-somatic effects of patient aggression on nurses: a systematic review. *Journal of Advanced Nursing*, **49**: 283–296.

Nijman HL, Palmstierna T, Almvik R, *et al* (2005) Fifteen years of research with the Staff Observation Aggression Scale: a review. *Acta Psychiatrica Scandinavica*, **111**: 12–21.

Nijman H, Bjørkly S, Palmstierna T, *et al* (2006) Assessing aggression of psychiatric patients: methods of measurement and its prevalence. In *Violence in Mental Health Settings: Causes, Consequences, Management* (eds D Richter, R Whittington). Springer.

Richter D, Berger K (2000) Physical and psychological consequences for employees after a patient assault: a prospective study in six psychiatric hospitals [German]. *Arbeitsmedizin-Sozialmedizin-Umweltmedizin*, **35**: 357–362.

Royal College of Psychiatrists (2005) *National Audit of Violence 2003–2005 Final Report*. Royal College of Psychiatrists (www.wales.nhs.uk/documents/FinalReport-violence.pdf).

Royal College of Psychiatrists (2007) *Healthcare Commission National Audit of Violence 2006–7: Final Report – Working Age Adult Services*. Royal College of Psychiatrists (http://www.rcpsych.ac.uk/pdf/WAA%20Nat%20Report%20final%20with%20all%20appendices.pdf).

Social Care, Local Government and Care Partnership Directorate (2014) *Positive and Proactive Care: Reducing the Need for Restrictive Interventions*. Department of Health.

Steinert T (2002) Prediction of inpatient violence. *Acta Psychiatrica Scandinavica*, **106** (Suppl): 133–141.

Steinert T (2009) Why are guidelines more irrational than meta-analyses [in German]. *Psychiatrische Praxis*, **36**: 238–242.

Steinert T, Lepping P (2009) Legal provisions and practice in the management of violent patients, a case vignette study in 16 European countries. *European Psychiatry*, **24**: 135–141.

Steinert T, Lepping P (2011) Is it possible to define a best practice standard for coercive treatment in psychiatry? In *Coercive Treatment in Psychiatry: Clinical, Legal and Ethical Aspects* (eds T Kallert, JE Mezzich, J Monahan). Wiley–Blackwell.

Steinert T, Lepping P, Bernhardsgrütter R, *et al* (2010) Incidence of seclusion and restraint in psychiatric hospitals: a literature review and survey of international trends. *Social Psychiatry and Psychiatric Epidemiology*, **45**: 889–897.

Stenbacka M, Moberg T, Romelsjo A, *et al* (2012) Mortality and causes of death among violent offenders and victims – a Swedish population based longitudinal study. *BMC Public Health*, **12**: 38.

Swanson JW, Swartz MS, Van Dorn RA, *et al* (2008) Comparison of antipsychotic medication effects on reducing violence in people with schizophrenia. *British Journal of Psychiatry*, **193**: 37–43.

Taylor PJ (2008) Psychosis and violence: stories, fears and reality. *Canadian Journal of Psychiatry*, **53**: 647–659.

Topiwala A, Fazel S (2011) The pharmacological management of violence in schizophrenia: a structured review. *Expert Reviews in Neurotherapy*, **11**: 53–63.

Whittington R, Richter D (2006) From the individual to the interpersonal: Environment and interaction in the escalation of violence in mental health settings. In *Violence in Mental Health Settings: Causes, Consequences, Management* (eds D Richter, R Whittington). Springer.

Whittington R, Shuttleworth S, Hill L (1996) Violence to staff in a general hospital setting. *Journal of Advanced Nursing*, **24**: 326–333.

Winstanley S, Whittington R (2004) Aggression towards health care staff in a UK general hospital: variation among professions and departments. *Journal of Clinical Nursing*, **13**: 3–10.

World Health Organization, Violence Prevention Alliance (2012) *Definition and Typology of Violence*. WHO (www.who.int/violenceprevention/approach/definition/en/index.html).

CHAPTER 3

Substance misuse emergencies

Derrett Watts

Over the last 15 years in England and Wales, the number of people who have used drugs at some point in their lives has increased, as has the number who have taken Class A drugs in the last year. However, the number who have used any illicit substance in the last year has fallen (Table 3.1). Levels of use for all three parameters are higher in the young adult (16–24 years) age group.

Cannabis was the most frequently used drug in the last year (6.8%), followed by cocaine powder (2.1%). While the overall reduction in use might be encouraging, the increase in Class A drug use might partially explain the increase in deaths related to drug misuse (1156 in 1996 v. 1784 in 2010). The most common cause was accidental poisoning (49.7%). Intentional self-poisoning or poisoning of undetermined intent was present in 302 cases (16.9%; NHS Information Centre, Lifestyles Statistics, 2011).

In an annual report into drug-related deaths, Ghodse *et al* (2010) also found an increase in the number of drug-related deaths, but questioned whether this might reflect changes in reporting practice rather than a true increase in the death rate. Opiate use, either alone or in combination with other drugs, was implicated in 60% of drug-related deaths, and overall there was a trend to multiple substances being involved. In England, 14.5% of the

Table 3.1 Levels of illicit drug use in England and Wales in 1996 and 2010–2011

Drug use	Adults (16–59 years)		Young adults (16–24 years)	
	1996	2010–2011	1996	2010–2011
Ever taken an illicit drug	30.5%	36.4%	48.6%	40.1%
Used ≥1 illicit drug in the last year	11.1%	8.8%	29.7%	20.4%
Used ≥1 Class A drug in the last year	2.7%	3.1%	9.2%	6.6%

Source: NHS Information Centre, Lifestyles Statistics (2011)

deaths were attributed to suicide, with women more than twice as likely as men to die in this way (Ghodse *et al*, 2010).

Drug-related presentations in A&E

The first aim of making a comprehensive assessment is to allow for 'treating any emergency or acute problem' (Department of Health (England) and devolved administrations, 2007). Although much has been made of the high rate of alcohol-related admissions to accident and emergency (A&E) departments (particularly at night), a study in Bristol found that 6.9% of all A&E patient attendances were directly or indirectly linked to illegal drug use (Binks *et al*, 2005). They presented with acute injuries, overdose and physical health complications of their drug use, and almost half required hospital admission. The lifetime illegal drug use in this sample was similar to that in the general population (36.2% v. 34.0%), but drug use in the last month was higher (16.1% v. 6.0%). In total, 9.9% had used drugs within the last 24 hours. The authors estimated that illegal drug use could be causing 1 million visits to A&E departments in England and 400 000 acute hospital admissions annually. A Canadian study (Palepu *et al*, 2001) identified similar issues. They looked at a group of 598 injecting drugs users over a 39-month period, and found that 440 (73.6%) visited the emergency department at some point during the study, with 265 (44.3%) attending three or more times and 91 (15.2%) ten or more times.

Drug-related hospital admission seems to be a growing problem. In 2009–2010, there were 5809 admissions to English hospitals with a primary diagnosis of a drug-related mental health and behavioural disorder – 2.5% higher than in 2008–2009. If we consider the primary or secondary diagnosis given for admissions, 44 585 admissions were linked to a drug-related mental health and behavioural disorder – 5.7% higher than in 2008–2009. Men were more than twice as likely to be admitted as women (NHS Information Centre, Lifestyles Statistics, 2011).

Concerns in this area have been reflected in the Royal College of Psychiatrists report into Psychiatric Services to A&E departments, which states 'These patients can cause particular management difficulties for medical and nursing staff and might receive inadequate treatment (e.g. because of premature self-discharge, etc.)' (Royal College of Psychiatrists, 2004).

Other settings for emergency presentations

Individuals with substance misuse problems will also present as emergencies in other settings. The link between substance misuse and severe mental illness is well known. Menezes *et al* (1996), reviewing 171 people with psychotic illness, found the 1-year prevalence of a drug problem to be more than one in seven; with young males (aged 20–29 years) the rate increased to 50%. Substance use as a whole (alcohol and/or illicit drugs) led to similar rates of admission, but admissions that were twice as long, and significantly greater use of psychiatric emergency services. Prior to this, Atkinson (1973) looked at more than 500 presentations at a psychiatric emergency admitting unit in California. Some degree of drug 'abuse' (meaning, in this study, alcohol or drug dependence) was found to be present in 20%, with combined alcohol and drug use in a further 12% percent, and felt to be the major factor in 14% of cases (drugs alone) and 10% (mixed drugs and alcohol). Substance misuse was found to be associated across the range of severity and psychiatric diagnostic categories of presentation and in every major diagnostic category. The study also found that over half the cases were not identified, and that drug testing might be 'indispensable where a good history is lacking'.

Section 136 of the Mental Health Act 1983 allows a police officer to take someone who is in a public place and displaying evidence of mental disorder such that they need to be in immediate care, to a place of safety where they can undergo an assessment of their mental health. Hampson (2011) states that the section 136 suites within psychiatric units should accept patients intoxicated with alcohol or drugs, rather than such patients being taken to a police custody suite or general hospital, 'unless they require urgent medical attention or their behaviour is too disturbed'. However, users and carers believe that too many patients are taken to custody suites, particularly if they are under influence of alcohol or drugs, while some police forces report refusals by staff in section 136 suites 'to take anyone who has consumed alcohol or drugs, regardless of their behaviour or degree of intoxication' (Hampson, 2011).

Linked to this issue is the management of drug misuse in police custody generally. In 2005–2006, 52% of all those who responded to the Arrestee Survey for England and Wales reported having taken one or more drugs in the month before arrest (Boreham *et al*, 2007). Cannabis was the most widely used drug, but 13% stated they had taken heroin, 11% crack cocaine and 8% ecstasy. Many substance misusers have negative perceptions of their medical management while in police custody, and there was considerable variation in practice (Gregory, 2007). A report on the management of people with substance misuse in police custody suggested that the number of these people in police custody is increasing, and 'Most of these detainees are vulnerable individuals and the recognition of their substance use problems is now perceived as important and is receiving local and national attention' (Royal College of Psychiatrists, 2011). A special area of consideration is the effect substance intoxication or withdrawal might have on fitness for interview and the validity of any confessions.

Diversity of substance use

In a UNICEF report, an anonymous user of drugs said, 'People will try anything if you tell them it will make them high' (Li, 2007). The range of drugs misused seems to be ever increasing: 41 new substances were reported in Europe during 2010, rising to 81 during 2013 (European Monitoring Centre for Drugs and Drug Addiction, 2011, 2014). It is thus important, particularly with acute presentations when it isn't always clear which substance has been used, that detailed histories are obtained, where possible also gaining collateral information from friends or relatives and, if necessary, contacting the National Poisons Information Service (in England and Wales via NHS Direct, and in Scotland via NHS 24). The National Poisons Information Service is a national service that provides expert advice on all aspects of acute and chronic poisoning. It is approved by the Department of Health and commissioned by the Health Protection Agency.

This chapter will focus on seven groups of substances, as derived from those identified within ICD-10 (World Health Organization, 1992):

- opiates
- cannabinoids
- sedative hypnotics
- cocaine
- other stimulants, including caffeine
- hallucinogens
- volatile solvents.

The prevalence of UK and European use of some of the most significant of these substances is summarised in Table 3.2.

In 2010–2011, it is estimated that 0.6% of the UK population used hallucinogens and 0.4% used tranquillisers (including benzodiazepines and barbiturates; Smith & Flatley, 2011). Figures on solvent use are harder to obtain, given its hidden nature, but in a survey of 11–15 year olds in England 3.8% reported sniffing glue, gas or other volatile substances in the last year (Fuller, 2011).

Types of emergencies

Individuals with drug misuse can present in emergencies for a variety of reasons: intoxication, withdrawal, complications of drug administration method, problems with prescriptions, or other reasons that might or might not be linked to their drug use. The nature of the reason for presentation will require specific responses from health professionals (Table 3.3).

General principles of assessment and treatment

Before looking at each of these types of emergencies, it is important to consider the general principles of assessment. The nature of emergency situations might mean that it is not feasible to complete a comprehensive assessment at the initial consultation, when management of risk might be paramount. However, assessments in these situations should still follow the basic principles of all assessments:

Table 3.2 Substance use in the UK and Europe

Substances	UK population[a] (18–59 years)		European population[b] (16–64 years)	
	Use in the last year (%)	Use in the last year (%)	Lifetime use (%)	Country variation in use in the last year (%)
Opioids	0.2	0.4	Not available[c]	0.36–0.44
Cannabinoids	6.8	6.7	23.2	0.40–14.30
Cocaine	2.2	1.2	4.3	0.00–2.70
Other stimulants				
Ecstasy	1.4	0.7	3.2	0.10–1.60
Amphetamines	1.0	0.5	3.8	0.00–1.10
GHB	0.0[d]	Not available	Not available	3.90–14.50
Ketamine	0.6	Not available	Not available	

a. Source: Smith & Flatley (2011)

b. Source: European Monitoring Centre for Drugs and Drug Addiction (2011)

c. Source: European Monitoring Centre for Drugs and Drug Addiction (2011; p. 73) discusses difficulties in deriving prevalence figures

d. 0.1% of UK 16–24 year olds had used GHB in the last year

- gathering a history (both from the patient and using collateral information if available – e.g. friends, family, health or other professionals);
- undertaking examinations (physical and mental state);
- conducting investigations (such as blood or drug screen tests);
- developing a formulation of the presentation.

A good assessment allows an effective treatment plan to be implemented. Proper recording of each step will greatly assist other professionals – perhaps from different agencies – who subsequently become involved in treatment. When considering behaviour, it is useful to remember the 'model of change' set out by Prochaska *et al* (1992), who identified five stages of change.

1 Pre-contemplation: no thought of change in the near future (next 6 months).
2 Contemplation: change is thought about but no action taken.
3 Preparation: a decision to make change is made, with the intention this will occur in the next month. Additionally there will have been some (unsuccessful) action to make change within the last 12 months.
4 Action: steps to make change are taken.
5 Maintenance: sustained change achieved for over 6 months (should be viewed as an active process rather than a static stage).

Table 3.3 Types of emergency drug-related presentations

Emergency	Explanation	Areas for further study
Intoxication	'A condition that follows the administration of a psychoactive substance resulting in disturbances in level of consciousness, cognition, perception, affect or behaviour, or other psycho-physiological functions and responses. The disturbances are directly related to the acute pharmacological effects of the substance and resolve with time, with complete recovery, except where tissue damage or other complications have arisen' (World Health Organization, 1992)	How to recognise, assess (history, examination, investigations) and treat
Withdrawal	'A group of symptoms of variable clustering and severity occurring on absolute or relative withdrawal of a psychoactive substance after persistent use of that substance. The onset and course of the withdrawal state are time-limited and are related to the type of psychoactive substance and dose being used immediately before cessation or reduction of use. The withdrawal state may be complicated by convulsions.' (World Health Organization, 1992)	How to recognise, assess and treat
Complications of methods of use	The principal methods of drug use are by inhalation, ingestion and injection. Each method in itself carries different risks – which might affect emergency presentations.	Range of methods used, complications from each method
Emergencies relating to sorting out prescriptions	Some emergency presentations might be linked to those not prescribed seeking prescriptions or those on prescriptions having difficulties with them.	Opiate substitution, benzodiazepine scripts
Emergencies in drug users that might or might not be directly linked to their drug use	Some presentations might be due to secondary effects of drug use or might not be directly due to the drug use but reflect higher incidence of range of conditions in those who misuse drugs	Physical, psychological and social problems

37

These can be viewed as a cycle of change, or a spiral; any assessment should aim to help the patient consider moving at least one step forward. The assessment should look at the following domains: drug and alcohol misuse, health and social functioning, and criminal involvement (Department of Health (England) and devolved administrations, 2007).

Even in emergency situations, the history should explore these areas:

- range of drugs used (including illicit, prescribed and over-the-counter preparations, nicotine and alcohol)
- age of commencing each substance, and how this has changed over time (including periods of abstinence or escalation of use)
- frequency and amount taken (e.g. quantity and cost)
- route(s) used (e.g. inhaled, oral or injected)
- social setting of use (location and whether accompanied or alone)
- effects of use (episodes of intoxication, physical or psychological effects of use, risks of harm to self or others, other changes in behaviour)
- intent of any overdose (accidental or deliberate).

The aim is to determine whether the drug use constitutes a harmful pattern of use or dependence syndrome, as per ICD-10 (World Health Organization, 1992). In this, Harmful Use is deemed to occur if there is clear evidence that substance use has resulted in clearly identifiable and specific harmful effects, that 'the pattern of use has persisted for at least 1 month or has occurred repeatedly within a 12-month period, and that the symptoms present could not be attributed to another condition'. For a diagnosis of dependence syndrome, three or more of the following symptoms must have been present concurrently for at least 1 month (or, if for shorter periods, 'have occurred together repeatedly within a 12-month period'; World Health Organization, 1992):

- compulsion to use substance
- inability to control substance use
- physical withdrawal symptoms
- development of tolerance to drug (the need to take more of the drug than previously to get the same effect)
- other interests dwindle because of the drug use
- drug use continues despite awareness of harmful effects of using.

The history should explore a number of other areas, as follows.

Physical and mental health

Physical examination should be systematic, with particular attention being paid to evidence of injected drug use, anaemia, and jaundice or other signs of liver disease, while mental state examination should especially help in assessing depressive or psychotic symptoms and areas such as risk and insight. Look for any conditions that might promote drug use (e.g. self-medication of uncontrolled pain or anxiety symptoms), be masked by drug use (e.g. insomnia, dental pain), be exacerbated by drug use (e.g. depressive or psychotic symptoms), or be apparently incidental to drug use (e.g. hypertension).

Social factors

Social factors include the resources available to the patient and difficulties experienced in areas such as education, employment, finances, housing and relationships.

Criminal justice

Note should be taken of any history of convictions, the nature of the crimes, and any pending court cases.

Risk assessment

An assessment should be made of the risk of exploitation and harm by others, self-neglect, suicide and deliberate self-harm, violence and harm to others (including children). It should take into account past history and current presentation.

Assessment of motivation to change

It is important to consider what actions the patient has taken to change drug use in the past, what their current plans are, and what are their future aspirations.

For all of these areas, it is important to know the patient's past and current involvement with other agencies and, where appropriate, to seek permission to share information with them in relation to your assessment.

Specific investigations looking for the presence of drugs – urine tests or mouth swabs – should be used to supplement the history, and confirm use of drugs. It is important to note some variation between drugs as to how long they will remain present in urine. For example, morphine/diamorphine will remain in the urine at detectable levels for around 48 hours, cocaine metabolites 2–3 days and cannabinoids up to 27 days (Department of Health (England) and devolved administrations, 2007).

The focus of treatment has altered over time. During the 1980s and 1990s, with the advent of HIV, efforts centred on reducing harm (e.g. needle exchanges). Later, the focus moved to reducing drug-related crime and helping patients engage and be retained in treatment. The UK Government drugs strategy for 2010 shows another, recent shift in emphasis, this time towards recovery, as indicated by its title 'Reducing Demand, Restricting Supply, Building Recovery: Supporting People to Live a Drug Free Life' (HM Government, 2010).

In an emergency situation, the short-term goal might be harm reduction and facilitating people to engage in treatment, but longer-term goals should not be restricted to this and patients should be encouraged to aim for recovery.

Intoxication and withdrawal

Effective management of intoxication is emphasised in the UK guidelines for drug treatment, which state that 'All services working with drug misusers should have an emergency protocol in place that covers the management of drug overdoses' (Department of Health (England) and devolved administrations, 2007). As emergency presentations linked to drug use might include both intoxication and withdrawal in one episode, we will consider these together. A further complication is that more than one substance might have been used, confusing the situation and increasing risk. In this regard, the use of alcohol alongside other substances should be especially noted. For each of the substance types discussed, we will consider how to recognise intoxication and withdrawal, any associated risks and what to do.

Opiates

The celebrated 17th-century English physician Thomas Sydenham recognised the value of opiates in the 'suppression of coughs and respiratory ailments, the treatment of diarrhoea and dysentery and the provision of deep and refreshing sleep', in addition to its 'unequalled' role in pain relief (Jay, 2010). He further stated, 'Among the remedies which it has pleased Almighty God to give to man to relieve his sufferings, none is so universal and so efficacious as opium' (Smith, 1995).

However, opiate use, either alone or in combination with other drugs, has been implicated in 60% of drug-related deaths (Ghodse *et al*, 2010). The *British National Formulary* lists 15 opiate preparations of varying strengths that can be prescribed, principally for their analgesic effects (Joint Formulary Committee, 2011). The more commonly used drugs include buprenorphine, various codeine preparations, diamorphine, fentanyl, methadone, morphine salts, oxycodone and tramadol hydrochloride. People who have been prescribed these medications or obtained them illicitly might present with intoxication or withdrawal; other opiate-related presentations might be due to illicit use of heroin preparations, either smoked or injected.

Four types of opiate receptors have been identified: mu (μ), delta (δ) kappa (κ) and ORL1-receptors (Corbett *et al*, 2006). Different drugs show varying levels of affinity for different receptor types. Most of the prescribed opiates are μ-receptor agonists. Methadone and morphine can be viewed as full agonists, but buprenorphine is a partial agonist at the μ receptor, has partial or full agonist activity at the ORL1 and δ receptors, and is a competitive antagonist at the κ receptor. Such issues can be clinically important when treating patients prescribed with different substances.

The symptoms and physical signs of opiate intoxication and withdrawal are detailed in Table 3.4, based in part on items from the Clinical Opiate Withdrawal Scale (COWS; Wesson & Ling, 2003), which was developed to allow objective assessment of the severity of withdrawal. A cautionary

Table 3.4 Symptoms and physical signs of opiate intoxication and withdrawal

Symptoms/signs	Opiate intoxication	Opiate withdrawal
Symptoms		
Level of consciousness	Drowsiness	Insomnia
Mood	Euphoria	Restlessness[a]
Anxiety	Calmness	Anxiety[a]/irritability[a]
Pain	Analgesia	Bone/joint aches[a]
Abdominal	Constipation if chronic use	Stomach cramps,[a] nausea/vomiting,[a] loose stools/diarrhoea[a]
Other	Slurred speech	Sweating,[a] rhinorrhea,[a] lacrimation,[a] yawning[a]
Physical signs		
Temperature	Hypothermia	Hyperthermia
Skin	Might have recent injecting sites	Piloerection[a]
Pupils	Meiosis	Mydriasis[a]
Respiratory rate	Decreased respiratory rate	Increased respiratory rate
Heart rate	Bradycardia	Tachycardia[a]
Blood pressure	Hypotension	Hypertension
Central nervous system	Hypokinesis	Tremor,[a] hyperreflexia

a. Assessed as elements of the Clinical Opiate Withdrawal Scale

note is that patients might have used more than one substance, which can confound the presentation to some degree. Specific key symptoms of opiate intoxication are reduced levels of consciousness, pinpoint pupils (meiosis) and a decreased respiratory rate.

A urine or mouth swab to test for opiates can help confirm the diagnosis, and is particularly useful if results are immediately available; however, more immediate treatment might be required. If the patient is unresponsive, use the A-B-C approach, checking airways (ensure no obstruction to airway), breathing (if not breathing, give two 'rescue' breaths) and circulation (if no pulse, will need to commence cardiac compressions).

Opiate overdose can be reversed by the opiate antagonist naloxone, which should be used if there is a coma or reduced respirations (Joint Formulary Committee, 2011; Taylor *et al*, 2012). It can be given intravenously, intramuscularly, subcutaneously, or through an endotracheal tube. Although onset of action will be slower via the intramuscular and subcutaneous routes, they might be the most accessible routes, depending on the situation. If there is no response to the first dose, it should be repeated at intervals of 2–3 min; where repeated doses are required, an intravenous infusion can be given. In these situations, care should be taken to ensure alternative causes of unresponsiveness (such as hypoglycaemia or head injury) have not been overlooked. The effects of naloxone will last for 20–40 min and, if intoxication has been caused by longer-acting opiates (such as methadone or dextropropoxyphene) or large amounts of heroin, symptoms of intoxication might recur when the naloxone effects have worn off. Patients and family members should be aware of this risk, and thus a period of monitoring or admission might be required (Clarke *et al*, 2005). It should also be noted that buprenorphine overdose might be only partially reversed by naloxone, because of buprenorphine's partial agonist properties.

Future developments in this area might include the extension of 'take-home' naloxone schemes, whereby doses of naloxone are given to patients who use opiates (or their families), along with training in the management of overdose (Strang *et al*, 2006). It is important that, following any emergency treatment, patients should be assessed and encouraged to engage in drug-misuse treatment services.

Cannabinoids

Cannabis was used by 6.8% of UK adults (aged 16–59 years) in 2010–2011, making it the most commonly used illicit drug. Among 16–24 year olds, use was estimated at 17.1%, and it was the most commonly used drug in this subgroup too (Smith & Flatley, 2011). It is derived from the Indian hemp, cannabis sativa, with the most important psychoactive ingredient being delta-9-tetrahydrocannabinol (THC). Various different preparations are used, with the most common being marijuana (crushed leaves and flower heads), hashish (cannabis resin) and hash oil (concentrated resin extract). All are normally smoked, and vary in THC content; marijuana (5% THC), hashish (20% THC) and hash oil (60% or more THC; Wills, 2005). Adverse effects seem to be more likely as THC content rises.

Cannabis is taken for its euphoric and relaxant properties. Normal perceptual experiences can also be intensified, such as eating and watching films. Acute adverse effects can include anxiety, dysphoria, paranoia, and cognitive (short-term memory and attention) and psychomotor (slowed reaction times and sedation) impairment (Hall *et al*, 2001). Physiologically, it will be accompanied by tachycardia, lowered blood pressure, dry mouth, increased appetite, and conjunctival injection and suffusion (Winstock *et al*, 2010). There have been no reported cases of fatal toxicity in humans (Hall *et al*, 2001). The acute effects generally ease after a few hours (Pope *et al*, 1995), and thus management should focus on treating any immediate risks, identifying any underlying psychiatric conditions and encouraging engagement with ongoing services if required. If psychotic symptoms persist, urgent psychiatric evaluation and treatment will be required.

Common withdrawal symptoms include anger, aggression, decreased appetite or weight loss, irritability, anxiety, restlessness, and sleep difficulties including strange dreaming (Budney, 2006). Treatment of withdrawal should involve a combination of advice (e.g. gradual reduction of quantity, delay first use until later in the day, sleep hygiene), psychoeducation, relapse prevention and possibly short-term analgesia, hypnotics or diazepam, at low dose for 3–4 days (Winstock *et al*, 2010).

Sedative hypnotics

Barbiturates were first synthesised in 1864, and were subsequently used for treating a range of conditions, including epilepsy and insomnia, and for the induction and maintenance of anaesthesia. Their use grew such that there were 135 000 barbiturate addicts in England by 1965 (Lopez-Munoz *et al*, 2005). However, the popularity of barbiturates declined as their role in fatal overdoses became apparent and newer drugs were produced.

Benzodiazepines were developed in the 1950s and a variety were introduced clinically in the following decade (Lader, 1991). The risk of dependence was established early on (initially for high doses but later more generally) and by the latter part of the 1980s around 1.2 million people in the UK were on long-term prescriptions for benzodiazepines, of which it was felt a third might have difficulties in withdrawal (Ashton, 1994). Although prescribing guidelines have sought to influence the issuing of scripts, the rise of the internet has compounded the problem, and they are frequently being taken with other drugs. Table 3.5 indicates the frequency with which various substances are mentioned on death certificates, either alone or in combination with other drugs. Benzodiazepines contribute to the risk of death by causing respiratory depression and lowering blood pressure.

In benzodiazepine intoxication, the patient will be drowsy, with symptoms such as confusion, poor concentration and impaired coordination. This might lead to an increased risk of falls, particularly in the elderly (Ashton, 1995). The benzodiazepine antagonist flumazenil can be used to reverse

Table 3.5 Number of deaths for which selected substances were mentioned on the death certificate in England and Wales in 2010

	Alone	In combination	Total
All drug poisoning deaths	1798	949	2747
Heroin/morphine	487	304	791
All antidepressants	157	227	381
Methadone	173	182	355
All benzodiazepines	35	272	307
Cocaine	59	85	144
Amphetamines	33	23	56
Mephedrone	2	4	6

Source: Office for National Statistics (2011)

the sedative effects of benzodiazepines. It can also be used with caution in overdose management. Although this is an unlicensed indication (Joint Formulary Committee, 2011), it can help to reduce the need for intubation and hence admissions to intensive care. It should only be used after a full assessment of the patient's general physical state and whether other substances have also been taken, and should be avoided if there is a history of epilepsy or dependency on benzodiazepines, or if drugs that lower the seizure threshold have been taken. It should be given slowly intravenously and only where full resuscitation equipment is immediately available (National Institute for Health and Clinical Excellence, 2004).

The most serious risks following sudden cessation of benzodiazepines are of seizures and confusional states, although a range of other symptoms might be evident, with headache and insomnia particularly common (Onyett, 1989). They can be divided into two groups (Ashton, 2005):

- symptoms common to all anxiety states (e.g. anxiety, panic attacks, insomnia, depression, muscle pain, palpitations, sweating)
- symptoms relatively specific to benzodiazepine withdrawal (e.g. perceptual disturbances, depersonalisation, visual and auditory hallucinations, formication).

Assessment should determine if there are physical or psychiatric complications of withdrawal and arrange monitoring in the community or in hospital if required. Given its longer half-life, diazepam is the preferred benzodiazepine, as withdrawal is typically more gradual than with other drugs. In emergency situations, clinicians should avoid an expectation being developed that any benzodiazepine prescriptions will be continued in the long-term – such a decision needs to be made by either a general practitioner (GP) or specialist substance-misuse practitioner who would be able to oversee a reduction regime coupled with psychosocial support. Thus, few prescriptions should be started in the emergency scenario, and ideally only after discussions with a GP or specialist involved in the patient's care.

Stimulants

Stimulants share the characteristic of increasing alertness and physical energy. The most commonly used illicit stimulants are cocaine, ecstasy (3,4-methylenedioxy-N-methylamphetamine, also known as MDMA) and amphetamines, although newer drugs are frequently emerging (e.g. mephedrone, also known as meow meow or MCAT). Differences occur in terms of the speed of onset of effects, with the crack form of cocaine giving a more rapid high. Adverse effects reported by stimulant users seem to be common and wide-ranging, including anxiety, depression, mood swings, paranoia and panic attacks, with sleep and appetite disturbances being most frequent. Generally these were mild but 30–55% reported one symptom as severe (Williamson *et al*, 1997). Emergency presentations for toxicity are most likely to involve cardiovascular issues (tachycardia, hypertension, cardiac arrhythmia, myocardial infarction, stroke), hyperthermia, and psychiatric symptoms (aggressive behaviour, confusional states and paranoid psychosis) (Seivewright *et al*, 2007).

A 1990 study found cocaine to be the most common illicit drug used by patients attending emergency departments in the USA, and one of the leading causes of drug-related deaths (Brody *et al*, 1990). The authors examined the records of 216 patients using cocaine who attended emergency departments and found the most common symptom to be chest pain. Although a wide range of physical and psychiatric symptoms was reported, they concluded that most were short-lived, only a small proportion required admission and the key aim of treatment should be to encourage engagement with drug treatment services. In terms of the general pharmacological approaches to management of stimulant misuse, Seivewright *et al* (2007) suggests that 'A pragmatic consideration is the preferable avoidance of benzodiazepines in managing drug users, because of the potential for misuse'. Antidepressants, particularly those with a serotonergic action, would be preferable, and given alongside psychosocial interventions. As there is no specific antidote, treatment of emergency presentations should be supportive and manage any complications that emerge, such as cardiac ischaemia. This means, despite the advice just stated, benzodiazepines might be required for agitation or anxiety, and higher doses than normally used might be required; beta blockers should be avoided (Lidder *et al*, 2008).

A review of stimulant psychosis found that 'a large enough dose of a stimulant drug can produce a psychotic reaction, usually lasting only hours and being self-limited in the majority of individuals' (Curran *et al*, 2004). The authors concluded that management should combine advice to stop using stimulants alongside antipsychotic treatment until the acute symptoms settle, and that antipsychotics should be continued at low doses for those who have experienced more than one episode of psychosis (Curran *et al*, 2004).

Kosten & Sofuoglu (2004) describe stimulant withdrawal in three stages; a 'crash' period (depression, agitation and intense drug craving), an intermediate phase (fatigue, loss of energy, decreased interest in surroundings) and a late phase (brief periods of intense cravings). During this late phase, antidepressants might be required if mood is lowered.

Ecstasy (MDMA) is a drug with both stimulant and hallucinogenic properties, the use of which, often in combination with other drugs, led to increasing emergency presentations from the end of the 1990s. The most common symptom was non-specific ('feeling strange, unwell, dizzy'), but there was also evidence of disturbances in behaviour and increased temperature ('Saturday night fever'; Williams *et al*, 1998).

The serious effects of dehydration and rhabdomyolysis led to users drinking large amounts of water after taking the drug, but this has led to an increased risk of hyponatraemia secondary to inappropriate secretion of the anti-diuretic hormone and an increased risk of cerebral oedema and seizures (Matthai *et al*, 1996). Less severe hyponatraemia responds to fluid restriction accompanied by monitoring of serum sodium levels, but the complications described above or serum sodium levels below 125 mmol/l will need more specialist input (Taylor *et al*, 2012).

Hallucinogens

Lysergic acid diethylamide (LSD) is the best known of this group, which also includes phenylcyclidine, magic mushrooms, mescaline and ketamine. LSD is a synthetic drug, taken orally, that within minutes of ingestion leads to physical symptoms such as nausea, headache, dilated pupils, raised pulse rate, changes in blood pressure and (sometimes) increases in body temperature (Ghodse, 2010). The 'trip' it induces leads to experiences such as emotional lability, time distortions, visual and auditory illusions, synaesthesia and depersonalisation (Wills, 2005). Because of the rapid onset of tolerance, withdrawal phenomena are not seen. Most episodes settle down within 12 hours, and patients tend to respond to supportive help in a calm environment and do not need medical intervention, although those in agitated states might require benzodiazepines (Giannini, 2000).

Volatile solvents

Four types of inhalants can be identified; volatile solvents, aerosols, gases and nitrites ('poppers'). Overall use seems to be increasing, with higher rates among women (Medina-Mora & Real, 2008). Potential acute adverse effects of use include burns, cardiac arrhythmia (including ventricular fibrillation), myocardial ischaemia, dyspnoea and pneumonia (Ridenour, 2005). Treatment will focus on the management of these complications.

Complications associated with methods of use

The principal methods of drug use are oral ingestion, inhalation and injection. Inhalation of drugs has been considered in the previous section, so this section will focus on injection. The risks of drug injection can relate to the sharing of equipment (e.g. blood-borne viruses such as hepatitis and HIV) or the injecting process itself (e.g. local infection, septicaemia, infected emboli, venous thrombosis), in addition to the toxic effects of the drug itself (Haber *et al*, 2009). This might mean that physical symptoms co-exist with drug withdrawal and thus care must be taken not to overlook the possibility of infection or blood clots, for example, in this scenario.

There are an estimated 15.9 million injecting drug users worldwide, of which 3 million might be HIV positive (Mathers *et al*, 2008). In the UK, HIV rates might be low in this group but approximately 40% are infected with hepatitis C (National Institute for Health and Clinical Excellence, 2009). From the late 1980s, increased awareness of the spread of blood-borne viruses via this route led to harm-reduction programmes being developed. Needle and syringe programmes (NSPs) provided sterile equipment and advice on safer injecting, and were available in a range of community settings. They sought to reduce the risk of contracting these conditions and reduce the rate of accidental overdose. This approach has been at least partially successful, as levels of injecting drug use have been falling in England, with estimates from the Government Home Office suggesting there were around 137 000 injecting drug users in 2004–2005, but only 117 000 in 2006–2007 (National Treatment Agency for Substance Misuse, 2010).

Emergency care of injecting drug users should provide information on how to access both local NSPs and hepatitis screening and immunisation services, in addition to encouraging engagement with services to reduce or stop drug use. This is particularly true for some groups that might not have easy access to NSPs, such as female drug users, the homeless, and those who use performance- and image-enhancing drugs or have only recently started to injecting (National Institute for Health and Clinical Excellence, 2009).

One increasingly concerning issue is that of the so-called 'drug mules', who 'transport different drug types and rely on multiple methods of concealment to avoid law enforcement detection' (European Monitoring Centre for Drugs and Drug Addiction, 2012), often internally. The physical risks of transporting drugs in this way include intoxication if the packages rupture and small bowel obstruction, and patients should be admitted for observation and possible surgical removal of the packages, depending on the nature of the packaging and clinical presentation (Kelly *et al*, 2007).

Emergencies in drug users that might or might not be directly linked to their drug use

People who misuse drugs are at risk of physical and psychiatric comorbidities that might not be associated with their drug misuse (Royal College of Psychiatrists, 2004). Engagement with other areas of healthcare provision might be poor, with barriers including stigma, ethnicity, socioeconomic status, gender, and the perception of services (National Institute for Health and Clinical Excellence, 2011). This lack of engagement will make emergency presentations more likely for a range of conditions, and thus it is important that services facilitate entry into treatment, for both acute and chronic care management.

One specific area that can prove difficult is that of pain management, especially in opiate-dependent patients. Haber *et al* (2009) describe a possible reluctance by clinicians to prescribe, as 'requests for analgesia may be interpreted as drug seeking', and outline a measured approach of ensuring the patient feels the pain has been acknowledged, using non-opioiate analgesia (such as paracetamol or non-steroidal anti-inflammatories) as first-line treatment, but if opiates are required then higher doses might be needed. Reassessment of baseline doses (possibly involving a titration process) might also be needed for methadone once the acute episode of pain has settled, and this would require joint working with the prescribing agency. A further complication comes with the increasing use of buprenorphine as an alternative to methadone for opiate substitution. Buprenorphine has partial opiate-receptor agonist activity, which means that patients on higher doses might not respond well to other opiates; therefore, non-opiates would again be preferred, but if pain cannot be managed this way, buprenorphine might need to be stopped and switched to full agonist preparations (i.e. methadone or morphine; Taylor *et al*, 2012).

Emergencies relating to sorting out prescriptions

Concern about drug seeking in emergency situations is evident in a Royal College of Psychiatrists report, which says that 'Less commonly, people who misuse substances without any obvious medical needs may access A&E departments solely in an attempt to obtain controlled drugs' (Royal College of Psychiatrists, 2004). The key drugs of concern are opiates and benzodiazepines and, in general, prescriptions for these should not be issued without discussion with the current prescribing agency (if already on a prescription) or primary care (if the patient is registered with a GP).

References

Ashton H (1994) The treatment of benzodiazepine dependence. *Addiction*, **89**: 1535–1541.

Ashton H (1995) Toxicity and adverse consequences of benzodiazepine use. *Psychiatric Annals*, **25**: 158–165.

Ashton H (2005) The diagnosis and management of benzodiazepine dependence. *Current Opinion in Psychiatry*, **18**: 249–255.

Atkinson RM (1973) Importance of alcohol and drug abuse in psychiatric emergencies. *California Medicine*, **118**: 1–4.

Binks S, Hoskins R, Salmon D, *et al* (2005) Prevalence and healthcare burden of illegal drug use among emergency department patients. *Emergency Medicine Journal*, **22**: 872–873.

Boreham R, Cronberg A, Dollin L, *et al* (2007) *The Arrestee Survey 2003–2006. Home Office Statistical Bulletin 12/07*. Research, Development and Statistics Directorate.

Brody SL, Slovis CM, Wrenn KD (1990) Cocaine-related medical problems: consecutive series of 233 patients. *American Journal of Medicine*, **88**: 325–331.

Budney A (2006) Are specific dependence criteria necessary for different substances: how can research on cannabis inform this issue? *Addiction*, **101** (Suppl 1): 125–133.

Clarke S, Dargan P, Jones A (2005) Naloxone in opioid poisoning: walking the tightrope. *Emergency Medicine Journal*, **22**: 612–616.

Corbett AD, Henderson G, McKnight AT, *et al* (2006) 75 years of opioid research: the exciting but vain quest for the Holy Grail. *British Journal of Pharmacology*, **147** (Suppl 1): S153–S162.

Curran C, Byrappa R, McBride A (2004) Stimulant psychosis: systematic review. *British Journal of Psychiatry*, **185**: 196–204.

Department of Health (England) and the devolved administrations (2007) *Drug Misuse and Dependence: UK Guidelines on Clinical Management*. Department of Health (England).

European Monitoring Centre for Drugs and Drug Addiction (2011) *Annual Report 2011: The State of the Drugs Problem in Europe*. European Monitoring Centre for Drugs and Drug Addiction.

European Monitoring Centre for Drugs and Drug Addiction (2012) *A Definition of 'Drug Mules' for use in a European Context*. European Monitoring Centre for Drugs and Drug Addiction.

European Monitoring Centre for Drugs and Drug Addiction (2014) *European Drug Report: Trends and Development*. European Monitoring Centre for Drugs and Drug Addiction.

Fuller E (2011) *Smoking, Drinking and Drug Use Among Young People in England – 2010*. Health and Social Care Information Centre (http://www.ic.nhs.uk/pubs/sdd10fullreport).

Ghodse H (2010) *Ghodse's Drugs and Addictive Behaviour. A Guide to Treatment*. Cambridge University Press.

Ghodse H, Corkery J, Ahmed K, *et al* (2010) *Drug Related Deaths in the UK: Annual Report 2010*. National Programme on Substance Abuse Deaths, International Centre for Drug Policy, St George's, University of London.

Giannini J (2000) An approach to drug abuse, intoxication and withdrawal. *Americal Family Physician*, **61**: 2763–2774.

Gregory M (2007) Characteristics of drug misusers in custody and their perceptions of medical care. *Journal of Forensic and Legal Medicine*, **14**: 209–212.

Haber P, Dermikol A, Lange K, *et al* (2009) Management of injecting drug users admitted to hospital. *Lancet*, **374**: 1284–1293.

Hall W, Degenhardt L, Lynskey M (2001) *The Health and Psychological Effects of Cannabis Use. Monograph Series No. 44*. Commonwealth of Australia.

Hampson M (2011) Raising standards in relation to Section 136 of the Mental Health Act 1983. *Advances in Psychiatric Treatment*, **17**: 365–371.

HM Government (2010) *Drug Strategy 2010 Reducing Demand, Restricting Supply, Building Recovery: Supporting People to Live a Drug Free Life*. Home Office.

Jay M (2010) *High Society: The Central Role of Mind-Altering Drugs in History, Science and Culture*. Thames & Hudson.

Joint Formulary Committee (2011) *British National Formulary* (61). BMJ Group and Pharmaceutical Press.

Kelly J, Corrigan M, Cahill R, *et al* (2007) Contemporary management of drug-packers. *World Journal of Emergency Surgery*, **2**: 9.

Kosten T, Sofuoglu M (2004) Stimulants. In *The Textbook of Substance Abuse Treatment* (3rd edn) (eds M Galanter, H Kleber). American Psychiatric Publishing.

Lader M (1991) History of benzodiazepine dependence. *Journal of Substance Abuse Treatment*, **8**: 53–59.

Li K (2007) *Maldives Launches First-Ever National Drug Abuse Prevention Campaign*. UNICEF (http://www.unicef.org/infobycountry/maldives_42327.html).

Lidder S, Ovaska H, Archer J, *et al* (2008) Doctors' knowledge of the appropriate use and route of administration of antidotes in the management of recreational drug toxicity. *Emergency Medicine Journal*, **25**: 820–823.

Lopez-Munoz F, Ucha-Udabe R, Alamo C (2005) The history of barbiturates a century after their clinical introduction. *Neuropsychiatric Disease and Treatment*, **1**: 329–343.

Mathers BM, Degenhart L, Phillips B, *et al* (2008) Global epidemiology of injecting drug use and HIV among people who inject drugs: a systematic review. *Lancet*, **372**: 1689–1695.

Matthai S, Davidson D, Sills J, *et al* (1996) Cerebral oedema after ingestion of MDMA ('ecstasy') and unrestricted intake of water. *British Medical Journal*, **312**: 1359.

Medina-Mora M, Real T (2008) Epidemiology of inhalant use. *Current Opinion in Psychiatry*, **21**: 247–251.

Menezes P, Johnson S, Thornicroft G, *et al* (1996) Drug and alcohol problems among individuals with severe mental illnesses in South London. *British Journal of Psychiatry*, **168**: 612–619.

National Institute for Health and Clinical Excellence (2004) *Self-Harm: The Short-Term Physical and Psychological Management and Secondary Prevention of Self-Harm in Primary and Secondary Care (NICE Clinical Guideline 16)*. NICE.

National Institute for Health and Clinical Excellence (2009) *Needle and Syringe Programmes: Providing People who Inject Drugs with Injecting Equipment (NICE Clinical Guideline 18)*. NICE.

National Institute for Health and Clinical Excellence (2011) *Psychosis with Coexisting Substance Misuse: Assessment and Management in Adults and Young People (NICE Clinical Guideline 120)*. NICE.

National Treatment Agency for Substance Misuse (2010) *Injecting Drug Use in England: A Declining Trend*. NTA (http://www.nta.nhs.uk/uploads/injectingreportnov2010finala.pdf).

NHS Information Centre, Lifestyles Statistics (2011) *Statistics on Drug Misuse: England, 2010*. Health and Social Care Information Centre.

Office for National Statistics (2011) *Deaths Related to Drug Poisoning in England and Wales, 2010*. ONS (http://www.ons.gov.uk/ons/rel/subnational-health3/deaths-related-to-drug-poisoning/2010/stb-deaths-related-to-drug-poisoning-2010.html).

Onyett S (1989) The benzodiazepine withdrawal syndrome and its management. *Journal of the Royal College of General Practitioners*, **39**: 160–163.

Palepu A, Tyndall MW, Leon H, *et al* (2001) Hospital utilization and costs in a cohort of injection drug users. *Canadian Medical Association Journal*, **165**: 415–420.

Pope H, Gruber A, Yurgelun-Todd D (1995) The residual neuropsychological effects of cannabis: the current status of research. *Drug and Alcohol Dependence*, **38**: 25–34.

Prochaska JO, DiClemente CC, Norcross JC (1992) In search of how people change: applications to addictive behaviors. *American Psychologist*, **47**: 1102–1114.

Ridenour T (2005) Epidemiology of inhalant use. *Current Opinion in Psychiatry*, **18**: 243–247.

Royal College of Psychiatrists (2004) *Psychiatric Services to Accident and Emergency Departments (Council Report 118)*. Royal College of Psychiatrists.

Royal College of Psychiatrists (2011) *Substance Misuse Detainees in Police Custody Guidelines for Clinical Management (4th edn) (College Report 169)*. Royal College of Psychiatrists.

Seivewright N, McMahon C, Egleston P (2007) Stimulant use still going strong. *Advances in Psychiatric Treatment*, **11**: 262–269.

Smith K, Flatley J (2011) *Drug Misuse Declared: Findings from the 2010/11 British Crime Survey England and Wales*. Home Office (http://www.homeoffice.gov.uk/publications/science-research-statistics/research-statistics/crime-research/hosb1211).

Smith R (1995) The war on drugs. *BMJ*, **311: 1655.**

Strang J, Kelleher M, Best D, *et al* (2006) Emergency naloxone for heroin overdose. *BMJ*, **333**: 614–615.

Taylor D, Paton C, Kapur S (2012) *The Maudsley Prescribing Guidelines in Psychiatry*. Wiley Blackwell.

Wesson DR, Ling W (2003) Clinical Opiate Withdrawal Scale (COWS). *Journal of Psychoactive Drugs*, **35**: 253–259.

Williams H, Dratcu L, Taylor R, *et al* (1998) "Saturday night fever": ecstasy related problems in a London accident and emergency department. *Journal of Accident and Emergency Medicine*, **15**: 322–326.

Williamson S, Gossop M, Powis B, *et al* (1997). *Adverse effects of stimulant drugs in a community sample of drug users. Drug and Alcohol Dependence*, **44**: 87–94.

Wills S (2005) *Drugs of Abuse*. Pharmaceutical Press.

Winstock A, Ford C, Witton J (2010) Assessment and management of cannabis use disorders in primary care. *BMJ*, **340**: 800–804.

World Health Organization (1992) *ICD-10 Classification of Mental and Behavioural Disorders*. WHO.

CHAPTER 4

Alcohol and psychiatric emergencies

Rob Poole

In recent decades, there have been major changes in the pattern of alcohol use in the UK. Through most of the 20th century, UK licensing laws tightly restricted the availability of alcohol. Alcohol duty (a specific sales tax) made alcoholic drinks expensive to consume, especially at home. From around 1980, the UK government lifted restrictions on the availability of alcohol and the relative cost was allowed to drop. It is well established from the international evidence that overall population consumption of alcohol within a nation is closely related to availability and affordability. As prices have dropped, there has been a considerable rise in per capita alcohol consumption. Rates of alcohol-related harm, including death, have steadily risen.

At present, the alcohol industry accepts the need to control alcohol-related harm. Their preferred method is educational. They use advertising campaigns to encourage the population to drink responsibly. They draw a sharp distinction between irresponsible drinkers, who drink in bad and harmful ways, and responsible drinkers, who, it is said, drink in moderate, harmless or even health-enhancing ways. The distinction between responsible and irresponsible drinking patterns has a commonsensical appeal. It echoes the popular idea of the 'alcoholic', who suffers from a disease of alcoholism, and drinks in a pathological fashion that is different to how other people drink. However, the distinction between 'responsible drinkers' and 'irresponsible drinkers' is hard to sustain on the basis of the scientific evidence (Bailey *et al*, 2011).

Levels and patterns of alcohol consumption are continuously distributed in the population. Harmful drinking differs from less harmful drinking as a matter of degree, not type. There is a syndrome of physical and psychological dependency (characterised by tolerance, withdrawal symptoms and a range of behaviours reflecting the salience of drinking over other activities), but a large proportion of those harmed by alcohol do not show this. Increases in alcohol consumption have affected everyone who drinks (about 95% of the UK adult population). It is not confined to 'problem' drinkers or the alcohol dependent. Rates of heavy drinking have increased especially quickly among women, who in general tend to consume less than men.

It is hardly surprising to find that psychiatric emergencies are frequently caused, precipitated or complicated by the effects of alcohol. It is important to recognise that this is not confined to heavy drinkers, and that assumptions about the type of person who does drink heavily can be misleading. The highest levels of alcohol consumption occur among the educated middle class. Heavy drinking among older people is more common than is generally appreciated (both *de novo* and as a continuing habit). At the other end of the substance misuse spectrum, illicit drug use and alcohol consumption are not separate phenomena. Much heavy alcohol consumption in clubs is accompanied by drug use. Chronic opiate dependency is commonly accompanied by heavy drinking.

The use of illegal drugs, especially cannabis, by people with serious mental illness has attracted a great deal of research attention. However, among the general population, alcohol use is more widespread than drug use. Despite the well-recognised association between schizophrenia and cannabis use, many studies show higher rates of problematic alcohol use (McCreadie, 2002). Alcohol use among people with bipolar affective disorder may be even more common.

Understanding and managing the interaction between alcohol use and mental disorder has been a challenge for psychiatry ever since the discipline formed. Some key clinical and scientific problems remain unresolved, such as the mechanism underlying chronic alcoholic hallucinosis. More troubling are the persistent difficulties that mental health services have in finding appropriate and helpful clinical responses to patients' alcohol use. The development of specialist functional teams and specific care pathways mean that people who are mentally ill and drink too much are at risk of being seen as the 'wrong kind of patient'. Service reconfiguration has not taken into account common combinations of problems (Burns, 2010). Hence people with mental illness who misuse alcohol can fall outside of the criteria of all available services, especially at times of crisis.

Psychiatric emergencies are protean. They occur when somebody is frightened (patient, family or professional) and it falls to a mental health professional to resolve the situation. Even after many years of practice, clinicians are routinely confronted with emergency situations that they have never previously encountered. Understanding and managing such situations depends on the application of principles, some of which are drawn out in this chapter.

Many of the problems of assessing and managing psychiatric emergencies where alcohol is involved come together in one scenario. The psychiatrist gets a call to attend a general hospital emergency department in order to assess someone who is drunk and threatening suicide. He attends with a sinking heart. The patient is distressed, intoxicated, disinhibited and tearfully insistent on suicidal intent. The psychiatrist has difficulty in assessing the patient. It is extremely trying to attempt to reason with someone who is distressed and drunk. Even when it is fruitful, it is hard to know whether plans and undertakings will be adhered to. In the background, the staff of the emergency department are likely to want the patient to be removed from the department as soon as possible, so that they can concentrate their attention on physically sick patients. The mental health home treatment team and the inpatient unit, following policies that focus on people who are unequivocally mentally ill, are unlikely to be keen to get involved in the immediate care of a drunken patient. Whether or not the patient is suffering from an underlying mental illness, there is meanwhile a degree of risk, at least until they sober up.

These situations tend to arise out of hours. It is not impossible to achieve a satisfactory outcome, but it can be difficult. There are numerous other types of mental health emergencies involving alcohol that are equally complicated and demanding for clinicians. However, I will return to this scenario as an example.

The relationship between alcohol use and psychiatric symptoms

There are real limitations to reductionism as a method of understanding the complexities of causation in psychiatry, but nonetheless it is helpful to have some clarity about the fundamental ways in which alcohol and psychiatric symptoms interact (Poole & Brabbins, 1996):

- alcohol-induced symptoms (e.g. depression due to heavy alcohol use)
- withdrawal states (e.g. delirium tremens, anxiety)
- physical disorder due to severe alcohol misuse (e.g. Wernicke–Korsakoff syndrome, subdural haemorrhage)
- pathoplastic effects (e.g. intoxication superimposed on symptoms of underlying mental illness) and relapse of mental illness associated with heavy drinking
- alcoholic hallucinosis
- alcohol combined with other psychoactive substances.

Alcohol-induced symptoms

Confronted with problems in their lives, a remarkably high proportion of the population come to rely on the healing power of ethanol. When mental health professionals suggest that drinking might be making matters worse, it can be frustrating to find that the patient insists that alcohol is the only thing that keeps them going.

One of the many attractive characteristics of alcohol is that it is strongly anxiolytic, an effect that has a very rapid onset. This is probably the main reason that people who are feeling stressed find alcohol comforting. However, it has an equally powerful effect in causing depressed mood. This depressant effect has a more gradual onset and is more persistent than alcohol's anxiolytic effects. Even a single exposure to a large quantity of ethanol can cause depressed mood; gloomy self-reproach can linger much longer than headache and nausea during a hangover.

The anxiolytic effects of alcohol offer immediate relief for tense, troubled people. The depressant effects of the drug insidiously undermine mental health, generating further anxiety. It is easy to enter a cycle whereby drinking is driven by the need to overcome the effects of previous drinking. This can occur without becoming physically dependent on alcohol and in the absence of significant alcohol tolerance. Many psychiatrists spend a substantial part of their working week trying to get patients to understand this process and to grasp that alcohol is part of the problem, not part of the solution.

Acute alcohol intoxication can be a cause (as opposed to a precipitant) of psychiatric crisis in some common and particular ways. The first situation involves a person who is struggling with relationship or other life problems. They show little evidence of a depressive illness per se and express no suicidal intention until they drink a large quantity of alcohol. They then become morose and disinhibited, and develop a strong and immediate desire to end their life. Attempts at severe self-laceration, hanging, carbon-monoxide poisoning or self-poisoning follow. Overdoses taken under these circumstances can be especially dangerous, owing to the combined effects of toxic levels of drugs and alcohol. Where the outcome is fatal, these deaths appear among open and narrative verdicts in coroners' inquests, as the deceased's intentions can be difficult to discern. When such suicide attempts fail and the person is seen for psychiatric assessment, it can be important to realise that a lack of clear intent does not imply a low risk of recurrence. People in this type of alcohol-induced crisis are often taken to hospital by their friends and relatives, creating a scenario of the type described in the introduction. On sobering up, some will be sheepishly apologetic and show little evidence of wanting or needing psychiatric assistance. Others will prove to be persistently troubled. However, at the point of presentation, people who are seriously intoxicated and who show a willingness to harm themselves are at high risk.

The next common situation is a variation of the first. The person at the centre of it is usually male, and intoxication releases his anger over a relationship problem. This leads to an act of aggression or violence, sometimes in a domestic setting, sometimes in public. The police are called and he is arrested. His situation has now objectively deteriorated, with a deepening of the relationship problem, and sometimes a threat to employment because of the arrest. His mood changes to an oppositional form of self-recrimination and remorse. He makes angry attempts to violently harm himself and is aggressive towards anyone trying to stop him from doing so. The police are increasingly reluctant to risk a death in their custody, and young men in this frame of mind are often brought to emergency rooms by police officers looking for a psychiatric disposal.

Another, rather different situation where alcohol is a primary cause is the person with a definite alcohol problem, often including physical dependence, who is seriously intoxicated and in a state of despair. They have previously been resistant to all efforts to help them stop drinking, but they have finally been persuaded by their friends or family to accept help. Patient and carers present themselves to emergency services (often a general hospital emergency department) requesting immediate admission for detoxification and alcohol rehabilitation. They are frustrated and angered by the response of services: that the patient cannot be assessed because they are too drunk ('But she's always drunk … that's her problem!'); that immediate admission is not indicated because the patient needs to show motivation to long-term sobriety ('But if we take her home, she'll change her mind!'); and that she'll be sent an appointment to see alcohol services at sometime in the future, and that in the meantime she shouldn't stop drinking abruptly ('So you're telling her to go home and carry on drinking? I don't believe this!').

Alcohol withdrawal

Alcohol is a powerful anticonvulsant that depresses neuronal membrane excitability via a number of different mechanisms. After the central nervous system (CNS) has functioned in the presence of high levels of ethanol over a long period of time, it adjusts through a kind of homeostasis to return neurones to an optimal level of excitability. Neuronal cell membranes become more excitable so that they operate in more or less a normal way in a high concentration of ethanol. This is alcohol tolerance, and behaviourally the consequence is that large amounts of alcohol might have little effect on the person's behaviour.

It should be noted that although liver enzymes are induced by ethanol, rapid metabolism of alcohol is not the primary mechanism for alcohol tolerance. There are other elements to tolerance, including learned behaviour, that are intrinsic elements of alcohol dependence. However, neuronal tolerance is the mechanism that underlies the main features of acute alcohol withdrawal. Essentially, once the CNS has become alcohol tolerant, abrupt discontinuation of alcohol consumption throws the brain into a state of hyper-excitability. Initial features are over-arousal, anxiety, jitteriness, tremor, and sleep disturbance. This can progress to frank delirium (delirium tremens or the DTs), where the previous features are accompanied by fluctuating clouding of consciousness, paranoid ideas, severe fearfulness, auditory (and sometimes visual) hallucinations, irritability and aggression. With or without other withdrawal symptoms, alcohol withdrawal can provoke epileptic seizures. These can be life-threatening.

Paranoid ideas with auditory hallucinations, agitation and fearfulness can seem superficially similar to acute schizophrenia, unless the history of heavy drinking is evident. The particular features of fluctuating clouding of consciousness, vivid visual hallucinations and marked behavioural responses to hallucinations should raise the suspicion of alcohol withdrawal. It is also important to remember that alcohol withdrawal can occur alongside functional psychosis, especially when people are hospitalised and forced to abstain.

Physical disorder due to severe alcohol misuse

There are no reliable figures on the prevalence of the Wernicke–Korsakoff syndrome, but there seems to be consensus among clinicians that it is becoming more common (Ramayya & Jauhar, 1997). It predominantly affects chronic heavy drinkers in their middle years. They tend to show evidence of advanced alcohol dependence, and a marked decline in social functioning and circumstances. Wernicke's encephalopathy and Korsakoff syndrome represent the acute and chronic ends of a single process, and either can be seen in the absence of the other.

The syndrome is due to thiamine (vitamin B_1) deficiency. Heavy drinkers are prone to thiamine deficiency for two main reasons. First, heavy drinkers tend to a have poor diet, with much of their calorific intake being ethanol and sugar in alcoholic drinks. Their diet tends to be low in thiamine. Secondly, ethanol inhibits thiamine absorption through the intestinal mucosa. The liver stores thiamine, which is used up during glucose metabolism. The moment of highest risk of acute thiamine deficiency for heavy drinkers is when they stop drinking and start eating. This is exactly what happens when they are admitted to hospital. Although Wernicke–Korsakoff syndrome can arise at any time in the life of a middle-aged heavy drinker, it is especially common in the context of medical intervention (often under circumstances where the person's heavy alcohol intake has not been identified or is not regarded as the primary problem).

Wernicke's encephalopathy is a medical emergency that commonly arises in psychiatric practice. It is intrinsically life threatening, as it can progress to coma, seizures and death. In addition, prompt diagnosis and treatment with parenteral thiamine can prevent or ameliorate subsequent Korsakoff syndrome. The main features are confusion, memory impairment, ataxia, ophthalmoplegia, and nystagmus. Generations of doctors were taught that it was characterised by a triad of symptoms: confusion, ophthalmoplegia and ataxia. This was unhelpful, because all three elements are present in only a small minority of cases, eye signs being the least common feature. Confusion, on the other hand, with or without ataxia, is almost invariable.

The diagnosis is clinical, and it is easily missed unless the possibility is actively considered whenever heavy drinking is suspected. The features can be confused with intoxication on one hand and withdrawal on the other. The symptoms might lead to medical attention being sought, through a fall or confused behaviour in the community, or they might emerge when the patient has been admitted to hospital for some other reason and is given a carbohydrate load that uses up inadequate thiamine stores.

In 1989, the Committee on Safety of Medicines issued a warning regarding anaphylactic reactions to parenteral thiamine. Prior to this, doctors had a low threshold for giving people parenteral thiamine where Wernicke's was suspected. Subsequently, we have probably become over-cautious (Thomson & Cook, 1997). The risk of anaphylaxis is low, and parenteral thiamine is most effective where it is administered promptly and in adequate quantities.

People who are drunk are prone to falling over. They are more likely than others to sustain injuries when they fall, because a general slowing of cognition prevents normal instinctive manoeuvres to protect themselves. A high proportion of facial injuries are sustained when intoxicated, because people who are drunk don't put their hands out to break their fall. Similarly, head injury is common amongst people with alcohol problems. A history of recent-onset confusion in a drinker should raise the suspicion of head injury and subdural haemorrhage. This can occur alongside Wernicke's encephalopathy, where ataxia leads to a fall and a head injury – two simultaneous brain pathologies, both of which require treatment.

The clinical picture of Korsakoff syndrome is dominated by a profound impairment of short-term memory in the absence of global dementia. There might be secondary features, such as confabulation and perseveration, but the inability to retain and recall new information creates a huge obstacle to social functioning and independence. Generally speaking, this means that the patients need 24 h care, either by family or within a residential care setting. This is difficult, as these relatively young people often have little insight into their condition. They usually have an underlying drink problem that leads them to seek out alcohol. Abstinence, thiamine supplementation and a proper diet can lead to significant improvement in memory function, but this is slow. Improvement can continue for 2 years or more. There is invariably a degree of residual memory impairment. Korsakoff syndrome is a catastrophe for the person and their family.

Pathoplastic effects and relapse of mental illness associated with heavy drinking

There can be little doubt that alcohol has a profoundly unhelpful effect on people suffering from major mental illness. Many people with chronic schizophrenia suffer from high levels of anxiety, and, just like many other people, they drink to try to cope with this. They often describe a marked worsening of auditory hallucinations the next day, which might be relieved by further drinking. This is another trap whereby people with a mental illness can come to believe that drinking is helpful.

Psychotic relapse is frequently associated with heavy drinking. It can be more or less impossible to work out causality: Does alcohol have an adverse physiological effect on the CNS that provokes relapse? Does drunkenness lead people to forget to take medication? Does the distress of psychosis provoke drinking? For practical purposes, it is just as well to assume that these and other mechanisms can all apply.

Heavy drinking certainly has an effect beyond exacerbation of common psychotic symptoms. Symptoms of anxiety and depression are more prominent where people with psychosis drink. Some people who are paranoid about those around them are more likely to take action related to their beliefs when intoxicated. There is a weak association between psychosis and violence, but there is a strong association between heavy drinking and violence. Alcohol misuse is an ominous risk factor for people with psychotic illness, with implications for the risk of serious self-harm and aggression.

Alcoholic hallucinosis

There is a dearth of high-quality research into alcoholic hallucinosis, a condition that causes clinicians considerable confusion. It is a chronic hallucinosis that arises in clear consciousness in the absence of schizophreniform features, although there may be explanatory (secondary) delusional beliefs. The main symptom is vivid auditory hallucinations that have a concrete quality similar to true perceptions. They occur alongside unimpaired reality testing. The person is aware, or rapidly realises, that the hallucinations arise from within themselves. Despite this insight, many people suffering from alcoholic hallucinosis shout back at the voices, as this can relieve the distress that they cause.

Alcoholic hallucinosis can start as a continuation of the hallucinations of DTs, or it can insidiously appear during periods of heavy drinking. The experiences may be relieved or exacerbated by taking alcohol. The hallucinations respond poorly to antipsychotic medication, but gradually disappear during periods of abstinence. This can take many months, though several weeks is more usual. There seems to be some kind of kindling effect, as the hallucinations tend to reappear as soon as drinking is resumed.

Alcoholic hallucinosis is increasingly seen in the young. The voices tend to be worse at night, when they may be accompanied by visual experiences. Insight may be less evident during darkness, but returns by day.

Intoxication with alcohol and other substances

As pointed out earlier, alcohol use is often accompanied by use of other psychoactive substances, both legal and illegal. Combined intoxications can have extremely unpredictable effects, and these do not always pass quickly. Two specific combinations can cause major problems in clinical practice.

The first is alcohol and opiates. The problem here is respiratory depression. The substances have a synergistic effect with a high risk of death due to complete loss of respiratory drive or, more commonly, aspiration of stomache contents due to suppressed gag reflex. There are a large number of opiates available, with a wide range of plasma half-lives.

When people report recent use of alcohol and opiates in combination, their current state of manifest intoxication may prove misleading. If there is a significant quantity of unabsorbed alcohol in their stomach, they may become much more intoxicated over subsequent hours. It is important that anyone looking after them is aware that snoring is not a sign of sound sleep; it is a consequence of respiratory distress. Snoring may be the only warning that the person is in a life-threatening state of respiratory depression.

The second especially troublesome combination is alcohol and stimulants. For these purposes, stimulants include cocaine, amphetamine, ketamine, MDMA (3,4-methylenedioxy-N-methylamphetamine) and analogues of these drugs, a grouping that is pragmatically useful but far from pharmacologically sound (neither ketamine nor MDMA is strictly a stimulant). The combination of these drugs with alcohol can induce confusion, fearfulness, hallucination, paranoia and, sometimes, suicidal ideas that can persist for several days. The use of these drugs is common, especially in city-centre clubs, and adverse reactions regularly occur in people with no previous psychiatric history.

Assessment and management

One of the difficult aspects of psychiatric emergencies is that assessment and management are tasks that have to be attended to simultaneously. Assessment has to continue whilst risk is contained. This is especially true where the patient is intoxicated, and this is one of the challenges in the scenario set out in the introduction to this chapter.

The key to all psychiatric assessment is to find out what has happened: in other words, to obtain a good history. This is an invariable principle. Mental state examination and investigations are important, but they are of little value in the absence of a proper history. Where the patient is intoxicated, history may be the only information available to guide decisions, and informants are then invaluable.

The role of alcohol in a psychiatric emergency might not be immediately obvious, and ascertaining whether the person has been drinking heavily is a part of all assessment in emergency and routine practice. It is particularly important to recognise that non-dependent drinking (for example, 40 units or 400 mL of alcohol per week, which corresponds to just over a half of a bottle of wine per day), which might not be evidently problematic to those around the person, can exacerbate a range of mental health difficulties.

Taking a history

I shall not attempt to set out the general principles of history taking here, as there is a range of good resources available (Poole & Higgo, 2006). There is little point in attempting to take an alcohol history in isolation. It is more meaningful to gather information about alcohol, tobacco and drug use, including use of over-the-counter and prescribed drugs, all of which are part of a more general enquiry about the patient's life.

There are standardised validated questionnaires that can be used to assess drinking, for example, CAGE and AUDIT (Bush *et al*, 1987; Saunders *et al*, 1993). However, there is no substitute for skilled clinical interviewing. Box 4.1, rather than being a list of questions to be mechanically asked of all patients, is a menu (by no means exhaustive) of the range of questions that might be asked when initial probes suggest that the person is drinking more than is desirable. Where the person is intoxicated and able to answer questions, asking them what they have drunk on that day is especially important, as well as the timing. Intoxication is not just a function of total volume consumed; the rate of consumption is also important. A bottle of spirits consumed by someone with minimal alcohol tolerance over 24 h will cause marked intoxication but no worse in most cases; the same volume consumed by the same person over 1h might prove fatal.

The concept of 'units of alcohol' was developed to improve general understanding of the relative strength of alcoholic beverages. A unit of alcohol is 10 mL of ethanol. Doctors quite often ask patients how many

---

Box 4.1   A menu of questions related to substance misuse

Alcohol

- At what age did you start drinking?
- Exactly how much did you drink yesterday, and at what times?
- Which brand, and what strength, of beer/cider do you drink?
- Do you drink wine as well? Do you ever drink spirits?
- Exactly what did you drink on your worst day this month?
- How much do you spend on alcohol? Where does the money come from?
- Have you ever been convicted of drink driving?
- Do other people think your drinking is a problem? Do you agree?
- Has your tolerance increased? Do you shake or retch in the mornings?
- Have you ever tried to give up drinking? What made you try?
- Have you had accidents when drunk or suffered from memory blackouts?
- Have you ever had a fit or hallucinations when you stopped drinking?

Drugs

- At what age did you start using drugs?
- What drugs have you ever used, and what do you use now?
- How do you pay for it? Do you owe a drug supplier money?
- Have you ever injected drugs?
- Have you ever had a bad drug experience? Or had withdrawal symptoms?
- Do you think that drugs cause you any problems?
- Which of the following do you use? Heroin, methadone, pharmaceutical opioids, benzodiazepines, cocaine, crack-cocaine, amphetamine, ketamine, LSD, magic mushrooms, ecstasy (and its analogues), cannabis, rarer drugs (e.g. khat)?

Source: reproduced with permission from Poole & Higgo (2006)

---

units of alcohol they drink each week, in order to compare this with national guidelines on safe drinking. However, simple calculations of units of alcohol can be misleading, as beverages vary widely in strength. The alcohol content of beer, for example, varies between 3.5% and 9%.

Many people who drink more than is desirable systematically underestimate their consumption. Although there is sometimes an element of deliberate 'improvement' of the facts (quite often to bring unit consumption within well-known safe limits), one of the remarkable aspects of alcohol misuse compared with, for example, cigarette addiction, is the way that users frequently seem to mislead themselves about their habit. It is more helpful to ask people exactly what they drink, with reference to consumption in the recent past (the day of assessment or the day before): how much of which particular drink of what strength within what time scale. It is useful to know something of the strengths of commonly available drinks (Table 4.1). This can present a problem for UK psychiatrists who come from cultures where alcohol is not used. The internet is a useful resource in this respect, as it allows rapid access to information on the strengths of different alcoholic products.

Wherever possible, the patient should be asked to describe quantities in specific terms. For example, many people who drink non-spirits heavily will describe drinking one glass of spirits before going to bed, often described as a 'double'. This implies the quantity sold as a double in pubs, which contains two units of alcohol. It is important to ask them to demonstrate the quantity between thumb and forefinger, as this is almost invariably far in excess of a pub double.

One of the major purposes in taking an alcohol history is to assess whether the person is physically dependent. This assessment rests on a description of tolerance to the effects of alcohol and withdrawal symptoms, of which coarse tremor is the most common. Some people drink so continuously that they never have the opportunity to develop withdrawal symptoms. There are some relative indicators as to whether the person is likely to develop withdrawal symptoms on discontinuation of drinking. The amount of alcohol drunk without marked effects such as slurring of speech, the time of day that the first drink is taken and the extent of craving provide some guide, though no indicators are truly reliable.

Table 4.1 Approximate alcohol content of commonly consumed beverages

Beverage	Quantity	Alcohol by volume	Units of alcohol
Spirits	1 bottle (700 mL)	40%	28
Wine	1 bottle (700 mL)	12–15%	8.5–10
Beer (cans/bottles)	1 can/bottle (330–500 mL)	3.5–9%	1–4.5
Beer (draught)	1 pint (570 mL)	3.5–5%	2–3
Cider	1 bottle (500 mL to 2 L)	2–7.5%	1–15

Physical examination can provide some confirmation of suspicions of heavy drinking in the form of a smell of alcohol, hepatomegaly or spider naevi, but the majority of heavy drinkers will not show these signs. Laboratory tests have a use, but they can be misleading. If blood gamma-glutamyl transferase (γ-GT) levels are very elevated, this frequently indicates heavy drinking. However, some heavy drinkers have normal γ-GT levels, and many commonly used medications, such as non-steroidal anti-inflammatory drugs, cause moderately elevated γ-GT. Other abnormalities in liver function tests might or might not be related to alcohol intake, but most drinkers show no liver dysfunction. Even when liver function tests are abnormal, they rarely indicate how advanced alcohol-related liver disease has become. In a full blood count, raised mean corpuscular volume is, strictly speaking, a relatively non-specific indicator of poor nutrition (through folate or B_{12} deficiency). However, it is generally the most sensitive blood-test indicator of heavy drinking. If a heavy drinker has a history of drug use, it is important test for hepatitis C. The combination of hepatitis C and heavy drinking can lead to rapidly progressive liver disease.

Fitness for assessment

It is always difficult to decide whether an intoxicated patient is fit for assessment or not. There is no doubt that assessment of someone who is very drunk can be seriously misleading. However, much conflict and distress is generated by rigid refusal to assess people who have been drinking to lesser degrees of intoxication.

Determining whether a patient is fit for assessment is based on clinical skills. There are no reliable tests or investigations that can supersede clinical judgement. Some services breathalyse patients, and decline to assess if they are over the UK limit for driving (a blood level of 80 mg/100 mL). This practice is irrational and difficult to support. The effects of alcohol vary according to tolerance and circumstances. For most people, the drink-driving limit is well below a degree of intoxication that would render assessment meaningless. This is not to suggest that breathalysers (and urine drug testing) have no role. They can be useful, for example, when repeatedly administered to determine whether blood alcohol levels are increasing or dropping. However, this is no substitute for trying to discover what the person has consumed by asking them (or any available informant). History is a better indicator of whether the person is likely to become more intoxicated (because of recent rapid consumption of spirits, for example) than any technical test.

The main features that suggest that a person cannot currently be fully assessed because of alcohol intoxication are significant aggression, muddled or incoherent speech, inability to converse (particularly perseveration of speech that obstructs dialogue), dysarthria, ataxia, nystagmus, and sedation. It should be noted that some of these features are similar to those of Wernicke's encephalopathy.

Cooper and colleagues (2010) have suggested that the most meaningful test is whether the person has mental capacity to make decisions about their care and treatment. Whatever approach is used, some face-to-face assessment is necessary in making the decision as to whether to proceed immediately with full assessment. Declining to assess without seeing the patient cannot be justified. It is therefore more appropriate to regard the process as an extended assessment rather than delayed assessment, where the interview with the patient can be resumed as soon as they have reached an appropriate level of sobriety. Meantime, there is a good deal that the psychiatrist can do to further the assessment. The patient's general practitioner might have useful information. The person might be known to the local alcohol team. Relatives and other informants should be interviewed. There is a risk that informants either collude through minimisation or exaggerate in desperation. This underlines the importance of gaining information from more than one source. Informants who live with the patient should be asked about domestic violence, which is relatively common and might require intervention in its own right. Women can be perpetrators of domestic violence.

In order to make appropriate assessments of intoxicated people, there have to be organisational systems and agreements that work. Emergency departments must be prepared to look after the patient until they are fit for interview, which they will normally accept if it is accompanied by the quid pro quo that the patient will be fully assessed promptly on becoming sober. Mental health teams that assess emergencies in the community need well-thought-through policies on how they will proceed if a patient, referred as an emergency, proves to be drunk. In all situations, patient and staff safety in the interim has to be actively managed.

Managing acute intoxication

A person who presents as a psychiatric emergency, but proves to be too intoxicated to fully assess immediately, is at risk. First, if they are entertaining suicidal ideas, they are quite likely to act on these. Second, they are unlikely to be able to guard themselves from harm. Third, they can act aggressively to those around them. Fourth, there is a risk of death due to compromised respiration.

These people need someone to look after them, and allowing them to leave hospital unaccompanied, or worse still, discharging them unaccompanied with instructions to return when sober, invites disaster. These situations are especially difficult in the community. There is a major dilemma when you attend someone's home and find them alone and too drunk to assess. Neither the police nor the mental health services are likely to be in a position to provide domiciliary care until they are sober. If there is no friend or relative available to attend to them, and if they fall below a legal threshold that would justify removal to hospital, there is no alternative but to leave them where they are. A prompt return is called for under such circumstances.

When people are intoxicated and behaviourally disturbed in a hospital setting, there is a temptation to use medication to control them. However, the combination of alcohol and benzodiazepines is potentially lethal, especially when the latter is administered parenterally. It can provoke disinhibition and paradoxical excitement. The combination of antipsychotics and alcohol is not necessarily safer, risking both sedation and epileptic seizures.

There is no role for medication in managing acute intoxication. The environmental measures that are effective in minimising disturbed behaviour caused by mental illness work equally well with people who are intoxicated. These include a quiet, comfortable setting that minimises emotional stimulation, with supportive staff present. Politeness and clarity as to when they going to be seen and what will happen next help a lot.

Most people who are seriously drunk will eventually lapse into unconsciousness or, perhaps, sleep. When this happens, it is tempting to leave them as they are. However, they should always be placed in the recovery position, because aspiration of stomach contents is a major risk. Regular nursing observations are essential. As previously mentioned, snoring is ominous under these circumstances.

After assessment

Once an assessment has taken place, the patient's alcohol consumption has to be addressed as part of an overall treatment strategy (Poole & Higgo, 2008). In a small minority of cases, it will be evident that the person is alcohol dependent and that this is the primary problem, in which case referral to alcohol treatment services is the obvious next step. There can be problems, however, in managing people who recurrently harm themselves when intoxicated but deny suicidal intentions when sober. This is a high-risk pattern of behaviour, but most mental health units and home treatment teams specifically exclude people who need treatment for substance misuse only. Although it is entirely correct that treatment for alcohol dependency is best conducted by specialists, few alcohol treatment services in the UK can respond quickly and effectively to a risk of this nature. Many people with this kind of problem decline intervention by substance misuse services. This is one example of the 'wrong kind of patient' syndrome mentioned previously. Services have developed in such a way that potentially treatable patients in a life-threatening situation can be excluded by service criteria from prompt and effective treatment. In my opinion, admission to a mental health unit for detoxification under these circumstances can be justified, although others will disagree. It can allow clarification of the nature of the problem and, where appropriate, plans can be developed for joint management with local substance misuse services.

Most patients whose alcohol consumption has an adverse effect on their mental health are not physically dependent. They are unlikely to meet criteria for alcohol treatment services. It is good practice to deal with substance misuse within generic mental health teams as far as is possible and safe, and this is the position set out in national guidelines on so-called 'dual diagnosis' (National Institute for Health and Clinical Excellence, 2011). The patient doesn't actually suffer from two problems (e.g. drinking and depression) they suffer from one problem with various aspects that should be dealt with as far as possible through a single strategic treatment plan executed by one team.

The main principles in managing non-dependent drinking are as follows.

- To provide the patient and carers with a plausible explanation of the role of alcohol in the mental health problem.
- To make a realistic estimate of the degree of improvement that is likely to occur through abstinence or reduced consumption.
- To get the patient to monitor their level of consumption and degree of distress in an alcohol diary.
- To get carers and others to provide a supportive environment by abstaining themselves and organising activities in alcohol-free settings.

Generic mental health professionals are more than capable of successfully overseeing a programme based on these principles, provided they regard doing this as part of their job.

Inevitably, some patients who present as a psychiatric emergency with alcohol involved will have to be admitted to a mental health unit. Many in-patient units have a standard detoxification regime agreed with the hospital pharmacy that is begun on admission for all patients who are known to drink heavily. There are serious problems with this practice. Detoxification should only be commenced if there is a reasonable likelihood that the person will suffer from withdrawal symptoms without it, and it is arguable that detoxification should only proceed when the person shows clinical signs of withdrawal. Detoxification is for people who are physically dependent on alcohol.

If detoxification is necessary, standardised regimes are rarely appropriate. They almost invariably involve a 3- to 5-day reducing regime of chlordiazepoxide, commencing at 20 mg four times a day, together with oral thiamine supplements. The regime is a compromise between safety and the organisational imperative of ensuring that admissions are as brief as possible. However, alcohol-dependent patients show wide variation in the dose of chlordiazepoxide needed to eliminate withdrawal symptoms. A surprisingly large number of people with marked tolerance to alcohol show no withdrawal symptoms on abstinence, and others have withdrawal symptoms that only respond to double the standard dose, or return unless the reducing regime is extended to 2 weeks or longer. For this reason, most specialist in-patient detoxification units use a sliding-scale regime based on nurse assessment of withdrawal symptoms using validated standardised instruments (e.g. the Clinical Institute Withdrawal Assessment for Alcohol scale; Sullivan *et al*, 1989). If physical withdrawal occurs, the dose of

65

chlordiazepoxide needed to control the symptoms is established in the first 24 h. The dose is reduced over the next 5–7 days, with daily assessment and some flexibility for people who prove to need a lengthier withdrawal regime.

It is sometimes unrealistic to expect generalist mental health units to deploy this kind of sliding scale regime successfully. However, a compromise is possible, with a standardised 7-day regime and daily medical review. If the patient shows signs of sedation, the dose of chlordiazepoxide is too high. If the patient shows a coarse tremor, agitation or other withdrawal symptoms, the dose is too low. Cautious adjustment of the dose will avoid an unpleasant or dangerous withdrawal experience. It is important to remember that good nursing care, with close attention to fluid intake and hydration, is an essential component of detoxification. Patients benefit from support and reassurance.

There is no harm in oral thiamine supplementation, but it will not prevent Wernicke's encephalopathy in the thiamine deficient. In each detoxification, a decision has to be made whether parenteral thiamine is justified as a prophylactic measure, bearing in mind the small but real risk of anaphylaxis.

Most patients undergoing detoxification in a general mental health unit are suffering from a mental illness. There is a difficult decision to be made as to whether to commence psychotropic medication during detoxification. As a general rule, it is best to wait. Where the patient is depressed, there is likely to be some improvement during detoxification, and the degree of this is unpredictable. Nearly all psychotropic drugs interact with benzodiazepines, and the high starting dose of chlordiazepoxide invites marked sedation. However, this is counsel of perfection. Many patients will already be on psychotropic medication, some of which cannot be discontinued (e.g. depot preparations). People with psychosis are often too unwell to allow any delay in treatment, in which case the introduction of antipsychotic drugs should be conducted carefully, with a low starting dose and daily review. It is particularly important to avoid prescribing more than one benzodiazepine, and to avoid p.r.n. benzodiazepine regimes after completion of detoxification.

Detoxification is not a treatment for alcohol dependence. It is a necessary first step to allow the patient to go safely from heavy drinking to being alcohol-free. If it is not followed by an intervention aimed at maximising the chances of sustained abstinence, then a return to heavy drinking is highly likely. This might be delivered within the community mental health team, if they have the expertise, or by a specialist alcohol team working in conjunction with the community mental health team, or by a voluntary sector organisation. Alcoholics Anonymous (AA) has a particular approach to addictions that does not suit everyone. However, they provide intense and long-term support. In cases where the programme resonates for the patient, AA can work very well.

Attitudes

The misuse of alcohol raises issues of morality, volition and stigma. Both science and society tend to understand 'alcoholism' either in terms of moral deficit (a failure of volition) or hereditary taint (a genetic predisposition). In our culture, drinking to excess is shaming. This goes some way to explain why many drinkers systematically underestimate their consumption, and the defensive reactions of most people when it is suggested that their drinking might be damaging their health.

Negative attitudes to uncontrolled drinking are held by mental health professionals as much as the rest of the population and this can be seriously counterproductive in treatment. People who feel accused of drinking, or blamed for it, will rightly feel that they have been subjected to a moral judgement rather than an objective appraisal of the nature of their problems. Being made to feel that they are the 'wrong kind of patient' and that their drinking makes them unsuitable for services can only exacerbate this.

Mental health professionals cannot detach themselves from social attitudes, but a degree of self-awareness can prevent those attitudes from causing problems in clinical practice. A calm, kindly, firm professional can explore alcohol misuse with patients, intoxicated or sober, and arrive at a point where the patient feels that this a person who is trying to help them, rather than trying to reprimand them for a personal failing. Of course, abstinence from alcohol does involve volition; the patient does have to believe that abstinence is possible and the right thing for them, and they must want to stop drinking. This is more likely in a therapeutic relationship that is supportive and takes a problem-solving approach.

Health organisations have to recognise that substance misuse accompanies or causes a wide range of health problems. It is not an unusual complication but an intrinsic part of the syndromes that we regard as mental illnesses. If we establish systems that regard mental illness and substance misuse as two diagnoses rather than one complicated problem, a substantial proportion of our clientele will be excluded from appropriate interventions.

Conclusions

This chapter has reviewed some of the common issues, principles and situations where a psychiatric emergency involves excessive alcohol consumption. To return to the scenario in the introduction, where a psychiatrist is called to assess a drunk, distressed patient: many psychiatrists would decline to see the patient at all, and arrange for assessment to be conducted 12 h later. The patient would then be nursed by emergency department staff, who might resent looking after 'the drunk in bed 4' while the mental health services, to whom they might feel the patient 'belonged', do nothing. After some sleep, and suffering from a hangover, with no plan in place, the patient might then decide to leave before assessment occurs. No problems would be solved and, at best, the entire sequence might be repeated a few days later.

This chapter has attempted to point to another, more appropriate, way of proceeding that is practically possible in contemporary practice. Extended assessment, proper detoxification, coordination of mental healthcare, and continuing support to abstinence (or controlled drinking for the non-dependent) are all possible, and are far more likely to help the patient to recovery.

References

Bailey J, Poole R, Zinovieff F, *et al* (2011) *Achieving Positive Change in the Drinking Culture in Wales.* Alcohol Concern (http://www.alcoholconcern.org.uk/publications/policy-reports/achieving-positive-change).

Burns T (2010) The dog that failed to bark. *The Psychiatrist*, **34**: 361–363.

Bush B, Shaw S, Cleary P, *et al* (1987) Screening for alcohol abuse using the CAGE questionnaire. *American Journal of Medicine*, **82**: 531–535.

Cooper P, Caulfield M, Mason T (2010) Developing a procedure to test for intoxication and mental capacity: the 'Under the Influence test' pilot study. *Mental Health Nursing*, **30**: 9–13.

McCreadie RG (2002) Use of drugs, alcohol and tobacco by people with schizophrenia: case–control study. *British Journal of Psychiatry*, **181**: 321–325.

National Institute for Health and Clinical Excellence (2011) *Psychosis with Co-Existing Substance Misuse: Assessment and Management in Adults and Young People (NICE Clinical Guideline 120).* NICE.

Poole R, Brabbins C (1996) Drug induced psychosis. *British Journal of Psychiatry*, **168**: 135–138.

Poole R, Higgo R (2006) *Psychiatric Interviewing and Assessment.* Cambridge University Press.

Poole R, Higgo R (2008) *Clinical Skills in Psychiatric Treatment.* Cambridge University Press.

Ramayya A, Jauhar P (1997) Increasing incidence of Korsakoff's psychosis in the east end of Glasgow. *Alcohol and Alcoholism*, **32**: 281–285.

Saunders JB, Aasland OG, Babor TF, et al (1993) Development of the alcohol use disorders identification test (AUDIT): WHO collaborative project on early detection of persons with harmful alcohol consumption – II. *Addiction*, **88**: 791–804.

Sullivan JT, Sykora K, Schneiderman J, *et al* (1989) Assessment of alcohol withdrawal: the revised Clinical Institute Withdrawal Assessment for Alcohol scale (CIWA-Ar). *British Journal of Addiction*, **84**: 1353–1357.

Thomson AD, Cook CCH (1997) Parenteral thiamine and Wernicke's encephalopathy: the balance of risks and perception of concern. *Alcohol and Alcoholism*, **32**: 207–209.

CHAPTER 5

Acute psychosis

Richard Hodgson and Santhusi Mendis

In this chapter, we will provide an overview of the assessment and short-term management of people of presenting with acute psychotic symptoms. Our aim is to focus on practicalities and to highlight real-world issues. In reality, it is not always possible to deliver what is considered best practice because of time and resource constraints. Decisions often have to be made on little information and clinicians need to be prepared to frequently review their management in the light of new information as the clinical picture unfolds. Cultural issues need to be borne in mind to avoid labelling culturally appropriate distress as mental illness.

Although it is crucial to share information among professionals (for example, when there are safeguarding concerns regarding children), confidentiality principles still apply. Thought will also need to be given to the use of the Mental Health Act 2007 or Mental Capacity Act 2005 in many cases.

This chapter will focus on urgent presentations, but it should be remembered that patients who have psychotic symptoms do not always present in crisis. With better psychoeducation, the routine use of relapse signature recognition, better access and other service developments it is not uncommon for patients to identify deterioration in their own mental health and seek help before a crisis response is needed.

Presentation

Patients suffering psychotic disorders often present in a distressed and agitated state, especially in a first episode. The majority of assessments take place in accident and emergency departments, custody suites, general hospital wards, the patient's residence and section 136 suites. Sometimes these presentations are voluntary – when the patient presents to find relief for his or her distressing experiences, or after being coaxed by their friends and family to seek help. Some of these voluntary presentations might be the result of delusional systems. For example, the subject might call the police to complain about a conspiracy or present to their general practitioner

(GP) requesting a surgical referral so that an implanted microchip that is controlling their mind can be removed.

There are little epidemiological data about the presentation of people with a psychotic disorder, as such data depend on other factors, such as the demographics of the local population and clinical practice. Penagaluri *et al* (2010) examined a sample of 206 consecutive patients seen in an emergency psychiatric service in a large, urban teaching hospital in an unspecified mid-sized city for the presence and intensity of hallucinatory experiences. Among the 191 for whom a diagnosis was attached, there were 26 (13.6%) patients with schizophrenia, 36 (18.8%) with major depression, 18 (9.4%) with bipolar disorder, 68 (35.6%) with primary substance dependence, and 43 (22.5%) with other diagnoses (including mood disorder not otherwise specified, adjustment disorder, generalized anxiety disorder and personality disorder).

The relationship between psychotic symptoms and behaviour

Psychotic patients have disturbed reality testing characterised by delusions, hallucinations and a lack of insight leading to erroneous ways of perceiving and relating to the outside world. These symptoms interact with the patient's cultural milieu and personality. For instance, an individual suffering from a delusion that his neighbours are persecuting him might become withdrawn and limit contact with the outside world. A more aggressive individual with the same delusions might be more proactive and attack his perceived persecutors.

Similarly, a delusion of grandeur that leads to a person mistakenly believing that she is a multi-millionaire could result in inappropriate expenditure. The behaviour exhibited can give clues to the underlying pathology. Grandiose delusions are more likely to be associated with mania than a depressive psychosis or schizophrenia. If a person with schizophrenia has grandiose delusions, the expected associated affect is often missing. It is therefore important to link the individual's behaviour to his or her psychopathology. By doing this we get a better understanding of the person's experiences, which will aid assessment and management.

Types of psychotic disorder

From a practical perspective, psychotic disorders can be divided into two major categories: organic and functional. Organic psychotic disorders arise as a result of an identified organic disturbance, which can be due to cerebral or non-cerebral causes. An example of a cerebral cause would be a person who develops acute psychotic symptoms as a result of temporal lobe epilepsy. Non-cerebral causes, such as low sodium levels, can also give rise to acute psychotic symptoms that occur in the context of delirium. Treatment should focus on the underlying disease, although treatment of psychotic symptoms might also be indicated. Symptomatic treatment, such as rapid tranquillisation, might be necessary in order to perform the necessary investigations to establish the correct diagnosis. Functional psychotic disorders are those conditions where there is, as yet, no recognised diagnostic organic pathology. This distinction is not absolutely reliable and psychoses related to substance misuse can be challenging.

From a purely clinical perspective, the key distinguishing factor between functional and organic psychoses is level of consciousness. In organic disorders, impairment is evident, as demonstrated by clouding of consciousness characterised by reduced attention and concentration. The patient might be disorientated in time, person or place. By contrast, in functional psychosis consciousness is clear, although clinical experience might be needed in judging the responses to enquiries regarding attention, concentration and orientation.

Organic psychotic disorders

Delirium

The classical presentation of an organic psychosis is delirium (acute confusional state). Elderly patients frequently present to emergency departments with the condition (Gower *et al*, 2012). This condition is not a normal manifestation of ageing and is indicative of an underlying organic pathology (Gower *et al*, 2012). Sometimes the cause is never determined and recovery occurs with supportive treatments. Delirium usually occurs acutely, and the cause can be cerebral or non-cerebral (Box 5.1). Infections, disturbances in electrolyte levels, liver failure and renal failure are some of the most common causes. Those whose cerebral function is already compromised by conditions such as stroke and dementia tend to be more vulnerable to delirium. Patients might also present with psychomotor disturbances. They might be hyperactive, hypoactive or have a mixed presentation (Martin & Fernandes, 2012). Patients exhibit clouding of consciousness and can be disoriented to time, place, and person. As a result of this disorientation, wandering behaviour is common. Poorly systematised delusions and hallucinations can also be experienced. The hallucinations can be both visual and auditory in nature.

The management of delirium consists of identifying and treating the underlying causes of the condition. It is often helpful for treatment to take place in a quiet, well-lit room, to keep the amount of external stimulation to a minimum. Patients who are disoriented often find it difficult to make sense of their external environment. For this reason, it is crucial to nurse them away from the hustle and bustle of an acute medical ward. As these patients are already physically compromised, pharmacological interventions should be considered only after behavioural interventions have failed. Treatment is normally with benzodiazepines or antipsychotics.

Box 5.1 Causes of delirium or organic psychosis

Neurological

- Space-occupying lesions
  - Haematoma
  - Tumour
  - Abscesses
- Degenerative diseases
  - Dementia
  - Huntington's chorea
  - Multiple sclerosis
  - Parkinson's disease
  - Wilson's disease
- Epilepsy
  - Inter-ictal confusional states
  - Ictal confusional states
  - Post-ictal confusional states
- Cerebrovascular accident
  - Embolism
  - Infarction
- Cerebral infections
  - Meningitis
  - Encephalitis

Non-neurological

- Organ failure
  - Renal failure
  - Hepatic failure
  - Heart failure
  - Respiratory failure
- Disturbances in electrolyte levels
  - Hypokalaemia
  - Hyperkalaemia
  - Hypontaraemia
  - Hypernatraemia
- Disturbances in plasma calcium
  - Hypocalcaemia
  - Hypercalcaemia
- Disturbances in blood glucose levels
  - Hypoglycaemia
  - Hyperglycaemia
- Endocrinological causes
  - Thyroid disease
  - Parathyroid disease
  - Adrenal disease

Other

- Poisons
  - Arsenic
  - Lead
  - Carbon monoxide
- Alcohol-related
  - Delirium tremens
  - Wernicke's encephalopathy
- Illicit substances
  - LSD
  - Ketamine
  - GHB
- Prescription drugs
  - Anti-cholinergic medication
  - Paracetamol and salicylate overdose
- Nuritional deficiency
  - Thiamine deficiency (can lead to Wernicke's encephalopathy)
  - Vitamin B_{12} deficiency
- Dehydration

Case study 1

Mrs Smith, a 76-year-old woman with a history of ischaemic heart disease, was admitted to the orthopaedic ward for a hip replacement. There was no evidence of dementia at admission and she was living on her own. Following surgery, she was lucid and coherent but staff noted that there was an acute change in her behaviour the next day. She seemed perplexed and agitated. She accused staff of trying to kill her and made numerous attempts to leave the ward. Her thoughts were muddled. She also claimed that she could see spiders crawling all over the ward. Her sleep pattern became disturbed. Her symptoms tended to fluctuate and they were worse at night. The doctor who examined her noted that she was disoriented to time, person and place. No relevant physical signs were noted and subsequent investigations were all negative. Her pre-admission medication was checked with her GP and it was noted that she normally took lorazepam 0.5 mg twice daily. Reinstatement of this medication resulted in a slow recovery.

Delirium tremens

This condition is an extreme form of alcohol withdrawal and occurs in those with alcohol dependence syndrome. The condition usually presents between the second and fifth day after cessation of alcohol. Therefore, if an accurate alcohol history is not obtained, or the patient denies excessive intake, the symptoms might be erroneously attributed to the reasons for the original admission. The condition often goes unrecognised and is a relatively common reason for a request for a psychiatric opinion from medical wards.

Case study 2

Mr Jones, a 56-year-old widowed man, was admitted with hypothermia after he was found lying in the streets. It was not possible to get a background history, as no relatives were contactable. His condition stabilised and he made a full recovery. However, 4 days after admission and just prior to discharge, there was a noticeable change in his behaviour. He became agitated and began to pace up and down the ward. He looked frightened, and claimed that there was a conspiracy to harm him. He claimed to see snakes on the ward, and demanded that something should be done about it. He was easily startled. He was disoriented and did not realise that he was on a medical ward, believing instead that he was in a torture chamber. Staff noted that he had a marked tremor. He began to sweat profusely, and his blood pressure and pulse rate were raised. His agitated state meant he was difficult to treat, and he was given large doses of diazepam. He gradually settled and further investigation revealed a history of alcohol misuse.

Like delirium due to other causes, delirium tremens occurs mainly in those who are physically compromised. The features are similar to those of delirium. Patients are agitated, disoriented and exhibit clouding of consciousness. Visual hallucinations are very common and are often Lilliputian (in which things seem smaller than in real life). Auditory and tactile hallucinations can also occur. Mood can be elated, depressed, or labile. As is the case with delirium due to other causes, the symptoms are worse at night. Tremor is a common symptom, and autonomic changes such as changes in blood pressure, temperature, and heart rate are seen. In some severe cases, the physiological changes can be so profound that cardiovascular shock can occur. Withdrawal seizures are another possible complication.

Left untreated, delirium tremens is associated with high morbidity and mortality. Treatment consists of benzodiazepines, usually chlordiazepoxide or diazepam. Lorazepam is used when the person's hepatic function is compromised. Parenteral thiamine is administered in order to address the thiamine deficiency that results from the neglect of nutritional requirements. Because of neglect of their nutritional needs, these patients are often deficient in glucose and carbohydrates as well. However, the prophylactic administration of glucose should only take place after vitamins are administered. If not, Wernicke's encephalopathy can develop.

Antipsychotic medication should be used with caution in this condition because of the risk of withdrawal seizures. Standard antiepileptic medication such as carbamazepine has been shown to be effective (Hughes, 2009).

Wernicke's encephalopathy and Korsakoff's syndrome

Wernicke's encephalopathy can occur in patients with alcohol dependence syndrome when they are withdrawing from alcohol. Patients become confused and struggle to engage in rational conversation. In addition to confusion, ophthalmoplegia, nystagmus, and ataxia are other features of the condition. The cause of the condition is widely believed to be thiamine deficiency. As in delirium tremens, withdrawal seizures are another complication. As it is associated with high mortality, treatment (benzodiazepines and parenteral thiamine) should not be delayed. If appropriate treatment is administered promptly, the condition is potentially manageable. However, if treatment is not administered, or if it is delayed, Korsakoff's syndrome can develop as a result of permanent cerebral changes. Usually there is global anterograde and retrograde amnesia with confabulation. In addition to impaired cognitive functioning, psychotic symptoms might also be present.

Drug-induced psychotic disorder

Although the term 'drug-induced psychotic disorder' is frequently used in clinical practice, it is not ideal. Certainly, illicit substances such as amphetamines could cause a release of dopamine and trigger an acute change in the sufferer's presentation with features resembling a psychotic illness. It is also the case that patients with schizophrenia experience an acute exacerbation of their symptoms following the use of illicit substances. However, in many cases it is not a true psychotic disorder.

Individuals suffering from an acute change in their mental state following the use of illicit substances present frequently as emergencies. Delusions of paranoia are common. These patients frequently experience auditory hallucinations that are derogatory in nature. If the presentation is due to intoxication, the symptoms should abate when the drug has been eliminated from the body. Therefore, the symptoms should resolve within a few hours to a few days. Until then the patient can remain distressed by their symptoms. For this reason, antipsychotics and benzodiazepines are often used to treat the symptoms.

Acute porphyrias

There are several types of porphyria, which result from a partial deficiency of the enzymes responsible for porphyrin synthesis. Porphyria attacks are often precipitated by alcohol, certain drugs and infection. The presentation is variable, with acute abdominal pain, peripheral neuropathy and seizures common. Psychiatric symptoms are a manifestation of this disorder and psychiatric patients have a higher rate of the illness when compared with the general population (Croarkin, 2002). The symptoms vary and can be mistaken for affective, psychotic or even stress-related illnesses. Delusions, hallucinations, mood changes and behavioural disturbances can be present in these conditions.

Wilson's disease

This is a recessive, inherited disorder of copper metabolism. Copper accumulates in the liver, brain, kidney, cornea, and bone. Deposits of copper in the cornea result in the characteristic Kayser–Flesicher ring. This neurological disorder is primarily a disorder of motor function, and tremor and rigidity are common early signs. Wilson's disease can also present with psychiatric symptoms. Wilson described psychiatric symptoms in 8/12 of his cases and 'schizophrenia-like psychosis' in two of the cases (Wilson, 1912). About 30–60% of patients with Wilson's disease present with depression (Akil & Brewer, 1995; Hesse *et al*, 2003). Furthermore, an association between bipolar disorder and Wilson's disease has been demonstrated, possibly explaining the frequent reports of symptoms such as irritability, sexual disinhibition and hyperactivity (Carta *et al*, 2012).

Functional psychotic disorders

Schizophrenia

Schizophrenia symptoms can be broadly divided into 'positive' and 'negative' categories. Delusions and hallucinations fall in the category of positive symptoms. The delusions and hallucinations that occur can be either congruent or incongruent with mood. Although delusions and hallucinations commonly occur in schizophrenia, they are absent in simple schizophrenia, which is a disorder characterised by prominent, debilitating negative symptoms. Apathy, poverty of thought, and blunted affect are examples of negative symptoms. The negative symptoms are not attributable to an underlying depressive disorder, or organic illness.

Catatonic symptoms can also occur in some patients. Catatonic symptoms can take the form of abnormal postures. Some patients, for example, lie mute and in a stupor for long periods. In other instances, they stand in positions that healthy individuals would find uncomfortable to hold for prolonged periods. It is sometimes possible to alter the individual's posture and for the individual to continue with it.

The onset of the illness is variable. One long-term follow-up study showed that about 50% of patients had an acute onset and 50% had a long prodromal phase (Ciompi, 1980). The course of the illness is also variable. For instance, about 20% of patients do not require readmission, even many years after discharge (Mura *et al*, 2012). On the other hand, patients might experience several episodes with complete or incomplete remission. In Ciompi's study (1980), for instance, about half of the patients had an undulating course with partial or full remissions followed by recurrences that occurred in an unpredictable manner. The course of the illness also varies according to country, with prognosis better in the developing world. A World Health Organization study showed that individuals with schizophrenia in developing countries were less likely to be chronically psychotic over the follow-up period and that they were more likely to be free of residual symptoms after 5 years (Cohen & Patel, 2008).

Delusional disorder

This disorder is characterised by the presence of a single or set of related delusions. The content of the delusions can vary, and examples include persecutory, grandiose, nihilistic, and jealous forms. Hallucinations and the negative symptoms of schizophrenia are absent in this condition.

Case study 3

Emily was convinced that her GP was in love with her. She would patiently wait outside his surgery until he finished his clinic and then follow him home. She would send him numerous letters expressing her love for him. Those letters would frequently end with the suggestion that he should marry her. Her constant stalking behaviour was noticed by others and was causing a tremendous amount of stress to the GP and his family. The doctor concerned was in fact a happily married man who maintained very professional relationships with his patients. His colleagues supported him in his assertions that he on no occasion behaved in any way that would suggest to Emily that he had any amorous feelings for her. Emily however refused to accept his assertion that there were no sexual feelings on his part towards her. In fact, she interpreted his avoidance behaviour as further proof that he was in love with her. Emily's behaviour gradually became so disruptive that the police were called and she was detained under the Mental Health Act 1983.

Affective functional psychotic disorders

Mania with psychotic symptoms

Manic mood can occur alongside psychotic symptoms such as delusions and hallucinations. When psychotic symptoms occur, they are mood congruent. For example, grandiose delusions frequently occur in this condition, in keeping with the elated mood. Paranoid delusions can occur alongside irritable mood. When hallucinations occur, they are also mood congruent.

Case study 4

Darren had a family history of bipolar affective disorder. He began to display features of the illness at 20 years of age. His friends noticed that over a few days he became irritable and argumentative. They were surprised at this, as he was usually a very placid man. He became overactive and would stay up till the early hours of the morning playing loud music. His speech became rapid and his friends found it difficult to follow his speech. Although previously a tidy individual, his flat became very messy. He would move from one task to another and found it difficult to complete any of them. The content of his speech became bizarre as well. He stated that he was the 'messiah' come to rid the world of all sin. He started to dress in white, stating that he was ordained by heaven to do so. He also said he could hear the voices of angels singing his praises. He finally came to the attention of the police after he caused a disturbance outside the local church. He said that he caused the disturbance as the vicar failed to recognise his spiritual significance.

Depression with psychotic symptoms

When psychotic symptoms occur in the context of depressed mood, they are mood congruent. Examples of mood-congruent delusions are delusions of nihilism and guilt. Similarly, any hallucinations that occur surround depressive themes such as worthlessness, hopelessness and suicidality.

Case study 5

Mrs M, an 80-year-old widowed woman who was living on her own, began to isolate herself. Neighbours had noted that she seemed low in mood and unlike her usual, bubbly self. After they had not seen her for over a month they informed the police, who forcibly entered her house to do a safe-and-well check. They found her flat to be in an unhygienic state. She appeared emaciated and it was obvious that she had neglected her food and fluid intake. She told everyone that she had restricted food as she was in financial ruin. Her nephew was convinced that this was not the case, as she had considerable amounts of money in her savings account. Her facial expression was blank and she kept rocking to and fro in her chair, claiming responsibility for a murder that had occurred recently. The police were incredulous, as the murderer had already been caught.

Assessment

The primary aim of assessment is to make a diagnosis and to instigate treatment (Table 5.1). However, many factors can impede a traditional medical assessment. The patient might be uncooperative, unable to furnish a history and resistant to physical examination and further investigations. Even if a patient is well known to services, an open mind should be kept about the aetiology of the current presentation. For example, diabetes is increasingly common in those with schizophrenia, and this could lead to confusion in diagnosis if the presentation is automatically attributed to a relapse in schizophrenia rather than, for example, hypoglycaemia. See Table 5.1 for psychiatric disorders than can be mistaken for psychotic conditions.

Safety

The assessment of a patient with what seems to be a psychotic illness should be regarded as a psychiatric emergency and should not be delayed unduly. A timely assessment reduces the likelihood of unexpected and unpredictable behaviours that might endanger the safety of the patient or others. Some interventions to reduce these risks, such as a police presence, might affect the assessment.

Before assessing the patient, it is important establish associated risks and these are often dependent on the assessment setting. Theoretically, risk should be minimised in a police cell compared with a home assessment. In whatever setting, it is important to conduct the interview in a quiet room with thought given to how a rapid retreat could be made if the situation deteriorates. The patient should not be between you and the door. Careful attention should be paid your communication style and manner. Patients with psychotic disorders are often very frightened and distressed, and careless or insensitive comments can unsettle them further. This might limit the taking of a full history, but the emphasis at this stage is to arrive at a working diagnosis and management plan.

In practice, assessments take place in less than ideal situations. For example, finding a quiet room that is not cluttered with potential weapons is not easy on a busy medical ward or emergency department. Home assessments might reassure the patient as they would be in their own environment, but the psychiatrist would not be and might have to contend with other issues, such as large dogs or uncooperative or intoxicated relatives.

When assessing these patients at home, it is sensible to do a joint assessment with another mental health professional such as a community psychiatric nurse or social worker. Personal attack alarms can be useful and it should be routine to notify another member of staff of where you are going and your expected time back at base.

Information gathering

The patient you have been asked to assess might have had previous contact with mental health services or might be a new referral. The referral source will highlight likely sources of information. For example, a referral from social services will indicate whether the patient has been detained before or has had any previous contact with local authority services. GP records are an invaluable source of information, but might not be accessible outside office hours. Local psychiatric records or at least a history of contact might be available 24 h. If the patient is known to other agencies, such as probation services, it is important to liaise with them. The referrer might be the key worker for that patient and be able to provide insights into the patient, their

Table 5.1 Psychiatric differential diagnosis of functional psychotic disorders

Disorder	Similarities to psychotic conditionss	Distinguishing feature/features from psychotic conditions
Anxiety	Psychomotor agitation. Inability to focus and engage in meaningful conversation, as in formal thought disorder.	Absence of psychotic symptoms such as delusions, hallucinations, and formal thought disorder.
Borderline personality disorder	Pseudohallucinations	The hallucinatory experiences are located in internal space, unlike those in functional psychotic illnesses, which are located in external space.
Paranoid personality disorder	Paranoid ideation	Although patients with paranoid personality have a tendency to be suspicious, this suspiciousness is not of delusional intensity.
Schizotypal personality disorder	Eccentric and bizarre behaviour and ideas	Although they exhibit eccentric and odd beliefs, these are not of delusional intensity.
Autistic spectrum disorder	Abnormalities in social interaction, and communication	These conditions fall under the category of pervasive developmental disorders, in that the impairments in social interaction, communication, and stereotyped and repetitive behaviour are manifest before the age of three years.
Malingering	Bizarre behaviour or speech	Malingering is behaviour that is consciously feigned for an obvious motivation. The symptoms of a psychotic disorder are not feigned. The conditions can be distinguished by observing the patient for a sufficient length, as feigned behaviour is unlikely to be sustained over a prolonged length of time.
Post-traumatic stress disorder	Increased arousal, irritability, and sometimes social withdrawal. Flashbacks are sometimes mistaken for psychotic experiences. Agitation can cause difficulties describing experiences.	This disorder is only seen following an exceptionally threatening or catastrophic event. Flashbacks, nightmares related to the event, autonomic hyper-arousal and emotional numbing are usually present.
Dissociative disorders	Loss of sense of personal identity and awareness of surroundings can result in the patient being perplexed.	These disorders occur following an extremely stressful and traumatic event. Unlike a psychotic disorder, they resolve spontaneously. They involve a temporary loss of the sense of personal identity and awareness of the surroundings, which does not occur in psychotic disorders.

79

previous history and management under similar circumstances, but this is not an excuse to blindly follow previous management plans.

Family members can be a valuable source of information, providing insights into the individual's pre-morbid mental state as well as the current mental state. You would preferably speak to them with the patient's consent, but this is not always forthcoming. In some circumstances, the patient might not have capacity to give consent to collateral information being gathered, and good medical practice dictates that a refusal should not necessarily be taken at face value. However, judgement is called for and not all relatives have the patient's best interests at heart. Care must be taken when sharing information in order to minimise the potential breach of confidentiality. Some patients have advance directives on how they should be managed if experiencing a relapse, including what treatments they would prefer and which relatives can be informed of an admission.

The interview

Ideally, the interview should be conducted in a quiet and safe environment. The main priority is to reassure the patient and develop a rapport. Questions should be open-ended and the patient given plenty of opportunity to talk without interruption. The interviewer should aim to gain a clear understanding of the underlying psychopathology and the effect it is having on both the patient and others. One aim is to understand the psychopathology from the patient's perspective. A risk assessment that incorporates risk to self and others is an important part of the process.

Once the information relating to the patient's mental state and associated risks has been gathered, the interviewer should ascertain the patient's level of insight. Does the patient regard his or her experiences as abnormal and part of a mental illness, and is he or she willing to accept the input of mental health services for follow-up and treatment?

Although a full history and examination is desirable, the interviewer must be prepared to adapt to the situation and focus on the most relevant areas. These will be dictated by information gathered beforehand and in the first few minutes of the interview, and from observation of the patient's behaviour. Do not assume that because the patient is initially obliging this situation will continue.

The first priority is to determine whether the patient has an organic or functional illness. Determining this can happen almost subliminally in many cases on the basis of prior information and the patient's presentation. Sometimes more than one diagnosis might have to be managed. For example, the initial assessment might suggest, correctly, that a diagnosis of major depression with psychotic feature is the primary issue. However, further enquiry or deterioration in the patient's level of consciousness could indicate that the patient has also taken an overdose. Even without a frank admission or obvious signs, the presence of discarded pills and containers would suggest a need for further observation or interview.

Aspects of the history can be checked immediately if you are in the patient's residence. They might say they are eating and drinking, but a lack of food in the fridge might contradict this. Likewise, the presence of unopened medication packets could indicate non-adherence despite the patient's protestations to the contrary. Most assessments will be straightforward but, unless other factors are considered, important features might be missed on the rare occasions they occur, such as acute porphyria.

An overview of management

Most assessments of acute psychosis will be multidisciplinary and the presence of a professional already known to the patient might facilitate management. Often, practical issues, such as getting the patient in an ambulance or arranging child or pet care, can provide the greatest challenges. Sympathetic handling of such matters can significantly affect the patient's demeanour. In addition to the involvement of mental health professionals, consideration should be given to the input of external agencies such as child protection teams or environmental officers.

Until relatively recently, the management of acute psychosis was predominantly done on an in-patient basis. The development of home treatment teams has changed this and some patients can be managed on a day-patient basis. Crisis houses also exist. The nature of the psychosis and any complicating factors will dictate the appropriate treatment location. Management should be holistic and adopt a multidisciplinary team approach to be effective.

The management plan should not be static. Instead, it should be reviewed regularly and updated as necessary. Patients should be encouraged to be active participants in devising their management plans in order to develop effective therapeutic relationships and to aid adherence. The patient should have a full understanding of their management plan and should receive a copy of it.

The principles underpinning the effective treatment of psychosis are early identification and treatment. Early-intervention teams target young people presenting with their first episode of psychotic illness. Active engagement is another important aspect of management. Assertive-outreach teams are specially set up to provide intense input to patients who have a history of disengagement from services.

Finally, the needs of the carers should not be ignored or overlooked. Carers often play a vital role in the treatment of patients. Caring for a loved one suffering from a psychotic illness can be challenging and carer stress often goes unrecognised. To prevent this from happening, carers should be offered an assessment that identifies their own needs and should be offered assistance to address them.

The management of a psychotic illness can be broadly divided into biological, psychological, and social components. The basic principles are outlined next, and focus mainly on the management of functional psychotic disorders.

Biological component

The biological component of management involves not only addressing the pharmacological management of the mental disorder, but also considering the individual's physical health needs. Patients presenting to psychiatric services often have undiagnosed physical health conditions. They also have poor access to healthcare (Bolton, 2011). In addition, psychotropic drugs are associated with various side-effects. These factors contribute to the high morbidity and mortality rates seen in this group of patients. Life expectancy is reduced by 20% among those diagnosed with schizophrenia, with physical illness accounting for 60% of the excess mortality (Newman & Bland, 1991).

For these reasons, it is important to do a thorough physical examination on every patient. In instances where the patient is too agitated or refuses to allow an examination, a general inspection should be conducted. It is possible to assess whether or not the patient is experiencing physical discomfort, whether their level of hydration is adequate and whether indicators of neurological problems, such as abnormal movements, are present. The findings should be clearly documented, and a more thorough physical examination should be deferred to a future date (Hodgson & Adeyemo, 2004).

Ideally, psychotropic medication should only be prescribed once a thorough evaluation has been undertaken of the patient's physical health and mental state. In addition to a physical examination, routine tests such as a full blood count, renal, liver and thyroid function tests, and glucose and cholesterol level checks should be performed. Psychotropic medications are associated with prolongation of the QTc interval and sudden cardiac death (Sumic *et al*, 2007), so an electrocardiogram might be needed to rule out cardiovascular problems. A drug screen might also be relevant. Pregnancy testing should be considered in women of childbearing age.

Neuroimaging should be conducted when a cerebral pathology is suspected. Cerebral pathology should be considered in individuals presenting with late-onset psychosis, neurological signs, a history of cerebral trauma or symptoms like fluctuating consciousness and olfactory and visual hallucinations. However, the National Institute of Health and Care Excellence (NICE; 2008) does not recommend routine neuroimaging in first-episode patients with functional psychoses.

NICE (2010) provides advice for the management of acute aggression. When a patient is agitated and at risk for causing harm to the self or others, a major tranquilliser such as haloperidol should be considered. This comes in oral and intramuscular form, but the oral route should be the first line of management. Administering intramuscular medication often requires restraint, and this is not only physically risky but can damage the therapeutic relationship. Haloperidol can be used in conjunction with a sedative such as lorazepam. Because of the extrapyramidal side-effects associated with a typical antipsychotic like haloperidol, an atypical antipsychotic such as olanzapine might be more appropriate. It is important to monitor the patient's vital signs after rapid tranquillisation.

Psychological component

A patient admitted to hospital is often very frightened. This fear often manifests as agitated and aggressive behaviour. By reassuring the patient and listening to their fears and anxieties, this agitation can be considerably decreased. Aggression in acute mental health wards could be minimised with the effective use of such de-escalation techniques. Access to a gym might help the patient vent their frustration. The role of supportive nursing should never be underestimated. It is important that the patient meets with a named key worker on a regular basis.

In-depth psychoanalytic work is generally not felt to be appropriate for those who are acutely psychotic. However, when the patient's symptoms have resolved to a sufficient extent, consideration could be given to psychological therapies. Cognitive–behavioural therapy has shown some efficacy in schizophrenia (Tarrier *et al*, 2004).

Social component

The psychiatric ward constitutes the social environment for an acutely psychotic patient admitted to an in-patient ward. It is important to ensure that this environment is safe and conducive to recovery. Patients should be offered the chance to participate in a variety of ward-based activities, which are intended to provide stimulation and make the in-patient stay a positive experience. Encouraging participation in group activities encourages socialisation with fellow patients. It is hoped that ward activities alleviate boredom, which can lead to agitated and disruptive behaviour. In addition to group activities, participation in physical activities should be encouraged when appropriate. Regular physical activity improves overall well-being and might encourage the patient to develop the habit of being physically active, thereby reducing their likelihood of developing conditions such as obesity. The individual's spiritual needs should be met as well, for instance by giving access to an area to pray in.

As the patient's symptoms resolve and the associated risks to the self and others decrease, it is crucial to integrate them back into the community. This is done by the process of giving the patient leave off the ward. After even a brief in-patient stay, the individual's confidence in living independently in the community might be diminished. This needs to be borne in mind when planning home leave. It is sensible to gradually increase the periods of leave. This gives professionals an opportunity to assess the patient's ability to cope.

After the patient is discharged from hospital, it is important to help them to achieve their maximum potential. Opportunities should be provided for them to engage in leisure and physical activities.

Potential pitfalls in the assessment and management of psychotic patients

Guarded patients

Some patients choose not to disclose their psychotic experiences to professionals. This poses problems in assessing the patient's mental state. In such instances, it is important to identify the reasons why the patient is being guarded. Clinicians should try to be warm and empathic. Questions should be open-ended to facilitate the development of rapport. Such rapport can take time to develop, so it might be helpful to see the patient over several sessions.

Failure to undertake an adequate risk assessment

Adequate, accurate risk assessment is crucial for the effective treatment of patients suffering from psychotic illnesses. A poor risk assessment is one that either overestimates or underestimates the risk patients pose to others or themselves. Patients experiencing command hallucinations telling them to harm themselves could act on them. There is also a danger that, as patients gain insight into their condition, they might contemplate ending their lives because of feelings of hopelessness.

Let us first look at instances where the risk posed might be overestimated. Sometimes factors such as poor verbal communication by professionals, an unsettled ward environment, and failure to listen could result in increasing distress in patients. This might translate into disruptive behaviour on the ward. In such situations, clinicians might attribute this behaviour to a propensity for violence rather than understanding the role played by external factors. What is known as 'institutional folklore' could also result in the overestimation of risk. This occurs when episodes falsely attributed to the patient enter the psychiatric case records and inform the management.

An underestimation of the risk posed by a patient might also occur when professionals fail to liaise with each other to communicate risk. Failure to listen to concerns about risk expressed by family members can lead to a failure to correctly assess risk.

Negative symptoms

Schizophrenia can involve negative symptoms, such as apathy and blunting of affect, that can be very debilitating. For instance, a previously outgoing and sociable young person could become withdrawn and disengaged from day to day life as a result of negative symptoms. In addition to being debilitating, negative symptoms could also result in unfair value judgements being made by professionals who have limited understanding of the condition. For instance, a person exhibiting apathy could be falsely accused of being 'lazy'. This is very unhelpful, as it precludes the patient from getting the help that he or she requires.

There is a danger of interpreting behaviour in a patient suffering from schizophrenia as being solely due to negative symptoms. Withdrawn behaviour, for example, could actually be due to a depressive condition or physical illness. These pitfalls highlight the importance of taking an enquiring approach when dealing with this group of patients.

Self test 1

You are asked to assess a 45-year-old married man at a police station. He had been arrested earlier for a severe assault on his wife, which resulted in her having to be admitted to hospital with several fractures. When arrested, he claimed that he was acting in self-defence. He says that he is convinced that his wife is having an affair, and that she and her alleged lover are trying to poison him. He claims that he knows that this is the case on the basis of his national insurance number. He admits to having followed her movements, checked her underwear for evidence of sexual activity, and opened her mail without her knowledge. He goes on to state that he has been assaulting her, in order to extract a confession. He also claims that he is not the father of his two small children. He seems calm during the interview, and is persistent in his beliefs. The police state that he has frequently been arrested for drunk and disorderly behaviour. You also find out that he is known to have disengaged from the mental health services, and that his compliance with his antipsychotic medication has been erratic.

Q1 What is the most likely diagnosis?

The belief that his wife is being unfaithful is firmly held, is based on irrational grounds, and is out of keeping with social norms. It is therefore a delusion of infidelity. The associated behaviour, such as the stalking behaviour, checking for sexual activity and domestic violence, shows how intensely this belief is held. The differential diagnoses include paranoid schizophrenia, delusional disorder, and Korsakoff's psychosis (in view of the difficulties with his alcohol intake).

Q2 What are the associated risks?

The risks are very high in such cases. He is at risk of causing serious bodily harm to his wife, or even murder. There is also the risk of harm towards his wife's supposed lover, which needs to be taken into consideration. As he is alleging that he is not the father of the children, there exists a possibility that he might harm them. Finally, in addition to the risks such patients pose to others, it needs to be borne in mind that such patients are might harm themselves out of despair.

Q3 How would you treat him?

Owing to the risks highlighted above, the first priority should be to ensure the safety of both the patient and others. As it is very likely that he is suffering from a mental disorder, it is imperative that he should be admitted to a psychiatric hospital. The police should investigate the history of domestic violence and intervene as necessary. A referral to child and family social workers should be made immediately to look into the child protection issues.

Once he is admitted to hospital, he should be further assessed for the risk he poses to himself and to others. If he is at risk of suicide, consideration should be given to placing him under close observation. A thorough examination should be carried out of his physical state before initiating treatment for his mental disorder. As there is a history of difficulties with alcohol use, he should be assessed for features of withdrawal and started on a detoxification regime if necessary. His urine should be tested for traces of illicit drugs. In view of his history of alcohol misuse, neuroimaging should be requested in order to rule out pathology.

When planning treatment for his mental disorder, it is important to find out the reasons for his non-adherence to his medication regime. If medication non-adherence and disengagement from treatment have been ongoing issues, the use of depot antipsychotics should be considered. Before re-starting antipsychotics, routine blood tests and electrocardiogram investigations should be performed to rule out underlying morbidity such as cardiac or metabolic disease, which can be exacerbated by antipsychotics.

A robust and assertive follow-up plan should be put in place by the mental health team following his discharge from hospital in order to prevent future episodes of disengagement. Provisions of the Mental Health Act 2007, such as a Community Treatment Order, might be useful. A referral to alcohol misuse services should be considered. The follow-up plan should incorporate close liaison with other agencies such as substance misuse services, law enforcement agencies, and child protection teams. A regular evaluation of the risks he poses to himself and to others needs to be conducted.

Self test 2

As a registrar in forensic psychiatry, you are asked to assess a 50-year-old man who has been remanded in prison after murdering his wife. He has had no previous contact with mental health services or the criminal justice system. It is reported that the police were called to his house after a woman's screams were heard by the neighbours. When the police arrived, they found his wife lying dead after having sustained a severe head injury. He had attempted to stab himself, but was prevented from doing so by the police. The neighbours reported that he seemed withdrawn and unlike his usual, jovial self in the months leading up to this incident. He had lost his job as a lorry driver because of turning up late to work. The neighbours were puzzled by this violence, as they reported that they had always given the impression of being a 'loving couple'.

You find him to be withdrawn. His face shows very little reactivity, and there is evidence of psychomotor poverty. He asserts that he killed his wife through an act of 'kindness'. He states that he is facing imminent financial ruin, and that both he and his wife would have ended up on the streets. He tells you that death would have been the preferable option for them both. You gather background information and find that this is not the case, as he has plenty of savings in his bank account. You present this information to him, and he remains adamant that this is not the case.

Q1 What is the most likely diagnosis?

The patient's belief in imminent financial ruin in the face of evidence to the contrary is an example of a nihilistic delusion. Nihilistic delusions can take other forms, for example an irrational belief that one's body organs are not functioning. Such patients complain that their heart or brain is not functioning, and persist in believing so when presented with the argument that human life is not sustainable under such circumstances.

He is likely to be suffering from low mood, as evidenced by his withdrawn behaviour and lack of facial reactivity. When nihilistic delusions occur in the context of depressed mood, they are called mood-congruent delusions. Other examples of mood-congruent delusions that occur in the context of low mood are delusions of guilt and delusions of hypochondriasis.

The most likely diagnosis, in view of the evidence of depression and nihilistic delusion, is a depressive disorder with psychotic symptoms. Other possible diagnoses include delusional disorder and paranoid schizophrenia.

Q2 How would you treat him?

As he is probably suffering from a mental disorder, it is important to divert the patient from prison to a secure mental health facility. Moving him should ensure that he gets an appropriate assessment and treatment for his condition. In addition to assessing his mental state, a careful risk assessment should be carried out, as he has already made an unsuccessful attempt to kill himself.

His physical health should be carefully assessed before beginning psychotropic medication, as this is associated with a number of side-effects. A detailed physical examination, routine blood tests, and electrocardiogram investigations should be conducted. As this is a late first presentation of a mental disorder, a computed tomography brain scan should be carried out to rule out cerebral pathology.

In terms of pharmacological treatment, an antipsychotic and an antidepressant are the most likely options. He should be fully informed of the benefits and side-effects of these medications. Response to treatment should be carefully assessed. As the symptoms of mental disorder resolve, there is typically a corresponding increase in the patient's degree of insight.

He may begin to experience tremendous feelings of guilt for murdering his wife, and this could increase his suicide risk. It might be necessary to increase the level of ward observations, not only to prevent him from harming himself, but to also provide him with emotional support. The input of a clinical psychologist might be beneficial.

References

Akil M, Brewer GJ (1995) Psychiatric and behavioural abnormalities in Wilson's disease. *Advanced Neurology*, **65**: 171–178.

Bolton P (2011) Improving physical health monitoring in secondary care for patients on clozapine. *The Psychiatrist*, **35**: 49–55.

Carta MG, Sorbello O, Moro MF, *et al* (2012) Bipolar disorders and Wilson's disease. *BMC Psychiatry*, **12**: 52.

Ciompi L (1980) The natural history of schizophrenia in the long term. *British Journal of Psychiatry*, **136**: 413–420.

Cohen A, Patel V (2008) Questioning an axiom: better prognosis for schizophrenia in the developing world? *Schizophrenia Bulletin*, **34**: 229–244.

Croarkin P (2002) From King George to neuroglobin: the psychiatric aspects of acute intermittent porphyria. *Journal of Psychiatric Practice*, **8**: 398–405.

Gower LE, Gatewood MO, Kang CS (2012) Emergency department management of delirium in the elderly. *The Western Journal of Medicine*, **13**: 194–201.

Hesse S, Barthel H, Hermann W, *et al* (2003) Regional serotonin transporter availability and depression correlated in Wilson's disease. *Journal of Neural Transmission*, **110**: 923–933.

Hodgson R, Adeyemo O (2004) Physical examination performed by psychiatrists. *International Journal of Psychiatry in Clinical Practice*, **8**: 57–60.

Hughes JR (2009) Alcohol withdrawal seizure. *Epilepsy and Behaviour*, **15**: 92–97.

Martin S, Fernandes L (2012) Delirium in elderly people: a review. *Frontiers in Neurology*, **3**: 101.

Mura G, Petretto DR, Bhat KM, *et al* (2012) Schizophrenia: from epidemiology to rehabilitation. *Clinical Practice and Epidemiology in Mental Health*, **8**: 52–56.

National Institute of Health and Clinical Excellence (2008) *Structural Imaging in First-Episode Psychosis (NICE Technology Appraisal 136)*. NICE.

National Institute of Health and Clinical Excellence (2010) *Schizophrenia: Core Interventions in the Treatment and Management of Schizophrenia in Adults in Primary and Secondary Care (NICE Clinical Guideline 82)*. NICE.

Newman SC, Bland RC (1991) Mortality in a cohort of patients with schizophrenia: a record linkage study. *Canadian Journal of Psychiatry*, **36**: 239–245.

Penagaluri P, Walker KL, El-Mallakh RS (2010) Hallucinations, pseudohallucinations, and severity of suicidal ideation among emergency psychiatry patients. *Crisis*, **31**: 53–56.

Sumic JC, Barric V, Billic P, *et al* (2007) QTc and psychopharmacs: are there any differences between monotherapy and polytherapy. *Annals of General Psychiatry*, **6**: 13.

Tarrier N, Lewis S, Haddock G (2004) Cognitive–behavioural therapy improves psychotic symptoms at 18 months in people with schizophrenia. *Evidence Based Mental Health*, **7**: 105.

Wilson SAK (1912) Progressive lenticular degeneration: a familiar nervous disease associated with cirrhosis of the liver. *Brain*, **34**: 295–509.

CHAPTER 6

Acute side-effects of psychotropic medication

Richard Hodgson and Roji Thomas

The modern era of psychopharmacology began in the 1950s, with the discovery of chlorpromazine. It gave new hope to those affected by mental illness and the use of other treatments such as leucotomy and insulin shock therapy declined. Drugs for a wide variety of psychiatric conditions were subsequently developed. However, the use of psychotropics is not without problems. In this chapter, we will examine common side-effects as well as some of the serious and potentially adverse events of specific drugs. It should be remembered that side-effects could present even if a patient has been on the same medication for many years. We aim to give a general overview and have avoided giving highly specific information regarding dosing, as this will change over time.

Good-practice guidelines when prescribing medication

When prescribing medication, safety should be maximised. The first task is to evaluate whether a drug is actually indicated following discussion with the patient. It must be remembered that the patient might have different priorities and that some side-effects might not be perceived as negative by the recipient. For example, depressed patients with prominent insomnia might welcome the sedative side-effect of some antidepressants. The leucocytosis associated with lithium might facilitate the prescription of clozapine in individuals with a low neutrophil count (Hodgson & Mendis, 2010). The efficacy of a medication will also determine whether a patient is willing to tolerate a medicine (Kinon *et al*, 2006).

Careful consideration of the evidence base, patient factors and pharmacological profile are all important in optimising pharmacotherapy. In patients on multiple drugs, only one drug or dose should be altered at a time in order to clearly evaluate the consequences. This is particularly relevant to drugs that induce or inhibit cytochrome P450 enzymes. This can affect the metabolism of other drugs and cause adverse effects even at therapeutic doses. It is important to have an up-to-date list of currently prescribed medication to avoid drug interactions. Getting this list might involve liaising with general practitioners or other medical teams that are involved in the patient's care (medicines reconciliation). Patients might also be taking over-the-counter preparations, complementary therapies, a relative's medications and drugs of potentially doubtful provenance obtained via the internet. Illicit substances might also be relevant, as well as tobacco and alcohol use.

Some of these difficulties can be negated if polypharmacy is avoided where possible. It is important to use medication within the guidelines set by the manufacturer's Summary of Product Characteristics and any deviation should be documented as off-label prescribing (Hodgson & Belgamwar, 2006). The *British National Formulary* provides guidance on the use of multiple antipsychotics and other aspects of polypharmacy.

Knowledge of the drugs a patient has previously taken will also improve prescribing. Recurrent side-effects can be avoided or reduced if a different titration regime is used. Patients might recall a particular drug as being beneficial (or unhelpful) in a previous illness. In treatment-resistant illness, this previous drug history is particularly important and careful enquiry might be needed to ensure that the patient has indeed completed a full therapeutic trial of previous agents.

Documentation is important and all prescribing decisions should be recorded. Ideally, the prescriber should document patient discussions regarding treatment choice, the rationale for the choice, that the risks and benefits were discussed with the patient and that the patient has made an informed capacitous decision to take the medication. Prescriptions must be written using generic names of drugs whenever possible and in clear handwriting to avoid drug errors. All prescriptions must be dated and signed. Baseline investigations are recommended for many psychotropics. Patients with pre-existing medical conditions such as renal or hepatic impairment need special consideration, as do women of childbearing age or those breastfeeding. Allergies, drug hypersensitivities and previous adverse events should be asked about and clearly documented in the case notes.

It is important to actively enquire about side-effects and adherence at review. Patients might not always volunteer information about side-effects – particularly sexual side-effects. A number of schedules exist for reviewing side-effects (Table 6.1).

Drug interactions

The majority of psychotropic drugs are metabolised by the liver. Exceptions include lithium and paliperidone, which are excreted largely un-metabolised in the urine. The cytochrome P450 (CYP) enzyme system is involved in the metabolism of most drugs. There are many different groups of enzymes within this system; of these, the CYP2D6 group is most commonly involved

Table 6.1 Side-effect rating scales

Scale	Type	Purpose
Liverpool University Neuroleptic Side-Effect Rating Scale[1]	Self-rating	Monitors general side-effects of neuroleptic medication
Simpson Angus Scale[2]	Clinician-rated	Monitors extrapyramidal side-effects of antipsychotics medication
Side-Effects Scale/Checklist for Antipsychotic Medication[3]	Clinician-rated	Monitors general side-effects of antipsychotics medication
Abnormal Involuntary Movement Scale[4]	Clinician-rated	Tests for the presence of dyskinesia in patients prescribed antipsychotics

[1]Day et al (1995), [2]Simpson & Angus (1970), [3]Bennett et al (1995), [4]Munetz & Benjamin (1988)

in the metabolism of approximately half of all psychotropic drugs. There are different mutant alleles within the CYP2D6 group, which results in varying capacity to metabolise drugs. Patients can be divided into poor, intermediate, extensive or ultra-rapid metabolism categories on the basis of CYP2D6 function. The CYP2D6 genotype can be determined using polymerase-chain-based assays (Hodgson et al, 2004).

CYP2D6 is affected by ethnicity. Up to 14% of the White population have at least two defective autosomal recessive alleles and are therefore 'poor metabolisers' (Hodgson et al, 2004). This might necessitate adjustment of drug dosages in these individuals to prevent adverse effects. The CYP2D6 enzyme can be inhibited by a number of drugs (Box 6.1). Co-administration of other agents with these drugs can result in increased risk of adverse effects.

The herbal remedy St John's Wort, often used for treating mild depression, can induce the CYP3A4 enzyme and the P glycoprotein pathway and therefore reduce the efficacy of co-administered drugs (Mannel, 2004). It is not recommended in combination with serotonergic drugs, as it can lead to serotonin syndrome.

Box 6.1 Drugs that inhibit CYP2D6

Antidepressants
- Fluoxetine
- Venlafaxine
- Paroxetine
- Duloxetine
- Amitriptyline

Antipsychotics
- Haloperidol
- Clomipramine
- Aripiprazole
- Risperidone
- Haloperidol
- Chlorpromazine

Others
- Atomoxetine
- Propranolol
- Metoclopramide
- Chlorpheniramine
- Donepezil
- Codeine

Discontinuation symptoms

Abrupt withdrawal of some antidepressants (e.g. paroxetine) can result in discontinuation symptoms, such as flu-like symptoms, insomnia, nausea, imbalance, sensory disturbances and hyperarousal (Warner *et al*, 2006). The condition is usually self-limiting and improves over a period of 1–2 weeks. If stopping paroxetine, it is advised to taper the dose. Management of the condition involves reassurance and, in severe cases, sometimes re-starting the drug to introduce a more gradual tapering regime.

Benzodiazepines can also cause severe discontinuation symptoms, including anxiety, nausea, tremor, photosensitivity, tachycardia, insomnia and, in severe cases, seizures and confusion. To prevent discontinuation symptoms, benzodiazepine dosage should be reduced gradually or the patient switched to a longer-acting benzodiazepine, such as diazepam, followed by a gradual withdrawal. Rapid lithium withdrawal can precipitate relapse, and patients should be counselled about this.

General side-effects

Psychotropic medication can give rise to many side-effects and affect all the major systems in the body (Table 6.2). Many side-effects can be predicted from knowledge of the receptor-binding profile of the drug. With advances in genetics and psychopharmacology, these predictions are likely to expand and ultimately be useful at an individual case level. The side-effects that are likely to occur in relation to individual receptor types and the drugs with the most affinity for these receptor types are shown in Table 6.3.

Acute dystonic reactions

Dopamine-receptor blockade is generally accepted as a key mechanism of antipsychotic function. However, blockade of nigrostriatal D_2 receptors can lead to side-effects. These particular side-effects are more likely to be associated with first-generation than second-generation antipsychotics. Now that second-generation antipsychotics dominate prescribing, many younger doctors have never seen these distressing side-effects.

A dystonic reaction is an acute movement disorder characterized by sustained muscular contractions affecting various muscle groups in the body, resulting in abnormal postures. It is most commonly caused by antipsychotics but it is also associated with antidepressants and other drugs such as metoclopramide, cinnarizine, carbamazepine, phenytoin, chloroquine, amodiaquine and cocaine. Half of all dystonic reactions occur within 48 h of initiation of the antipsychotic and 90% occur within 5 days.

Table 6.2 Side-effects of psychotropics

System	Side-effects	Drugs
Central nervous system	Headache Tremor Agitation Sweating Drowsiness Dizziness Sleep abnormalities Movement disorders such as akathisia, dystonia and tardive dyskinesia Confusion Ataxia	Antipsychotics Antidepressants Benzodiazepines Carbamazepine
Cardiovascular system	Tachycardia QTc prolongation Myocarditis Cardiomyopathy Postural hypotension Arrhythmias Cerebrovascular accidents	Citalopram Clozapine Venlafaxine Sertindole Other antipsychotics
Haematological	Neutropenia Agranulocytosis Anaemia Eosinophilia	Clozapine Carbamazepine Olanzapine
Gastrointestinal system	Nausea Diarrhoea Hypersalivation	SSRIs Clozapine
Genito-urinary system	Impotence Anorgasmia Decreased libido Menstrual irregularities	SSRIs First-generation antipsychotics
Endocrine system	Hypothyroidism Gynaecomastia	Lithium First-generation antipsychotics
Metabolic system	Impaired glucose tolerance Hyponatremia	Olanzapine Clozapine SSRIs
Dermatological system	Hypersensitivity reaction Toxic epidermal necrolysis Stevens–Johnson syndrome Photosensitivity Acne Hirsuitism Skin discolouration	lamotrigine Carbamazepine Valproate

SSRIs: selective serotonin-reuptake inhibitors

The following risk factors are associated with dystonic reactions:

- male gender
- younger age
- use of high-potency psychotropic medication
- learning disability
- treatment with electroconvulsive therapy
- cocaine use
- previous history of acute dystonic reactions.

The cranial and cervical musculatures are often affected in acute dystonia. The various types of movement disorders that can occur are

Table 6.3 Receptor types, medications and common side-effects

Receptor types	Common side-effects	Medications
Dopamine (D1–D5)	Extrapyramidal side-effects such as dystonic reactions and Parkinsonism	First-generation antipsychotics such as haloperidol, stelazine
	Hyperprolactinaemia causing gynaecomastia, lactation and sexual dysfunction	Second-generation antipsychotics such as risperidone and amisulpiride
Serotonin (5-HT$_{12}$ subtypes)	Sexual dysfunction, agitation, anxiety, panic attacks	Clozapine, olanzapine, serotonergic antidepressants
	Stimulation of 5-HT$_3$ receptors can cause nausea, vomiting, diarrhoea and abdominal cramps	
	5-HT$_{2A}$ stimulation by serotonergic antidepressants can lead to reduced dopamine transmission in the basal ganglia causing akathisia and mild Parkinsonism	
Noradrenaline (alpha 1 and 2)	Postural hypotension, tachycardia, sedation	Quetiapine, clozapine, reboxetine (norepinephrine-reuptake inhibitor), venlafaxine (serotonin/norepinephrine reuptake inhibitor), tricyclic antidepressants
Acetylcholine (muscarinic type)	Blurred vision, constipation, urinary retention, dry mouth, confusion, cognitive impairment, diabetes, dyslipidaemia	Clozapine, olanzapine, quetiapine, tricyclic antidepressants such as amitryptiline and dothiepin
Histamine	Sedation, weight gain	Clozapine, olanzapine, quetiapine, tricyclic antidepressants

shown in Table 6.4. Patients are usually very distressed by this side-effect and acute dystonic reaction should be suspected in any patient with a recent history of treatment with antipsychotic drugs who presents with features as described above. However, it should be remembered that dystonia can be confused with or be a feature of conversion disorders and hyperventilation (with subsequent tetany). Hypocalcaemia and hypomagnesaemia can result in dystonic movements. Neurological disorders such as Wilson's disease, Huntington's chorea, epilepsy and meningitis can confuse the clinical picture. Strychnine poisoning is an extremely rare cause.

Reassurance is important in the treatment of acute dystonic reactions, because of the associated distress. Parenteral procyclidine is the drug of choice, and intravenous administration is associated with a faster speed on onset and is also the route of choice if laryngospasm is suspected. Diazepam is sometimes used as an adjunct to relieve anxiety.

Akathisia

Akathisia refers to a subjective feeling of restlessness and symptoms of dysphoria such as panic and anxiety (Halstead, 1994), as well as motor manifestations such as rocking, restless legs, an inability to sit still and pacing. It is a common side-effect, particularly with high-potency antipsychotics but is also seen with antidepressants and metoclopramide. The prevalence of this condition varies from 11% in an in-patient population to 18% in a community sample (Barnes, 2003).

Table 6.4 Abnormal movement disorders seen in acute dystonia

Disorder	Explanation
Oculogyric crisis	Eyes deviating conjugately up and to one side
Trismus	Inability to open the mouth due to spasm of the masticatory muscles
Opisthotonic crisis	Tonic contraction of the paravertebral muscles, causing hyperextension of the spine
Tortipelvic crisis	Contraction of the muscles of the abdominal wall, hip and pelvis, causing distorted posture
Torticollis	Spasm of the neck musculature
Camptocormia	Flexion of the thoracolumbar spine
Buccolingual crisis	Protrusion of the tongue, forced jaw opening and facial grimacing
Laryngospasm	Contraction of the laryngeal muscles
Pisa syndrome	Truncal flexion towards either side
Lordosis or scoliosis	Abnormal curvature of the spine

This condition is often very distressing for the patient and can result in non-adherence to treatment and suicidal ideation. The motor manifestations can result in patients being misdiagnosed as showing increasing agitation or mania, prompting an increase in dosage of antipsychotic medication, which worsens the symptoms.

The most effective management strategy is withdrawal or reduction in antipsychotic dosage. These strategies might initially worsen akathisia because of receptor supersensitivity (Hodgson *et al*, 1994). Beta-blockers have been found to be useful and benzodiazepines might help as adjunctive treatment.

Pseudo-Parkinsonism

Blockade of dopamine receptors in the nigrostriatal pathway can cause Parkinsonian symptoms such as slow tremor or 'pill rolling' action of the hands, shuffling gait, mask-like facies and stooped posture. Bradykinesia or slowness of movement is another feature commonly seen. This condition is commonly known as pseudo-Parkinsonism or drug-induced Parkinsonism. Elderly women, patients on high-potency antipsychotics, and patients with coexisting tardive dyskinesia or other extrapyramidal symptoms are more at risk of developing this side-effect (Thanvi, 2009). The condition should be explained to patients and they should be reassured that is potentially reversible upon stopping the offending drug, although in some cases it can take many months to see improvement (Thanvi, 2009).

It is important to differentiate this condition from idiopathic Parkinson's disease. The presence of bilateral, sub-acute onset of symptoms closely linked to the addition of antipsychotics with early postural tremor and co-existent orobuccal dyskinesia is what differentiates pseudo-Parkinsonism from idiopathic Parkinson's disease (Alvarez & Evdiente, 2008). The absence of resting tremor and presence of action tremor (postural and kinetic) is also more likely to occur in this condition rather than in Parkinson's disease (Hirose, 2006).

Case study 1

A 25-year-old man was admitted to an acute psychiatric unit with a history of auditory hallucinations and persecutory ideas. He was agitated on the ward and was given a dose of oral haloperidol 5 mg. Two hours later, he assaulted a member of staff and had to be restrained. He was given a further dose of haloperidol (5 mg), this time intramuscularly. He was placed on close observation and vital signs were monitored regularly. He subsequently developed stiffness of the neck, followed by torticollis and oculogyric crisis. His blood pressure was 130/80 mmHg. Pulse rate was 102/min. Respiratory rate was 25/min. He was diagnosed with an acute dystonic reaction and was prescribed intramuscular procyclidine 10 mg. Within 30 min, his symptoms abated and he was subsequently put on a prophylactic dose of procyclidine (5 mg twice daily), which was stopped when his antipsychotic medication was changed to quetiapine.

Neuroleptic malignant syndrome

Neuroleptic malignant syndrome (NMS) is a rare but potentially life-threatening condition usually associated with an idiosyncratic reaction to high-potency first-generation antipsychotics. However, many other drug classes have been implicated, including lithium, antidepressants and second-generation antipsychotics. It is characterized by autonomic dysfunction, hyperthermia, altered mental state and muscle rigidity. Delay *et al* (1960) first used the term. Incidence rates range from 0.01–0.02% (Stubner *et al*, 2004) to 2.2% (Hermesh *et al*, 1988). It has been suggested that some of the earlier studies showing higher incidence rates lacked rigour in terms of diagnostic criteria. The average reported mortality ranges from 11 to 38% (Jahan *et al*, 1992). It is widely agreed that there has been a decrease in incidence rates as well in mortality rates over the last 20 years. This decrease is probably due to a more careful use of high-potency antipsychotic drugs and increased awareness of the condition (resulting in earlier treatment).

Dopamine blockade seems to be a trigger for the development of NMS and explains the key manifestations of NMS. For instance, dopamine blockade in the thermoregulatory centre in the hypothalamus results in pyrexia. Mental-state changes are explained by dopamine blockade in the mesocortical pathways. As dopamine acts as an inhibitor of sympathetic flow at the spinal cord level, blockade at this level can result in the autonomic dysfunction seen in NMS (Lindvall *et al*, 1983). Muscular rigidity can occur when dopaminergic transmission is affected at the corpus striatum.

NMS is characterized by a tetrad of symptoms: muscle rigidity, hyperthermia (temperature above 38 °C), autonomic dysfunction and mental-status changes (Table 6.5). Serious complications include myoglobinuria, renal failure and respiratory depression. Characteristic laboratory findings in NMS include raised creatinine phosphokinase levels due to rhabdomyolysis. However, this is not found in all cases and can be present in many other conditions. Recent intramuscular injections can also raise creatinine phosphokinase levels, as can bruising.

Differential diagnoses of neuroleptic malignant syndrome include conditions such as heatstroke, central nervous system infections, serotonin

Table 6.5 Features of neuroleptic malignant syndrome

Symptom	Examples
Muscle rigidity	Cog wheel rigidity, lead pipe rigidity mostly affecting the limbs, and (rarely) myoclonus, dysphagia and dysarthria
Fever	Pyrexia ($\geq 38°C$) or hyperpyrexia ($\geq 41°C$)
Autonomic dysfunction	Changes in blood pressure, diaphoresis, tachycardia, incontinence
Mental-state changes	Altered consciousness, confusion

syndrome, drug-induced extrapyramidal symptoms, lithium toxicity and anticholinergic crisis (Table 6.6).

Treatment

Neuroleptic malignant syndrome is a medical emergency. Renal failure is a common cause of death. Other complications include rhabdomyolysis, respiratory depression, pulmonary embolism and seizures. All neuroleptic drugs must be discontinued upon diagnosis. Supportive measures, such as maintaining fluid and electrolyte balance, are vital in treatment. Specific drugs such as dantrolene (a muscle relaxant) and bromocriptine (a dopamine agonist) have been shown to reduce mortality. Dantrolene works by inhibiting the release of calcium from the sarcoplasmic reticulum and reduces muscle rigidity and pyrexia. Benzodiazepines can act as adjuncts by working as muscle relaxants and relieving anxiety. Measures to prevent renal failure, such as alkaline diuresis, might be necessary in severe cases.

Table 6.6 Differential diagnoses of neuroleptic malignant syndrome (NMS)

Differential diagnosis	Similarities to NMS
Heatstroke	Heatstroke can present many of the features of neuroleptic malignant syndrome, however it can be distinguished by lack of muscle rigidity and autonomic disturbances.
Central nervous system infections	Central nervous system infections such as meningitis and encephalitis are important differential diagnoses that need to be ruled out early. They present with a history of prodromal illness, focal neurological deficits and positive findings in laboratory investigations of the cerebrospinal fluid and blood.
Serotonin syndrome	Serotonin syndrome can present with several features similar to NMS, such as fever, autonomic dysfunction and diaphoresis. However, this condition is more likely to present with features such as hyperreflexia, myoclonus, dilated pupils and diarrhoea than NMS (Birmes *et al*, 2003).
Drug-induced extrapyramidal side-effects	Extrapyramidal side-effects, particularly in patients with co-existing infection causing fever, can mimic many of the features of NMS and comprise the most common differential diagnosis (Kohen & Bristow, 1996). However they are less likely to cause autonomic dysfunction, confusion and altered consciousness. In the absence of co-existent infection, pyrexia is also unlikely to be seen.
Lithium toxicity	Nausea, diarrhoea, and fine resting tremors distinguish lithium toxicity from NMS. It is also more likely to present with hyper-reflexia and polyuria.
Anticholinergic crisis	Anticholinergic crisis presents with many of the features of NMS but can be distinguished by the presence of flushing, whereas rigidity, diaphoresis and elevated creatine phosphokinase are less likely to be seen in this condition.

Serotonin syndrome

Serotonin syndrome is a life-threatening condition caused by excessive serotonergic activity within the brain. It was first described in 1959 in a patient with tuberculosis who was prescribed pethidine. It can be caused by therapeutic doses of drugs, overdose or more commonly by interactions between serotonergic drugs.

Pathophysiology

Serotonin syndrome results from an increase in the amount of intrasynaptic serotonin in the brain. Many drugs have been implicated in serotonin syndrome and not all are psychotropics (Table 6.7).

Diagnosis

The diagnosis of serotonin syndrome is clinical, being based on history and a physical examination of the patient. The clinical features are seen in a number of different systems within the body (Box 6.2).

Various explicit criteria have been developed, including the Sternbach criteria (Sternbach, 1991) and Hunter's criteria (Dunkley *et al*, 2003), as shown in Box 6.3. Hunter's criteria were found to be simpler, more sensitive (84% *v.* 75%) and more specific (97% *v.* 96%) than Sternbach's criteria (Dunkley *et al*, 2003).

Differential diagnosis

The principal differential diagnoses are neuroleptic malignant syndrome, meningitis, heatstroke, encephalitis and anticholinergic overdose. Neuroleptic malignant syndrome is a key differential diagnosis of serotonin syndrome. NMS develops slowly following the addition of an antipsychotic drug. Tremor and hyperreflexia are less likely to occur. Rigidity and hyperthermia, when present, are more severe than in serotonin syndrome.

Table 6.7 Drugs causing serotonin syndrome

Drug	Mechanism of action
Selective serotonin-reuptake inhibitors	Serotonin-reuptake inhibitor
Tricyclic antidepressants	Serotonin-reuptake inhibitor
Monoamine-oxidase inhibitors	Inhibits serotonin metabolism
Tramadol	Serotonin-reuptake inhibitor
LSD	Serotonin agonist
Buspirone	Serotonin agonist
Amphetamine	Increases serotonin release
Lithium	Unknown

Box 6.2 Clinical features of serotonin syndrome

Cognitive	Autonomic	Neurological
• Anxiety	• Hyperpyrexia	• Muscle rigidity
• Agitation	• Tachycardia	• Tremor
• Disorientation	• Diaphoresis	• Hyperreflexia
• Lethargy	• Tachypnoea	• Bilateral Babinski
• Seizures	• Hypertension	sign
• Hypomania	• Dilated pupils	• Ataxia
• Hallucinations	• Diarrhoea	• Nystagmus
		• Shivering

Autonomic dysfunction is more common in NMS. There is a greater risk of diarrhoea in serotonin syndrome (versus ileus in NMS).

Heat exhaustion is less commonly associated with autonomic dysfunction and presents with flaccid muscular tone. The skin is often dry and hot. Infections such as meningitis and encephalitis can be differentiated by prodromal illness and positive findings in cerebrospinal fluid and blood.

Treatment

Serotonin syndrome can be life-threatening. However, the majority of cases are self-limiting. Discontinuation of the causative drug and supportive measures are the mainstay of treatment. Hyperthermia is treated with tepid sponging, fans and misting. Muscle rigidity and seizures can be treated with benzodiazepines. In severe cases, treatment with oral cyproheptadine (an antihistamine with 5HT-antagonist and anticholinergic properties) can be used.

Case study 2

A 51-year-old man was brought to an emergency department with a history of overdose of paroxetine. He had ingested paroxetine 3000 mg the night before. On examination, his blood pressure was 150/100 mmHg with pulse rate of 102/min, respiratory rate of 28/min and a temperature of 39°C. He presented with diaphoresis, shivering and hyperreflexia. Blood investigation showed a raised creatinine kinase level of 1500 IU/L (normal is 0–125 IU/L) and normal serum electrolyte levels. A provisional diagnosis of serotonin syndrome was made and supportive treatment measures started. Tepid sponging and cooling reduced his temperature. Fluid and electrolyte balance was maintained. The patient recovered within 48 h.

Anticholinergic side-effects

Anticholinergic (antimuscarinic) side-effects can occur with some first- and second-generation antipsychotic drugs, as well as with many tricyclic antidepressants. The most common side-effects are dry mouth, constipation,

Box 6.3   Sternbach and Hunter's criteria

Sternbach criteria

Recent addition or increase in a serotonin agent and no recent addition of neuroleptic agent.

At least three of the following symptoms:

- Mental status changes
- Agitation
- Myoclonus
- Hyperreflexia
- Diaphoresis
- Shivering
- Tremor
- Diarrhoea
- Incoordination
- Fever

Hunter's criteria

Recent addition or increase in a serotonin agent.

At least one of the following:

- Spontaneous clonus
- Inducible clonus plus agitation or diaphoresis
- Ocular clonus plus agitation or diaphoresis
- Tremor and hyperreflexia
- Hypertonia
- Temperature above 38°C plus ocular clonus or inducible clonus

blurred vision and urinary difficulties that can result in retention. Memory impairment and confusion can also occur, especially in older patients with underlying organic brain disorders. Management of these side-effects involves stopping the offending drug or switching to another drug with lesser anticholinergic effect. An anticholinergic crisis is an uncommon side-effect of psychotropic medication and is a medical emergency. The mnemonic 'red as a beet, dry as a bone, blind as a bat, mad as a hatter, and hot as a hare' refers to the symptoms seen in this condition, such as flushing, mydriasis, confusion and pyrexia. An anticholinergic crisis needs to be differentiated from other conditions such as serotonin syndrome, neuroleptic malignant syndrome and heatstroke. In severe cases, management can involve the use of cholinergic agents such as atropine.

Hyperglycaemia and weight gain

Patients with schizophrenia are more likely to develop metabolic syndrome in the long term than the general population. In part, this relates to lifestyle, but the disorder itself is associated with diabetes and other metabolic abnormalities (Kohen, 2004). Antipsychotic medication is also implicated.

In the short term, hyperglycaemia is associated with the use of second-generation antipsychotics, such as olanzapine, clozapine, risperidone and quetiapine. Antipsychotics differ in their propensity to cause hyperglycaemia. Olanzapine and clozapine in particular have been associated with worsening of pre-existing diabetes mellitus and new-onset diabetes mellitus. There have also been reports of the development of ketoacidosis in patients treated with olanzapine. Case reports have indicated the onset of hyperglycaemia in as little as 3 days with olanzapine use (Kohen *et al*, 2008). The mechanism of action was thought to be a secondary effect of weight gain, but the rapid onset of hyperglycaemia and reports of hyperglycaemia in patients who do not gain weight suggest a more direct effect on the pancreatic cells. One possibility is that because olanzapine and clozapine are both potent anticholinergic antagonists, they act on the muscarinic M3 receptors, reducing cholinergic stimulated secretion of insulin in the pancreas (Johnson *et al*, 2005).

Rapid weight gain is associated with some antipsychotics such as clozapine, olanzapine and quetiapine and might be an indicator to switch to a drug less associated with weight gain.

Case study 3
A 50-year-old man was admitted with acute psychotic symptoms. Treatment was initiated with olanzapine (10 mg daily). Fasting blood glucose was 14 mmol/L 2 months later. Glycaemic control was established with diet and metformin (500 mg twice daily). Olanzapine was subsequently discontinued and the patient was started on aripiprazole. Metformin was discontinued 2 weeks later, as his blood sugar continued to decrease. Weight gain during treatment with olanzapine was 2 kg.

Drug hypersensitivity

Psychotropic drugs are associated with a number of hypersensitivity reactions, ranging from urticarial skin rash to more serious adverse effects such as Stevens–Johnson syndrome and toxic epidermal necrolysis. Photosensitivity reactions are also common.

Hypersensitivity reactions commonly present as urticarial rash and angioedema. Stevens–Johnson syndrome and toxic epidermal necrolysis are considered to be parts of the same syndrome. Toxic epidermal necrolysis is the more severe illness, with a mortality rate of up to 35%, whereas Stevens–Johnson syndrome has a mortality rate of up to 15%. They are immune-mediated hypersensitivity reactions causing widespread lesions on the skin and mucous membranes in the mouth, gastrointestinal tract and the respiratory system, as well as systemic complications such as fluid electrolyte imbalance and sepsis. These conditions are most commonly associated with anticonvulsants such as lamotrigine, carbamazepine and valproate. Management involves immediate cessation of any drugs that might be causing the condition and urgent referral to medical care.

Drug hypersensitivity syndrome is a term used to describe a syndrome characterized by cutaneous lesions, lymphadenopathy, pyrexia and visceral involvement (e.g. hepatitis, nephritis). It has a mortality rate of 10% and is most commonly seen following treatment with anticonvulsants such as phenytoin and carbamazepine. Almost 90% of cases are associated with eosinophilia, giving rise to the acronym DRESS (drug reaction with eosinophilia and systemic symptoms).

Hyponatraemia

Hyponatraemia is defined as a plasma sodium level of <130 meq/L. It is most commonly associated with the use of SSRIs. The reported incidence of hyponatraemia associated with antidepressant use varies between 0.5 and 32% (Jacob, 2006). It is more likely to occur in women, the elderly and those with low body weight. It is also more common in patients with acute psychotic symptoms.

It has been postulated that SSRIs cause hyponatraemia by potentiating the action of antidiuretic hormone. The mechanism involved in acute psychosis seems to be multifactorial and include impaired thirst perception and increased secretion of antidiuretic hormone at low plasma osmolality (Goldman, 1988). It is usually asymptomatic and can present with non-specific symptoms such as nausea, headache and malaise. In severe cases, drowsiness, confusion and seizures can occur. Severe hyponatraemia (<102 meq/L) is a medical emergency and immediate referral to a medical unit should be made.

Rapid correction of hyponatraemia can result in osmotic demyelination syndrome, with extensive lesions in the pons and the sensory tracts resulting in flaccid paralysis and dysphagia. The neurological complications can be permanent. This can be prevented by slow correction of sodium imbalance and the use of corticosteroids.

Specific drug issues

Some medications have unique concerns associated with their use.

Lithium

Lithium was first used as a treatment for mania by Australian psychiatrist John Cade following a serendipitous observation that lithium urate had a tranquillizing effect on guinea pigs. Although the mechanism of action of lithium in bipolar disorder is not fully understood, it is known to modify the production and metabolism of serotonin and might also block dopamine receptors. It also affects ion transport and postsynaptic signal transduction mechanism involving second-messenger systems.

Lithium is prescribed as either carbonate or citrate salt. These preparations are not dose-equivalent and bioavailability varies between branded products. Therefore, a specific branded preparation should be prescribed. Lithium has a narrow therapeutic window of between 0.7 and 1.0 mmol/L but it should be remembered that the range does vary depending on indication and toxicity can occur even with plasma levels of lithium in the so-called normal, therapeutic range (West & Meltzer, 1979).

Before prescribing lithium, it is recommended that baseline measurements are taken, including thyroid and renal function tests and serum calcium level. Some authorities also recommend an electrocardiogram. The rationale for these tests relates to potential long-term adverse events such as hypothyroidism, renal abnormalities and hyperparathyroidism (McKnight *et al*, 2012). These adverse events are likely to present insidiously, so regular testing is recommended.

The main concern with using lithium is toxicity. Lithium is excreted unchanged by the kidneys. Therefore, any factor that compromises renal function or alters fluid balance might give rise to lithium toxicity. Patients should be issued with safety cards that highlight these factors and illustrate the symptoms of early toxicity.

Patients taking lithium should be advised to keep well hydrated. Conditions such as diarrhoea, vomiting, colds, influenza and urinary infections can alter the fluid balance. Patients will also need to drink more in hot weather. If the patient is unable to maintain hydration, monitoring of serum lithium level is advised and in extremis discontinuation of the drug should be considered. However, discontinuation should not be undertaken lightly, as abrupt discontinuation is associated with an increased risk of relapse.

Patients started on lithium can develop polydipsia and polyuria without biochemical evidence of altered renal function, which might be inconvenient or worse for the patient. Judicious dosage choice and timing might mitigate this adverse event.

The cardinal features of lithium toxicity, which can be fatal, are shown in Table 6.8. Cases of lithium toxicity can be mild, moderate or severe. Many of the symptoms are non-specific and overlap with the potential cause of the toxicity episode, such as diarrhoea. In addition, some acute features might already be present (e.g. tremor). Therefore, a high index of suspicion is required. Patients are unlikely to be asymptomatic if suffering from toxicity, which should be remembered when a very high lithium level is phoned through urgently by the laboratory when the cause is iatrogenic due to the use of the wrong blood bottle (lithium heparin).

Unfortunately, lithium toxicity can arise by interaction with many commonly prescribed drugs, several of which are available over the counter (Table 6.9). Patients need to be repeatedly reminded of this and instructed to inform other prescribers that they are taking lithium.

Treatment will vary depending on severity and many cases resolve quickly on cessation of the drug (to be followed by careful reintroduction

Table 6.8 Features of lithium toxicity at different levels of severity

Severity	Symptoms
Mild	Nausea, diarrhoea, fine resting tremor, drowsiness, polyuria
Moderate	Hyper-reflexia, myoclonic jerks, choreoathetoid movements, urinary or faecal incontinence, agitation, stupor, confusion, hypernatraemia
Severe	Renal failure, circulatory collapse, seizures, cardiac arrhythmias and coma

Table 6.9 Drug interactions of lithium

Drug	Mechanism of action
Non-steroidal anti-inflammatory drugs	Reduces lithium excretion
Diuretics	Both thiazide and loop diuretics can decrease lithium clearance
Haloperidol	Neurotoxicity has been reported with concomitant treatment
Antidepressants	Antidepressants with a serotonergic effect (e.g. selective serotonin-reuptake inhibitors, tricyclic antidepressants, venlafaxine) have been reported to cause neurotoxicity in combination with lithium
Angiotensin converting enzyme (ACE) inhibitors	ACE inhibitors decrease excretion of lithium and can precipitate renal failure
Carbamazepine	Neurotoxic reactions have been reported with the use of carbamazepine in combination with lithium

and monitoring). Gastric lavage can be considered in cases of acute poisoning with non-slow-release preparations. However, it is of little use in chronic accumulation. The treatment of choice in severe cases is haemodialysis. It is the most effective means of rapidly lowering the blood lithium concentration. However, rebound increases in serum lithium can occur after treatment and, therefore, prolonged or repeated treatments might be necessary.

Case study 4

A 50-year-old man was admitted to a medical ward with a history of confusional state. He had a history of bipolar disorder and was prescribed lithium carbonate (1000 mg once daily). He had recently been on holiday. He suffered diarrhoea and vomiting of 3 days' duration and had signs of dehydration including dry mouth and reduced urine output. In addition to this, he developed tremors, hyperreflexia and myoclonus. He also showed impaired consciousness. His serum lithium level was 4 mmol/L. Arterial blood gases were normal. Urea was raised at 6 mmol/Lm, sodium 5.5 mol/L and creatinine 50 umol/L. A diagnosis of lithium toxicity was made. He was the taken to the medical intensive care unit and given 24 h nursing care. Over the course of the next 48 h, he was given three haemodialysis procedures, after which his serum lithium level fell to 1.5 mm/L. He became alert and nasogastric tube feeding was initiated. He was extubated on the fourth day but was found to have a raised serum lithium level at 2.5 mmol/L. He showed impaired consciousness again. Haemodialysis was resumed. On the sixth day, he regained full consciousness and was transferred to a general medical ward.

Clozapine

Clozapine is an atypical antipsychotic drug licensed for treatment-resistant schizophrenia. It has a mechanism of action characteristic of second-generation antipsychotics, in that it has a widespread affinity for receptors other than dopamine D2receptors, such as serotonin and D4 receptors. In fact, the affinity for D4 receptors is much greater than for D2 receptors and, since the D4 receptors are less prevalent in the basal ganglia, clozapine is less likely to cause extra-pyramidal symptoms.

The use of clozapine is restricted because of concerns that it is associated with an increased risk of agranulocytosis. The cumulative incidence rate of agranulocytosis over a 1-year period for patients treated with clozapine is 0.8 per cent (Atkin *et al*, 1996). It is only available under special monitoring conditions. Clozapine is manufactured under different trade names and the manufacturers have their own monitoring centres but the monitoring schedule has been harmonised across the United Kingdom. The schedule for monitoring involves estimation of the white blood cell count and neutrophil count on a weekly basis for the first 18 weeks and then every two weeks until one year when four- weekly testing can be started. The increased testing interval is based on a higher risk of neutropenia and agranulocytosis in the first year. Although late cases do occur, approximately 50% of cases occur within six months and 75% by one year. Younger and African–Caribbean patients are at greatest risk. The neutrophil count at testing dictates the course of action to be taken, which ranges from a simple retest to immediate cessation of treatment and haematology referral. Patients must be warned to report any condition that might be suggestive of compromised immune function.

Other severe adverse events related to clozapine relate to cardiac abnormalities such as myocarditis and cardiomyopathy. Myocarditis or cardiomyopathy should be suspected in patients presenting with tachycardia, fever, malaise, chest pain or tachypnoea, particularly in the first 2 months of therapy. ECG changes such as ST depression can occur along with radiological signs such as enlarged heart and eosinophilia (Taylor *et al*, 2009). Patients suspected of suffering from cardiomyopathy or myocarditis should be referred to a cardiologist and clozapine should be stopped.

Clozapine is also associated with other side-effects which although not life threatening can cause distress. Hypersalivation can occur acutely and the treatment is not always satisfactory as the mechanism is not clearly understood.

Monoamine oxidase inhibitors

Monoamine oxidase inhibitors are now rarely used but were the first antidepressants to be developed. Monoamine oxidase exists in two forms: MAO-A and MAO-B. MAO-A is involved in the catabolism of serotonin and noradrenaline, whereas MAO-B acts on amines such as phenylethylamine. Both forms of monoamine oxidase metabolise dopamine and tyramine. Inhibition of MAO-A increases the availability of serotonin and noradrenaline in the brain, thereby providing an antidepressant effect.

Their use has declined partly because of the availability of newer antidepressants and partly because of potentially serious side-effects, such as hypertensive crisis and serotonin syndrome. Guidelines from the British Association of Psychopharmacology recommend that the use of monoamine oxidase inhibitors be restricted to after failure of first-line antidepressants and in patients with atypical depression (Anderson *et al*, 2000).

Tyramine is a sympathomimetic amine that is commonly found in food. It acts as a releaser of noradrenaline. An excess of noradrenaline can increase blood pressure by its action on presynaptic alpha 1 receptors. However, noradrenaline is kept within normal limits by the action of monoamine oxidase, which metabolises noradrenaline to vanillylmandelic acid.

Monoamine oxidase exists in the walls of the intestines and effectively metabolises any tyramine ingested via food. Any tyramine that gets absorbed is then metabolised by monoamine oxidases in the liver and in the sympathetic neurons. Monoamine oxidase inhibitors reduce the body's ability to handle dietary tyramine. If a patient treated with monoamine oxidase inhibitors ingests substantial quantities of tyramine through foodstuffs, this can cause an increase in the level of noradrenaline in the body and lead to a hypertensive crisis (also known as a tyramine crisis or 'cheese reaction'). Signs and symptoms that characterize a hypertensive crisis include headache, epistaxis, faintness, chest pain, dyspnoea and neurological deficits.

Patients should be advised to avoid foods containing high quantities of tyramine, including certain cheeses, alcohol, Marmite, broad bean pods and processed meats. This list is not exhaustive.

In an effort to reduce these undesirable effects, reversible monoamine oxidase inhibitors such as moclobemide were developed. In the presence of high quantities of noradrenaline, the reversible monoamine oxidase inhibitors are activated again and work to reduce noradrenaline to normal levels. This mitigates the risk of hypertensive crisis.

Benzodiazepines

Benzodiazepines are used in a variety of psychiatric conditions for the short-term relief of anxiety and to provide sedation. Because of their addictive potential, they should be used sparingly and for a maximum of 4 weeks. Use of benzodiazepines is associated with side-effects such as drowsiness, confusion, ataxia and muscle weakness.

In rare cases, a paradoxical increase in aggression and anxiety can occur with the use of benzodiazepines. The young and the elderly are more at risk of these types of reactions, as are patients with poor impulse control and a history of aggression. The incidence of such reactions varies: Dietch & Jennings (1988) reported an incidence of 1%, but other studies have reported incidences as high as 58% (Taylor *et al*, 2009). Upon diagnosis of these paradoxical reactions, benzodiazepines should be stopped and de-escalation techniques used to calm the patient. Flumazenil can be used as treatment in severe cases. Flumazenil has a short half-life, so repeated doses might be necessary.

References

Alvarez MV, Evidente VG (2008) Understanding drug-induced parkinsonism: separating pearls from oysters. *Neurology*, **70**: e32.

Anderson IM, Nutt DJ, Deakin JFW (2000) Evidence-based guidelines for treating depressive disorders with antidepressants: a revision of the 1993 British Association for Psychopharmacology guidelines. *Journal of Psychopharmacology*, **14**: 3–20.

Atkin K, Kendall F, Gould D, *et al* (1996) Neutropenia and agranulocytosis in patients receiving clozapine in the UK and Ireland. *British Journal of Psychiatry*, **169**: 483–488.

Barnes T (2003) Barnes Akathisia scale – revisited. *Journal of Psychopharmacology*, **17**: 365–370.

Bennett J, Done J, Harrison-Read P, *et al* (1995) Development of a rating scale: checklist to assess the side effects of antipsychotics by community psychiatric nurses. In *Community Psychiatric Nursing* (eds C Brooker, E White) Chapman & Hall: 1–19.

Birmes P, Coppin D, Schmitt L, *et al* (2003) Serotonin syndrome: a brief review. *Canadian Medical Association Journal*, **168**: 1439–1442.

Day JC, Wood G, Dewey M, *et al* (1995) A self-rating scale for measuring neuroleptic side-effects. Validation in a group of schizophrenic patients. *British Journal of Psychiatry*, **166**: 650–653.

Delay J, Piicht P, Lemperiere T, *et al* (1960) A non-phenothiazine and non-resperpine major neuroleptic, haloperidol, in the treatment of psychoses [French]. *Annales Medico-psychologiques*, **118**: 145–152.

Dietch JT, Jennings RK (1988) Aggressive dyscontrol in patients treated with benzodiazepine. *Journal of Clinical Psychiatry*, **49**: 184–188.

Dunkley EJ, Isbister GK, Sibbritt D, *et al* (2003) The Hunter Serotonin Toxicity Criteria: simple and accurate diagnostic decision rules for serotonin toxicity. *QJM*, **96**: 635.

Goldman MB, Luchins DJ, Robertson GL (1988) Mechanisms of altered water metabolism in psychotic patients with polydipsia and hyponatremia. *New England Journal of Medicine*, **318**: 397–403.

Halstead SM (1994) Akathisia: prevalence and associated dysphoria in an in-patient population with chronic schizophrenia. *British Journal of Psychiatry*, **164**: 177–183.

Hermesh H, Aizenberg D, Lapidot M, *et al* (1988) Risk of malignant hyperthermia among patients with neuroleptic malignant syndrome and their families. *American Journal of Psychiatry*, **145**: 1431–1434.

Hirose G (2006) Drug induced Parkinsonism. A review. *Journal of Neurology*, **253: 22–24.**

Hodgson RE, Murray D, Puranik A (1994) Blepharospasm after long term neuroleptic treatment. *Midlands Medicine*, **19**: 117–118.

Hodgson R, Smith, SE, Strange RC, *et al* (2004) Service innovations: pharmacogenetics clinics in psychiatry: a clinical reality? *Psychiatric Bulletin*, **28**: 298–300.

Hodgson RE, Belgamwar R (2006) Off-label prescribing by psychiatrists. *Psychiatric Bulletin*, **30**: 55–57.

Hodgson RE, Mendis S (2010) Lithium enabling use of clozapine in a patient with pre-existing neutropenia. *British Journal of Hospital Medicine*, **71**: 535.

Jacob S (2006) Hyponatremia associated with selective serotonin-reuptake inhibitors in older adults. *Annals of Pharmacotherapy*, **40**: 1618–1622.

Jahan MS, Farooque AI, Wahid Z (1992) Neuroleptic malignant syndrome. *Journal of the National Medical Association*, **84**: 966–970.

Johnson DE, Yamazaki H, Ward KM, *et al* (2005) Inhibitory effects of antipsychotics on carbachol-enhanced insulin secretion from perifused rat islets. Role of muscarinic antagonism in antipsychotic-induced diabetes and hyperglycemia. *Diabetes*, **54**: 1552–1558.

Kinon B, Liu-Seifert H, Adams DH, *et al* (2006) Differential rates of treatment discontinuation in clinical trials as a measure of treatment effectiveness for olanzapine and comparator atypical antipsychotics for schizophrenia. *Journal of Clinical Psychopharmacology*, **26**: 632–637.

Kohen D (2004) Diabetes mellitus and schizophrenia: historical perspective. *British Journal of Psychiatry Supplement*, **47**: 64–66.

Kohen D, Bristow M (1996) Neuroleptic malignant syndrome. *Advances in Psychiatric Treatment*, **2**: 151–157.

Kohen I, Gampel M, Reddy L, *et al* (2008) Rapidly developing hyperglycemia during treatment with olanzapine. *Annals of Pharmacotherapy*, **42**: 588–591.

Lindvall 0, Bjorklung A, Skagerberg G (1983) Dopamine containing neurons in the spinal cord: anatomy and some functional aspects. *Annals of Neurology*, **14**: 255–260.

Mannel M (2004) Drug interactions with St John's Wort: mechanisms and clinical implications. *Drug Safety*, **27**: 773–797.

McKnight RF, Adida M, Budge K *et al* (2012) Lithium toxicity profile: a systematic review and meta-analysis. *Lancet*, **379**: 721–728.

Munetz MR, Benjamin S (1988) How to examine patients using the abnormal involuntary movements scale. *Hospital and Community Psychiatry*, **39**: 1172–1177.

Simpson GM, Angus JW (1970) A rating scale for extrapyramidal side effects. *Acta Psychiatr Scand Suppl*, **212**: 11–9.

Sternbach H (1991) The serotonin syndrome. *American Journal of Psychiatry*, **148**: 705–713.

Stubner S, Rustenbeck E, Grohmann R, *et al* (2004) Severe and uncommon involuntary movement disorders due to psychotropic drugs. *Pharmacopsychiatry*, **37**: 54–64.

Taylor D, Paton C, Kerwin R, *et al* (2009) *The Maudsley Prescribing Guidelines* (10th edn). Informa Healthcare.

Thanvi B (2009) Drug induced Parkinsonism: a common cause of Parkinsonism in older people. *Postgraduate Medical Journal*, **85**: 322–326.

Warner CH, Bobo W, Warner C, *et al* (2006) Antidepressant discontinuation syndrome. *American Family Physician*, **74**: 449–456.

West AP, Meltzer HY (1979) Paradoxical lithium neurotoxicity: a report of five cases and a hypothesis about risk for neurotoxicity. *American Journal of Psychiatry*, **136**: 963–966.

CHAPTER 7

Emergencies in child and adolescent psychiatry

Ken Ma and Vishu Bhadravathi

This chapter will discuss the types of psychiatric emergencies that commonly present to child and adolescent mental health services (CAMHS) in the UK, paying particular attention to community tier 2/3 CAMHS (Box 7.1). We have tried to adopt a systems approach to the assessment and management of such emergencies, which may variously involve input in the community (including the involvement of crisis-resolution or home-treatment teams), short-term admissions to the local paediatric ward or admissions to regional tier 4 child and adolescent psychiatric units, as well as the involvement of other agencies, such as education, social care and the police.

From the outset, we would like to point out that this chapter is not a comprehensive text on common child and adolescent psychiatric conditions. Indeed, a basic knowledge of these conditions is presumed of the reader: the knowledge expected of a medical graduate. The uninitiated reader is referred to a number of excellent child and adolescent psychiatry textbooks currently available (Goodman & Scott, 2005; Turk *et al*, 2007; Rutter *et al*, 2008). Although this chapter is primarily aimed at psychiatric trainees working in the UK (especially higher specialty trainees), we hope it might also be of some use to general practitioners (GPs), GP trainees, doctors working in emergency departments and paediatricians. For this last group, we hope that they might gain a greater appreciation of how CAMHS clinicians approach and manage emergency assessments.

In this chapter, we will draw out some of the themes that we, as consultant child and adolescent psychiatrists in a busy urban CAMHS, face on a regular basis when managing emergency presentations. We will begin with a discussion on what constitutes an emergency in CAMHS. We will then examine the different pathways in which emergencies might become known to us, and how the clinician's response might vary depending on the pathway. We shall look at the different systems in which any child or adolescent presenting with a mental health emergency will invariably be situated, systems that present their own problems and issues but also potential for facilitating change for the patient. Next, the assessment

---

Box 7.1 Child and adolescent mental health services (CAMHS) tiers

CAMHS is organised in a 4-tiered model:

- Tier 1: primary care services
- Tier 2: individual specialist or uni-professional care, such as clinical psychologists and community paediatricians
- Tier 3: multidisciplinary teams in a community child mental health clinic or child psychiatry out-patient service
- Tier 4: tertiary services such as in-patient units, highly specialist out-patient teams and day hospitals

The term 'specialist CAMHS' generally refers to services at the tier 2 to tier 4 level, depending on the locality.

Source: Department of Health (1995)

---

process will be described, taking into account these different systems, which will in turn inform any management decision. After a discussion of the management process, we will present composite case scenarios that we hope will illustrate some of the issues discussed. Because of the dearth of UK research on the topic, we have necessarily included some research from other English-speaking countries.

It is worthwhile to note, especially for doctors and trainees working outside of child and adolescent psychiatry, that the configuration of CAMHS will differ according to region, and it is important when interacting with the local tier 2/3 CAMHS to be aware of what they are able to offer and, equally importantly, what other services exist outside of specialist CAMHS.

What constitutes a CAMHS emergency?

What constitutes an emergency in child and adolescent psychiatry can differ, depending on who is doing the defining (Edelsohn & Gomez, 2006). An 8-year-old boy with chronic behavioural problems who has just been aggressive again towards his socially isolated mother might be viewed as an emergency by his mother and the assessing emergency-department doctor, but not necessarily by the on-call child and adolescent psychiatrist. This point is important as it can potentially lead to disagreement between CAMHS clinicians and other health professionals working across different settings (GP surgeries, paediatric wards, emergency departments); other health professionals might not always realise the constraints within which CAMHS clinicians have to work or, indeed, what CAMHS actually do. In our clinical experience, CAMHS is sometimes incorrectly seen as the first port of call for problems that would be more appropriately managed by other agencies.

111

Edelsohn & Gomez (2006) write:

> '...a situation becomes an emergency when the typical systems in the community cannot handle it...typically reflect system failures of access, of quality and of engagement with the youth and family.' (p. 198)

The definition of what constitutes a CAMHS emergency might therefore be driven by the various elements in the network of a child or young person (CYP): the CYP themselves, their family, education, social care, the criminal justice system, health professionals. Of two patients with similar psychopathology and objective functional impairment, one might be seen as an emergency and the other not, simply because they have different combinations of extraneous circumstances. Factors not directly intrinsic to the child's actual psychopathology might be the trigger for an urgent referral (e.g. imminent expulsion from school, parental inability to cope when life events unrelated to the child supervene). This phenomenon should be well known to all psychiatrists. One of the core, everyday clinical skills is to analyse a particular situation and decide which elements of a patient's network should be mobilised, and to what end, in managing an emergency presenting to CAMHS (e.g. an urgent foster placement rather than admission to a tier 4 unit, if that is the most appropriate course of action).

Factors defining CAMHS emergencies

Edelsohn & Gomez (2006) adapted Rosenn's (1984) classification of psychiatric emergencies in children and adolescents into four categories:

- class 1: potentially life-threatening emergencies
- class 2: states of heightened disturbances that require urgent intervention, but are not life-threatening
- class 3: serious conditions that require prompt, but not immediate, intervention
- class 4: situations deemed by someone as an emergency but that are, in fact, not medically urgent.

In our everyday clinical practice, and in the face of limited resources, one of the challenges is distinguishing between class 1 emergencies (those we would try to respond to within 24–48 h) and class 2 emergencies, even though our criteria may not necessarily equate exactly to those of Edelsohn & Gomez (2006). Class 4 emergencies have been called 'pseudo-emergencies' in the past. Edelsohn & Gomez include in this group families who might be unaware of the proper mental health channels, those who might wish to bypass the lengthy waiting lists for routine appointments, families involved in interagency struggles, and CYPs with chronic antisocial behaviour. Garralda (1983), in one of the few UK papers on the subject, found that, although psychopathology seemed to be the major differentiating factor between emergencies and controls in an out-patient sample, parental self-ratings of depression were also positively correlated with emergencies. Peterson *et al* (1996) found that, over a 10-year period, in emergency-department presenters with a mental health issue and below 16 years of age, suicidality was associated with increasing age, being female and presentation on weekdays and during the school year. Aggressive children were more likely to present at weekends than during the week.

The following are all relevant factors when considering whether a referral is an emergency, and, if it is, why has it happened now?

Risks

Relevant risks include the risk of suicidal acts and the risk of harm to other people. For CYPs presenting after a self-harm attempt, the carers can often be mobilised to provide close monitoring and supervision – more often, perhaps, than is the case in adult mental health. Other risks that need to be considered include those of neglect and abuse (physical, sexual, or emotional) although these latter risks often call for interventions from agencies other than CAMHS.

It cannot be emphasised enough that the management of risk is a collective responsibility shared out among the different elements of a child's network, including family members themselves. There are some cases where the condition in itself may not ordinarily indicate a need for urgent assessment, but where risks increase the urgency (e.g. a child with probable ADHD who is engaging in high-risk impulsive behaviours, such as fire-setting).

Clinical symptoms

There are some clinical presentations that necessitate a more urgent response so that risk can be contained, early treatment implemented and further deterioration prevented, or at least delayed. These presentations include severe depressive disorder with significant biological features, anorexia nervosa (especially where there is a significantly low body mass index, rapid weight loss and/or incipient physical compromise) and psychotic illnesses. With reference to the last, it is worth noting that in children and adolescents 'hearing voices' alone, in the absence of other concerning features, might not necessarily be indicative of psychosis or another severe mental illness.

Factors extraneous to the CYP

Managing a CYP's mental disorder will often involve different systems (e.g. education, social care), as well as resources within the CYP's family network. When the patient's needs exceed what can be met by the available resources, an emergency presentation can result. This is sometimes accompanied by pressure to act from other agencies that, because of resource constraints, might not always be able to fulfil their own responsibilities and roles. In this connection, it is important to note that resource constraints within CAMHS might also lead to avoidable crisis presentations.

Types of emergencies seen

The types of CAMHS emergencies seen will vary according to the setting in which patients present and also the source of referral. In our everyday practice, we mainly see CAMHS emergencies within three settings: the out-patient department, the emergency department and paediatric wards. CAMHS emergencies are not nearly as common outside of normal working hours as those in adult mental health. However, anecdotally, when the former arise, they also take longer to assess and manage, compounded by a frequent lack of access to urgent tier 4 placements, should these be necessary (see below).

In our region, we run a consultant, out-of-hours, on-call system supported by junior psychiatry trainees (in some regions, higher specialist trainees in child and adolescent psychiatry also form part of the rota). As consultants, we recognise that some of our junior trainees will have had minimal exposure to CAMHS. As a point of good practice, junior trainees assessing a CAMHS emergency should always at least discuss a case with the on-call consultant before any management decisions are made. Furthermore – and perhaps contestably – we believe that child and adolescent psychiatry consultants should have a lower threshold for reviewing the patient themselves than general adult psychiatry consultants might. Trainees, unless they have done a CAMHS placement, will often have had less experience working with the CYP group.

Out-patient department

In most cases, urgent referrals will come from GPs and school nurses. Referred cases typically marked as urgent by referrers include suicidality with or without previous self-harm, psychosis, severe mood disorders, eating disorders and severe behavioural disturbance (including significant aggression or impulsivity). In all cases, we request as much relevant information as possible to be included in order to help with prioritisation. For example, a suicidal young man with significant depressive symptoms might represent a higher risk than a teenager who has threatened to kill herself during an argument with her boyfriend. Ideally, we would expect a preliminary assessment of any psychiatric symptoms, a basic mental state examination and an indication of the likely risks as part of any referral. However, we recognise this is not always feasible, especially if the referral comes from non-health professionals.

In one UK study (Healy *et al*, 2002), the characteristics of 107 consecutive presentations to an inner-London emergency CAMHS (including cases through the local hospital emergency department) were described. Deliberate self-harm was the presenting problem in a third of the presentations, although half were deemed not to have a mental health disorder after assessment. Other presenting problems included psychosis, adjustment and other anxiety-related disorders, problems related to intellectual difficulties, problems with conduct, and depression. About two-thirds presented out of hours.

Emergency department referrals

In the US literature, a significant increase was identified in the 1990s in mental health-related visits to paediatric emergency departments, an increase that was felt to be partly due to the nationwide decrease in mental health services capacity (see Grupp-Phelan *et al*, 2009). Grupp-Phelan *et al* found that, among their series of emergency department attenders under 20 years of age, the following chief complaints were the most common: suicidality (47%), aggression/agitation (42%) and anxiety/depression (27%). It is an illustration of the significant differences between the US and UK health contexts that in their series, 52% were admitted (93% of these to a psychiatric bed). Overall, 67% had received prior out-patient psychiatric care. The mean age was just under 13 years.

Starling *et al* (2006) found that, in 239 children aged 2–17 years presenting with emotional and behavioural disorders to a teaching hospital emergency department, physical presentations with suspected psychological factors represented the largest group (49%), followed by those with acute emotional disorders (32%) and behavioural disorders (18%). The second group included the deliberate self-harm and overdose cases as well as those with acute emotional distress and suicidal ideation, and the last group included those with aggression. The average age at first presentation was just under 12 years. Males were over-represented in those with behavioural disorders; females were more common in the group with acute emotional disorders.

Lee & Korczak (2010) described a series of referrals from emergency-department physicians to their Paediatric Psychiatric Crisis Clinic, which aimed to assess all clients within 72 h and frequently within 24–48 h. They saw more boys than girls and found a mean age of about 12 years. The most frequent reasons for referral were suicidality (26%), behavioural difficulties (24%) and depression (17%). After psychiatric assessment, adjustment disorder was the most common diagnosis (29%), followed by mood disorder (17%) and anxiety disorder (17%). Of note, the emergency-department physicians' discharge diagnoses and diagnoses made by the crisis clinic were only in agreement 21% of the time. The authors attributed this low agreement to a number of factors, including the more limited time emergency-department physicians have to assess patients and their lack of specialty expertise. Emergency-department physicians seemed more likely to suggest a mood, anxiety or psychotic disorder.

Across these three studies, suicidal acts and behavioural difficulties (including aggression and mood problems) seemed to be the major problems for children and adolescents presenting to emergency departments with a mental health issue; by comparison, psychosis was relatively uncommon. Although the studies came from English-speaking countries outside the UK, anecdotally the results do resonate with our experience, both as consultants and (previously) as higher specialist trainees. Our service is fortunate to have a good working relationship with the local paediatric wards and, apart from the self-harm and overdose cases, a number of psychiatric emergencies do get admitted there for assessment and/or preliminary treatment. These include patients who are feeling acutely suicidal but have not actually harmed themselves, patients who are presenting with possible psychotic symptoms and low-weight anorexic patients.

Police station assessments

These happen infrequently. In our local experience, young people under 16 years of age are only rarely detained under Section 136 of the Mental Health Act 1983.

CAMHS in-patient units

Although the focus of this chapter is on CAMHS emergencies that present in the community, urgent situations can obviously still arise in an in-patient setting. However, these do not tend to differ significantly from those that arise in other psychiatric in-patient settings, such as the following:

- extreme aggression or agitation;
- significant self-harm that occurs on the ward, including overdoses;
- side-effects of medication (e.g. acute dystonia) – neuroleptic malignant syndrome is rare in this age group, but a high index of suspicion needs to be maintained (see Neuhut *et al*, 2009);
- physical emergencies (e.g. occurrence of the refeeding syndrome in anorexic patients);
- catatonia (this is very rare).

Assessment process

We do not propose to reinvent the wheel and describe the standard assessment process in CAMHS for routine cases; the reader is referred to the relevant chapters in the aforementioned child and adolescent psychiatry textbooks if they do not already have a basic idea of the process. Suffice to say that CAMHS clinicians often pride themselves on the comprehensiveness of their assessments, which as a rule collate information drawn from multiple sources (e.g. the CYP, family or carers, education, social care if relevant). Such an assessment clearly takes time, and in our routine out-patient work it is unusual for us to come to a definitive diagnosis after the first appointment.

During an emergency assessment, time is often at a premium, so we have to focus our attention on the most pressing questions. For example, when we are asked to assess a patient urgently in the emergency department, the questions that follow will often be uppermost in our mind. (That is, of course, not to say that other issues are unimportant; rather, they can be looked into in due course, when more time is available.)

- What is the nature of the child's psychopathology? Is there in fact a potential psychiatric diagnosis to be made? Although some CAMHS colleagues from other professional backgrounds might object to the emphasis on diagnosis, we would argue that in an emergency situation, working with diagnoses – including the question of whether there even is one – can often afford a level of much needed clarity.
- If there is a preliminary psychiatric diagnosis, what is the severity?
- Are there potential organic causes for the CYP's presentation that have not been considered by the referring doctor?
- What are the risks (e.g. risk to self, risk to others, risk of being abused or exploited, risk of accidental injury)? Equally importantly, to what extent are the risks related to the mental disorder rather than to other factors (e.g. the social situation)? This is where CAMHS can sometimes get into rather heated debates with other agencies.
- At the end of the assessment, can the CYP go home? If so, what measures need to be put in place and by whom (the family, CAMHS, other agencies)? In some regions, CAMHS-specific crisis-resolution or home-treatment teams are available, thus theoretically reducing the need for in-patient psychiatric admissions.
- What are the family's strengths? More broadly speaking, what are the protective factors in play? In an emergency situation, it is sometimes easy to forget this important aspect, leading families to become inadvertently disempowered in the process.
- If the CYP cannot go home, what are the options? If there is a mental illness that cannot be managed in the community, are we looking at a tier 4 in-patient placement? Or, in the absence of any other options, is admission of an acutely ill older adolescent to an age-inappropriate adult psychiatry ward necessary? (Patients under 16 years of age should never be admitted to an adult psychiatric ward. For patients 16 –17 years of age admitted to an adult ward, hospital managers have a duty to ensure that their ward is suitable for patients in this age group; McDougall *et al*, 2009). To what extent can the local paediatric ward function as a 'holding place' while a more appropriate psychiatric facility is identified or other strands of the management plan are put in place? It is worth noting that sometimes a brief stay on a paediatric ward in itself can defuse a crisis situation and clarify the severity of any psychiatric symptoms and the diagnostic picture. The cooperation and willingness of paediatric staff is instrumental in such a situation.
- If the CYP's reasons for not being able to go home are not mainly to do with mental health issues, what are the options? Do the extended

family need to be involved, or an emergency residential placement arranged? In this scenario, it is crucial to have the involvement of social care.

- Last, but certainly not least, are there any child protection/safeguarding issues? (See Chapter 9 on safeguarding.)

Admittedly, some of the above questions fall more under the heading of management than assessment, and we will return to them in the next section. However, we have included them here because, for us, they represent a useful scaffold for the direction that the emergency assessment should take. Furthermore, in CAMHS and indeed in other branches of psychiatry, the assessment itself and the way it is conducted can often carry therapeutic value.

Quite beyond the expert knowledge that they bring to the table, in an emergency situation one of the roles of the CAMHS clinician (and certainly of the consultant psychiatrist) is to contain the anxiety of others – the CYP, the family and the network around them (including other healthcare staff). This is a point not often mentioned in textbooks. The appearance of being in calm command of the situation is crucial, even if you are not quite sure of how the situation might resolve. Although we often try to work in a collaborative way, where we acknowledge families to be the experts on themselves, in an emergency situation it can be more helpful to be seen as the expert with solutions to the immediate difficulties. Particularly as, during crises, any pre-existing communication dysfunctions within families can become accentuated, limiting their problem-solving capabilities.

It is worth noting at this point which emergency assessments can be carried out by non-medical members of a CAMHS team and which need to be performed by psychiatrists. The arrangement does differ across regions; we know of some teams where all emergency assessments are carried out by medical members, but we do not feel that this is necessarily helpful. If nothing else, other team members might become deskilled in managing urgent risks. In our team, most deliberate self-harm and overdose assessments are carried out by non-medical clinicians. Our psychiatrists will get involved in the following urgent situations:

- cases where significant suicidality is apparent
- complex risk assessments for cases that might proceed to in-patient care
- cases where medication might be required as a matter of urgency
- probable psychotic illness.

In an emergency situation, it is easy to forget the four-by-three psychiatric formulation grid that should be well-known to all trainees (Fig. 7.1). However, even if it is not always recorded explicitly, it should be retained as a mental framework to guide assessment in all cases. This is critical, as it will inform any management plan that is made.

	Biological domain	Psychological domain	Social domain
Predisposing factors			
Precipitating factors			
Perpetuating factors			
Protective factors			

Fig. 7.1 Aetiological formulation grid.

Managing emergency presentations

Before we look at the management of emergency presentations in greater detail, it would be worthwhile to highlight the context in which child and adolescent psychiatrists are functioning nationally.

Historically, CAMHS in England and Wales has suffered from a lack of in-patient beds and an uneven distribution of these beds (Worrall & O'Herlihy, 2001; Gowers & Cotgrove, 2003; O'Herlihy *et al*, 2003). Littlewood *et al* (2003), in a survey of consultant child and adolescent psychiatrists in the UK and Ireland looking at recruitment, retention, job satisfaction and job stress, found that only 29% had safe access to in-patient beds during working hours; this fell to 15% overnight and at weekends. The authors felt that the lack of beds was of significant concern. Locally, we feel that the situation has improved somewhat since then. However, although we do now have a protocol in place for out-of-hours in-patient admissions in the West Midlands, the lack of any guarantee that, as tier 3 consultants, we can locate an in-patient bed as and when necessary can still cause us anxiety. This is compounded by the fact that colleagues working outside of CAMHS might not always be aware of these constraints, for example when CAMHS patients admitted to paediatric wards become seen as bed blockers. Additionally, other professionals do not always understand why in-patient admission is not indicated in a particular situation.

As noted already, when managing CAMHS patients, it is important even in an emergency to remember that the CYP is always embedded in many different systems. Fig. 7.2 shows a schematic representation of the different systems in which a CYP can be located – systems that might usefully be engaged in a management plan (to varying degrees). Fig. 7.3 provides a useful framework for planning the management of a psychiatric case, which is forgotten in an urgent scenario at the clinician's peril. The aim

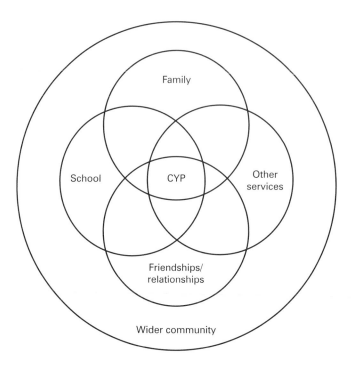

Fig. 7.2 The different systems in which a child or young person (CYP) might be embedded.

is to alleviate or eliminate as many of the predisposing, precipitating and perpetuating factors as possible, while trying to mobilise and enhance the protective factors. Of course, one of the tasks of the clinician is to decide, in collaboration with the CYP and their family, the most pressing tasks to be carried out in the short term. In an emergency scenario, discussion about medium- and long-term strategies might have to wait until the urgent situation has resolved.

Possible management strategies used in emergencies

Biological

- Apparent psychiatric presentations can have an underlying organic cause. (See Box 1 in Guerrero (2003) for a useful 12-step approach to general medical assessment in child and adolescent psychiatric emergencies.) Guerrero presents the scenario of an 8-year-old boy with hallucinations and disorganised speech after an upper respiratory infection; the boy turns out to have encephalitis. If the psychiatrist feels that not all the necessary physical investigations have been undertaken before the patient was referred, they should liaise with the referring clinician (e.g. paediatrician or GP).

	Biological domain	Psychological domain	Social domain
Short term			
Medium term			
Long term			

Fig. 7.3 A framework for planning the management of a case.

- It is uncommon for us to prescribe medication at an initial assessment, even if this is an urgent situation. We virtually never start stimulant medication without a more comprehensive assessment, or indeed antidepressant medication. In our experience, once a crisis situation resolves, an apparent depressive disorder that seemed severe at the time might prove to be less concerning than anticipated.
- The judicious short-term use of melatonin to alleviate insomnia might be indicated in some cases.
- In the uncommon situation of a florid psychosis, an atypical antipsychotic might need to be considered from an early stage. We recommend whichever one the clinician believes will be most effective over the longer term while producing minimal side-effects.
- Opinions differ as to whether extreme aggressive behaviours presenting urgently in the absence of a specific diagnosis (e.g. hyperkinetic disorder, autistic spectrum disorder) should be treated by pharmacological means. Different factors need to be taken into account. What is the probable explanation for the aggression? What are the actual risks to others? Would the short-term use of, for example, low-dose risperidone mean the patient could be stabilised at home until a more comprehensive assessment can be carried out? What would the risks be to the patient if medication were started? There is no easy answer in such a scenario. However, we would advise against the use of benzodiazepines, except in an in-patient psychiatric setting, because of the risk of a paradoxical increase in aggression and the potential for dependence.

Psychological

- As already noted, one of the main functions of a CAMHS clinician is to contain the anxiety of others.
- In the presence of a severe psychiatric disorder, the patient might require urgent admission to a CAMHS in-patient unit to contain

risks. This is more likely when support from a crisis-resolution team is unavailable. However, as also noted above, in-patient psychiatric admission is not indicated where the risks are related to care and control issues rather than being psychiatric in nature.

- When starting work in a new locality, it is crucial to find out early on what the process for CAMHS in-patient admission is, as arrangements can vary by area.
- Other alternatives to full in-patient admission do exist nationally (McDougall *et al*, 2008). These include day services and home-based, intensive treatment (so-called 'tier 3½' services). But again, the availability of these alternatives will vary nationally.
- Even during an emergency assessment, it is possible to apply psychotherapeutic techniques (e.g. cognitive–behavioural, systemic) to the consultation, with benefit to the patient and their family. Some clinicians find a solution-focused approach useful. The patient and their family might be reassured simply by the perception that someone is taking their problems seriously and offering useful suggestions.
- The resilience of the patient and their family can be enhanced through a discussion of appropriate coping strategies and distraction techniques. After an episode of deliberate self-harm, the family need to be advised on the safe storage of medication and potential self-harm objects as a matter of course.

Social

- Identify any child protection concerns and act accordingly. Trainees should always seek the advice of more senior colleagues.

Case studies

The following case scenarios highlight some of the issues we have discussed.

Case study 1

A 15-year-old girl, Z, has presented to the local emergency department with thoughts of suicide. She is well known to the local CAMHS team and is on medication for depression.

At this stage, the paediatric doctor assesses the girl, admits her to a ward and makes a referral to the local CAMHS team (or liaison service if there is one) for a fuller assessment and management.

One of the nurses on the team assesses the patient. Z has presented to the emergency department four times in the last year with overdoses of 5–8 paracetamol tablets each time. She also has a history of self harming by cutting her arms. She is known to go on different social networking sites to discuss her overdoses.

This information could have an impact on the clinician's attitude towards the client. It might give rise to 'doubts about the current intent' or a 'sense of hopelessness' in the clinician, possibly leading to a biased risk assessment. It is crucial to recall that, although the historical information is important, risks are dynamic and need to be assessed at every presentation.

> When seen by the CAMHS clinician, Z reports suicidal ideation with what seems to be a well-thought-out plan to end her life. She feels that she would act on these thoughts were she to be sent home. She is unable to identify any positive aspects to her life. Objectively, there are some mild to moderate depressive symptoms.

At this stage, the clinician might feel a different mixture of emotions (e.g. anxiety, frustration, feelings of being manipulated). However, despite what might be construed as previous low-risk self-harm and suicide attempts, her current reported intent to end her life needs to be taken seriously. The crucial element here is a prompt and consistent crisis response, which often helps to keep patients such as Z, and the network around them, contained. At this stage, involvement of the parents or carers is imperative.

> Her mother is unable to be present at the assessment. Z has had no contact with her father since she was 1 year old. Her mother has problems with alcohol and Z is her main carer.

This information signals a need for social-care colleagues to conduct an assessment on the mother's ability to keep Z safe. The option of admitting Z to an adolescent in-patient psychiatric unit for the short term to manage the crisis should be considered. In conjunction with Z's current mental state, the lack of social support and recurrent risk-taking behaviour with elements of a mental illness should prompt the clinician to consider in-patient assessment and management. At this point, one of the team psychiatrists will need to be involved, in order to conduct a psychiatric mental state examination and risk assessment and to facilitate the referral to the local in-patient unit.

> After assessing Z on the paediatric ward, the consultant at the local adolescent psychiatric unit does not feel that the patient would be best placed with them; she feels that Z's presentation is more to do with the patient's social adversity than with a psychiatric emergency.

It is the duty of tier 3 clinicians to decide whether to refer a patient for in-patient care, and the prerogative of tier 4 clinicians to decide whether this course of action should be pursued. In our experience, it is rare that tier 3 and tier 4 clinicians cannot agree on an appropriate management plan.

The tier 3 and tier 4 psychiatrists in this scenario agree that a multi-agency response is needed for Z. After their initial assessment, if there are no safeguarding concerns, social care might suggest a Common Assessment Framework (CAF) process, to look at the multiple needs of the young person. The CAF is a process whereby practitioners can identify the CYP's needs early, assess them holistically and deliver coordinated services to help address these needs. The process is entirely voluntary and informed consent is mandatory. The CAF is offered to children who have needs additional to those being met by universal services. CAF meetings involve all professionals who are or should be working with the CYP and their family. After assessment by the in-patient consultant, Z feels a little safer and agrees to be discharged home, with her mother finally admitting to her alcohol problem and agreeing to seek help. Z is followed up at the local CAMHS for individual work on coping strategies and emotional regulation. Through the CAF, her mother starts accessing the local substance-misuse service and Z is put in touch with a young carers project. She is also assigned a mentor at school. Z's mother agrees to be more proactive in monitoring Z's use of social networking sites.

Case study 2

A 10-year-old boy, C, has become agitated at school and starts throwing furniture around. The school phones his parents, who collect C and bring him to the GP surgery. At the GP surgery, the boy is restless and pacing. He was not previously known to CAMHS.

At this stage, the GP needs to seek other relevant information. He might consider behavioural problems or bullying. He might also be considering a referral to CAMHS.

C has a 2-month history of attacking pupils and has been threatening to do the same today. He has already been temporarily excluded on two occasions, and the head teacher is now considering permanent exclusion. Yesterday, C threatened to stab his 18-year-old cousin, who has been living with them, and brandished a kitchen knife in the cousin's direction. C's parents are very worried.

The additional information raises the GP's anxiety and leads to an emergency-department referral. The emergency-department consultant then makes an urgent referral to CAMHS, and C is seen by the psychiatrist on duty.

It is necessary to evaluate whether this is a real psychiatric emergency, as opposed to what Edelsohn & Gomez (2006) have described as a class 4 emergency (see page 112). Naturally, an assessment of the short-term risks is imperative. However, the assessment and the management plan at this stage also need to take into account the anxieties in the systems around the child (the school, the parents, the GP). There is anxiety on the school's part about other pupils being at risk, whereas the parents are concerned about the risk C poses to his cousin as well as the risk of C being permanently excluded from school.

A functional analysis of the presenting problem needs to be undertaken (the antecedents, behaviour and consequences). How relevant is the fact that C's cousin is living with the family? Is this a new arrangement? The information gathered might indicate a recent change in the child's environment. Has C always been resistant to changes in his routine? If so, this might indicate the need for a more in-depth assessment of his social communication.

> The psychiatrist discovers that the cousin moved in 2 months ago, as he has just started at the nearby university. He is sharing a room with C, which the parents now recognise might have been inappropriate, as C has always needed his own space from an early age for his toy car collection. The cousin has also been making fun of C regarding this collection, calling C 'babyish'.

The parents agree to a further assessment of C at CAMHS and decide to revise the living arrangements in the house. They agree to take C home after the psychiatrist advises them on the safe storage of sharp objects and potential weapons. C calms down after his parents decide that the cousin should temporarily sleep downstairs in the living room while a longer-term arrangement is considered. An early follow-up at CAMHS is offered.

The above scenario indicates what often occurs in our experience. The assessment itself, carried out in a calm and authoritative manner, can allay much anxiety and enable the family to identify relatively low-key solutions. For the psychiatrist themselves to have become caught up in the anxiety would have been most unhelpful. This anxiety might, for example, have led to the injudicious (in this situation) prescription of an antipsychotic.

Conclusions

Although we might not come across emergencies as frequently as our adult psychiatry colleagues, we believe that the practical focus on systems in child and adolescent psychiatry affords an approach to emergencies that can be helpfully transported into all areas of mental healthcare. If the non-specialist reader comes away with a greater appreciation of this, and also of some of the challenges and complexities of managing CAMHS emergencies, we shall consider our job done.

References

Department of Health (1995) *Child and Adolescent Mental Health: Together We Stand*. TSO (The Stationery Office).

Edelsohn G, Gomez J (2006) Psychiatric emergencies in adolescents. *Adolescent Medicine Clinics*, **17**: 183–204.

Garralda M (1983) Child psychiatric emergencies: a research note. *Journal of Child Psychology and Psychiatry and Allied Disciplines*, **24**: 261–267.

Goodman R, Scott S (2005) *Child Psychiatry* (2nd edn). Blackwell.

Gowers S, Cotgrove A (2003) The future of in-patient child and adolescent mental health services. *British Journal of Psychiatry*, **183**: 479–480.

Grupp-Phelan J, Mahajan P, Foltin G, *et al* (2009) Referral and resource use patterns for psychiatric-related visits to pediatric emergency departments. *Pediatric Emergency Care*, **25**: 217–220.

Guerrero A (2003) General medical considerations in child and adolescent patients who present with psychiatric symptoms. *Child and Adolescent Psychiatric Clinics of North America*, **12**: 613–628.

Healy E, Saha S, Subotsky F, *et al* (2002) Emergency presentations to an inner-city adolescent psychiatric service. *Journal of Adolescence*, **25**: 397–404.

Lee J, Korczak D (2010) Emergency physician referrals to the pediatric crisis clinic: reasons for referral, diagnosis and disposition. *Journal of the Canadian Academy of Child and Adolescent Psychiatry*, **19**: 297–302.

Littlewood S, Case P, Gater R, *et al* (2003) Recruitment, retention, satisfaction and stress in child and adolescent psychiatrists. *The Psychiatrist*, **27**: 61–67.

McDougall T, Worrall-Davies A, Hewson L, *et al* (2008) Tier 4 Child and Adolescent Mental Health Services (CAMHS) – inpatient care, day services and alternatives: an overview of Tier 4 CAMHS provision in the UK. *Child and Adolescent Mental Health*, **13**: 173–180.

McDougall T, O'Herlihy A, Pugh K, *et al* (2009) Young people on adult mental health wards. *Mental Health Practice*, **12**: 16–21.

Neuhut R, Lindenmayer J, Silva R (2009) Neuroleptic malignant syndrome in children and adolescents on atypical antipsychotic medication: a review. *Journal of Child and Adolescent Psychopharmacology*, **19**: 415–422.

O'Herlihy A, Worrall A, Lelliott P, *et al* (2003) Distribution and characteristics of in-patient child and adolescent mental health services in England and Wales. *British Journal of Psychiatry*, **183**: 547–551.

Peterson B, Zhang H, Santa Lucia R, *et al* (1996) Risk factors for presenting problems in child psychiatric emergencies. *Journal of the American Academy of Child and Adolescent Psychiatry*, **35**: 1162–1173.

Rosenn D (1984) Psychiatric emergencies in children and adolescents. In *Emergency Psychiatry: Concepts, Methods, and Practices* (eds E Bassuk, A Birk). Plenum.

Rutter M, Bishop D, Pine D, *et al* (eds) *(2008) Rutter's Child and Adolescent Psychiatry* (5th edn). Wiley–Blackwell.

Starling J, Bridgland K, Rose D (2006) Psychiatric emergencies in children and adolescents: An emergency department audit. *Australasian Psychiatry*, **14**: 403–407.

Turk T, Graham P, Verhulst F (2007) *Child and Adolescent Psychiatry: A Developmental Approach*. Oxford University Press.

Worrall A, O'Herlihy A (2001) Psychiatrists' views of in-patient child and adolescent mental health services: a survey of members of the child and adolescent faculty of the College. *The Psychiatrist*, **25**: 219–222.

CHAPTER 8

The psychiatric intensive care unit

Faisil Sethi, Roland Dix and Stephen Dye

The psychiatric intensive care unit (PICU) has been defined as a service that provides care for 'patients compulsorily detained usually in secure conditions, who are in an acutely disturbed phase of a serious mental disorder. There is an associated loss of capacity for self control, with a corresponding increase in risk, which does not enable safe, therapeutic management and treatment in a general open acute ward' (Department of Health, 2002). PICUs allow immediate response to critical situations (both within the PICU and in liaison with interface services) and PICU staff have become well versed in responding to emergency conditions within psychiatry.

PICUs evolved pragmatically within general adult psychiatry to provide safe, therapeutic care for patients displaying particularly disturbed or sustained high-risk behaviour that necessitates some security in their treatment. Because they developed unsystematically, at first the care provided seemed haphazard, with much disparity in clinical practice, governance and unit protocols (Zigmond, 1995; Beer *et al*, 1997; Pereira *et al*, 1999). In 2002, England's National Association of Psychiatric Intensive Care Units (NAPICU), in conjunction with the Department of Health, developed national standards for PICUs (Department of Health, 2002). Since these standards were published, funding was allocated to upgrade PICU physical environments (Pereira *et al*, 2005a), a national governance network established (Dye *et al*, 2005), and an accreditation scheme measuring units against set criteria developed (Cresswell *et al*, 2009). Since then, national standards have been updated (NAPICU, 2014). This has given managers, clinical staff, patients and relatives a benchmark upon which to base further improvements.

The concept of psychiatric intensive care has expanded to settings other than general adult psychiatry. Similar units have developed within forensic psychiatry, women's services and adolescent services. In the future there might be further developments: perhaps PICUs for older adults, patients with intellectual disabilities and those with personality disorder. Whatever the variant of PICU, all units have a similar ethos of providing intensive, comprehensive, multidisciplinary care for mentally unwell patients whose presentation in an acute phase of illness poses increased risks to themselves or others. Figure 8.1 displays the central positioning of the PICU within the adult mental health service framework.

Until recently, there were no nationally defined and accepted levels of staffing for PICUs. The Department of Health (2002) outlined the range of core professional staff required to operate a PICU, which at the time included nursing, medical, pharmacy, psychology, occupational therapy and social work. In recent years, activity coordinators, physical health

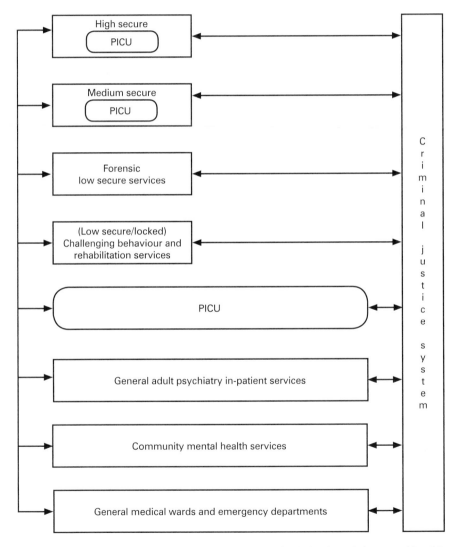

Fig. 8.1 The psychiatric intensive care unit (PICU) within the adult mental health service.

specialists (e.g. sports recreational therapists, physiotherapists), associated therapists (e.g. psychotherapists, art therapists), security specialists and police liaison officers have also come to be regarded as integral members of the extended, multidisciplinary team in many PICUs.

The revised clinical standards (NAPICU, 2014) state than an an average-sized PICU of ten beds would generally require a minimum nursing shift pattern of six staff in the morning, six staff in the afternoon and four to five staff at night. Staffing of a PICU is proportionally higher than that of a general adult psychiatry in-patient ward; this enables intensive and responsive multidisciplinary treatment in the shortest period of time to achieve maximal improvement in psychiatric symptoms, behavioural disturbance, risk management and the global functioning of the patient. PICUs also require a defined process by which they can increase staffing levels at times of increased need (e.g. to respond to an acute need for more intensive observation and engagement).

Admission criteria and patient typing

The general admission criteria for a PICU should include the following.

- Behavioural difficulties seriously compromising the patient's or others' physical or psychological well-being that cannot be safely assessed or treated in an open, acute in-patient facility.
- Significant risk of aggression, absconding with associated serious risk, risk of suicide or vulnerability in the context of a serious mental disorder.
- A new episode or an acute exacerbation of the patient's mental disorder.
- Multidisciplinary management strategies in the referring acute admission unit have not succeeded in effectively containing the presentation.
- Mutual agreement between the referrer and PICU on positive therapeutic benefits expected from the time-limited PICU admission.
- Patients who require conditions of security by virtue of their position within the criminal justice system (e.g. patients detained under section 48/49 of the Mental Health Act 1983).

Until relatively recently, little was known about the types of patients cared for in PICUs, but data have been accumulating (Pereira *et al*, 2005b, 2006a; Brown *et al*, 2008). Patients are predominantly involuntarily detained males in their mid-thirties with low rates of employment and close personal relationships, a high prevalence of chronic psychotic illness, complex needs including substance misuse, and personality difficulties. These studies noted that the primary diagnosis was a schizophreniform disorder, but a significant proportion of patients were diagnosed with an affective disorder (mainly mania). More controversially, studies have found that Black patients are over-represented and White and Asian patients are correspondingly under-represented (Feinstein & Holloway, 2002; Brown & Bass, 2004). There is considerable debate about the reasons for this disproportionate representation (Bowers *et al*, 2008).

The main reasons for admission to a PICU are violence to others or property (as opposed to self-harm), absconding behaviour, and alcohol or substance misuse prior to admission. Most patients are transferred from acute psychiatric wards, but a significant minority come directly from the community or police custody (mostly having been brought to hospital under section 136 of the Mental Health Act 1983). It is essential that PICUs respond to emergency episodes outside of PICUs as well as within them. This requirement was emphasised in 2006, when the Department of Health made £130 million available as part of an initiative to improve PICU provision and develop alternatives to police cells as section 136 places of safety.

Whatever the path of admission to a PICU, a standard admission process is required to ensure staff are familiar with procedures in what can be a fraught period for the patient and the team. Good practice requires a pre-admission assessment, but this is often a circumscribed affair in response to a psychiatric emergency. PICU referrals and pre-assessments allow for high-quality, effective, multidisciplinary treatment plans to be formulated at the outset.

The development of pathways is an integral part of the evolving 'payment by results' programme (Department of Health, 2013). The pathways are based on care provision for different patient types, which are defined using HoNOS (Health of the Nation Outcome Scales) evaluation. This can be refined within the PICU by introducing patient needs typing: robustly defining both patients and the services caring for them by combining the techniques of lean management and product family analysis (Kearney & Dye, 2010). Patients admitted to PICUs have similar presentations and thus, as a specialist service, only a limited number of patient types and care pathways will need to be outlined. Other factors, such as staffing resources, PICU environment and local protocols, will influence how pathways take shape and how specific underlying clinical processes are managed. By identifying specific needs for each patient type, patients are more likely to receive appropriate and effective care in a timely manner, leading to shorter length of PICU stay and speedier recovery. Examples of the proposed patient types moving through a PICU are shown in Fig. 8.2.

The national standards state that 'length of stay must be appropriate to clinical need and assessment of risk but would not ordinarily exceed 8 weeks in duration' (Department of Health, 2002; NAPICU, 2014). In an examination of 170 PICUs, Pereira *et al* (2006a) found that the average length of stay was 26 days, but over a quarter of all patients were defined as being delayed for discharge (i.e. remaining on the unit for longer than clinical need dictated). A study of 329 successive admissions to seven

English PICUs described a significant difference between units: 22% of patients were admitted for less than a week, 44% for 1–4 weeks, 14% for 4–8 weeks and 20% for more than 8 weeks (Brown *et al*, 2008).

The most common route of discharge is to acute psychiatric wards, but a small but significant proportion of patients are discharged directly into the community (mainly in the form of supported accommodation with

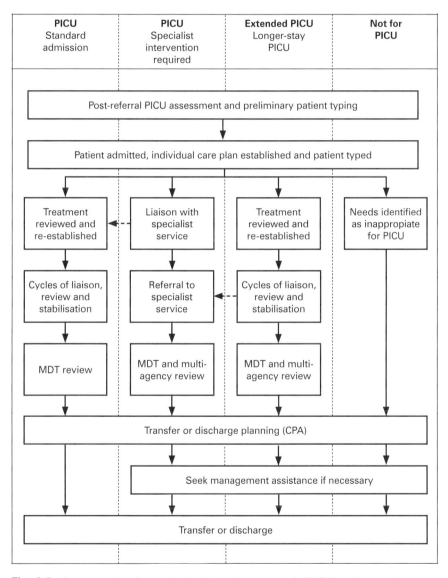

Fig. 8.2 An example of psychiatric intensive care unit (PICU) patient typing. Adapted with permission from Kearney & Dey (2010).

aftercare arrangements with a home treatment team or community mental health team). Others are transferred to more specialised services, either in the form of a rehabilitative low-secure setting for those needing continuing security within recovery or, if risks are continuing and significant, to forensic psychiatric services. A small minority of patients are transferred to the criminal justice system.

Most patients would be expected to achieve significant improvements in mental state, behaviour and global functioning during a PICU stay. Only a little over a quarter of those studied by Brown *et al* (2008) achieved a 50% reduction in Brief Psychiatric Rating Scale scores, which indicates a clinically meaningful improvement in psychiatric symptoms (Leucht *et al*, 2005). It would therefore seem appropriate that the majority of patients continue treatment on a less intensive ward.

PICU security parameters

The PICU is a discrete unit and should not be considered or situated as a service within a non-PICU ward. It differs from a general psychiatry open ward in its structure, functions, operations and treatment philosophy. The provision of a degree of security is one of its primary functions, and this has to be balanced against the need for a therapeutic milieu and homely environment. PICUs generally operate along four dimensions of a matrix: physical, procedural, relational and treatment-model security. These four dimensions are interdependent and should be managed jointly.

Physical security

General adult PICUs are often designed with a need to treat patients at the level of low security in mind (as opposed to medium or high security levels). Physical security includes all aspects of PICU unit design, including use of equipment and technology. PICU design has developed over the past decade and there is guidance available in the form of national standards and academic literature (Department of Health, 2002; Dix *et al*, 2005; Dix & Page, 2008a; Cresswell *et al*, 2009; NAPICU, 2014).

Some examples of physical security standards pertain to the building design: PICUs should be on the ground floor of a hospital, have clear lines of sight in clinical areas, have a secure perimeter with access to an outside space, and have a main entrance airlock. In relation to internal design, many products have been specifically designed for acute mental health in-patient settings (including PICUs), such as anti-ligature fixtures and fittings and furniture designed to partially withstand multiple modes of attack and be less likely to be an effective weapon.

Technology is playing an increasing role in physical security, with PICUs typically having a system of emergency alarms linked to within-PICU and within-hospital emergency response systems. More innovative design and technology is being used in the form of CCTV, sensory rooms and acoustic ceilings. Current developments include electronic-glazing partition screens and infra-red CCTV in seclusion rooms.

Procedural security

Procedural security is the system by which safety and security is maintained and involves effective application of policies, clinical and operational protocols, and practice guidelines. It allows staff to engage in safe practice with confidence and consistency.

Examples of standard operational procedures in most PICUs include the following:

- procedures for the use of the emergency alarm system
- procedures for the management of escorted and unescorted leave
- seclusion room operational procedures
- procedures for the control of illegal substances (e.g. searches)
- procedures controlling access to visitors and facilitative engagement with family and friends (e.g. via telephone)
- protocols regarding access to fresh air and smoking breaks
- multi-level and multi-agency procedures for managing aggression and violence
- procedures for monitoring rapid tranquillisation
- observation and engagement procedures
- operational interface with the criminal justice system.

Relational security

Relational security is about understanding the patient and their environment; most importantly, it is about translating that understanding into care. The PICU team should work well together and foster therapeutic relationships with patients. Good relational security is associated with a high staff-to-patient ratio, continuity within the team, effective multidisciplinary working, a well-trained clinical team with a suitable skill-set, an approach based on individualised care and commitment to a therapeutic programme in the PICU. A model for thinking about relational security, applicable to all mental health services, has been developed by the Department of Health (2010).

Treatment model security

The treatment model is part of the security matrix; this applies to all mental health services, but is overtly visible in the PICU. The model of intensive and dynamic clinical and risk assessment and management should be considered on an equal footing with the other security dimensions. This treatment model sits within a treatment philosophy that strikes a fine balance between containment and therapeutic recovery.

Risk assessment and management

In the UK, most PICU multidisciplinary teams use the structure of the Care Programme Approach, incorporating a risk assessment and management scheme. Most PICU clinicians cover the following areas in their baseline investigation of risk.

- Nature of the risk scenarios leading to PICU admission.
- Vulnerability factors (e.g. illicit drug use, intellectual disability, sexual or financial exploitation, intimate partner violence).
- Risks to self (e.g. untreated physical health disorder, self-harm, overdose, suicidality).
- Risks to others. These commonly include property damage, harassment and violence. Risks requiring more specialised assessment by the PICU team include the use of weapons, sexual assault, fire-setting and stalking. The object at risk could be a specific person, people in general, a health professional, or a particular place or building.
- Risks to children and other vulnerable adults. Risks of this nature that form part of the presenting psychopathology should not be taken lightly. However, for patients who are parents, the impact of the acute behavioural disturbance and the lead-up to PICU admission should be considered when assessing the well-being of dependents. Child welfare is paramount and other agencies (e.g. child and family social services, police) might need to be involved.
- Risks associated with current psychopathology (e.g. command hallucinations and threat/control-override symptoms).
- Past contact with psychiatric services indicating risk and historical indicators of effective risk management strategies. These would include past contact with secure or semi-secure services. Past PICU admissions could provide useful information in terms of which clinical interventions were effective.
- Criminal history indicating risk. Any contact with the criminal justice system should be explored, given that forensic and non-forensic populations are often managed in PICUs.

Most PICUs operate this kind of clinical risk assessment in a more or less unstructured fashion. It might be of indeterminate reliability and validity; given the nature of PICUs it is also susceptible to what can best be described as a counter-transference bias. However, it is a baseline and given the nature of PICU work, there is an expectation that risk assessment is regularly updated by the multidisciplinary team.

More specialised (actuarial) risk assessment tools are sometimes used in PICUs in the areas of aggression, violence, stalking, sexual violence, suicide risk, malingering, psychopathy and personality disorder. Actuarial risk assessments should be conducted by clinicians with appropriate expertise, training and clinical experience. However, this kind of risk assessment might not be ideal for PICUs, given the rapid behavioural changes seen during the acute phase of mental disorders. Some PICUs use structured assessment tools focusing on the short-term prediction of aggression or behavioural disturbance. At present, there is little clear evidence of their superiority over structured clinical judgement. Examples of such tools include the Overt Aggression Scale (Yudofsky *et al*, 1986), Bröset Violence Checklist (Almvick & Woods, 2003), Staff Observation of Aggression Scale – Revised (Nijman & Palmstierna, 2002), and Nursing Observed Illness Intensity Scale (Bowers *et al*, 2011). This is an area of ongoing research, and PICUs might provide a clinical platform for future innovation in this challenging area of clinical assessment.

PICU interventions

Engagement and observation

Graded observation in mental health in-patient units has occupied central ground for over a century. Although some studies have shown that observation can be useful in maintaining a safe environment, others have illustrated the superiority of engagement over observation in maintaining safety and the quality of experience (Bowles, 2002).

Graded observation offers a familiar format within which the activity of a person is observed and recorded during specified time intervals. Observation should not be a custodial pursuit; it should provide an opportunity for the team to interact with the patient in a therapeutic manner. An example of a PICU gradation schedule is shown in Table 8.1.

Engagement is a process in which patients and staff are meaningfully occupied in a shared interest. In mental health facilities in Bradford (UK), almost totally replacing observation with engagement produced significant improvements in the quality of relationships between staff and patient populations, at the same time decreasing adverse events (Bowers *et al*, 2003). This survey also showed that an increase in containment behaviours

Table 8.1 Graded observation schedule

PICU observation type	Timing	Checks
General observation	Every 30 or 60 min	Engagement, location
Intermittent observation	Every 15 or 30 min	Engagement, location, movements, behaviour
Enhanced observation (within eyesight)	Continuous (one nurse)	Engagement, location, movements, behaviour
Enhanced observation (within arm's length)	Continuous (one nurse)	Engagement, location, movements, behaviour

by staff (i.e. observation, seclusion, restraint) did not proportionally result in reduction of adverse incidents.

Engagement should be the first objective of all units, with the aim of providing close awareness and periodic supervision of the activities of a given patient group. The introduction of specific teams to mental health in-patient units charged with managing engagement, activity and physical health can result in significant improvement in activity engagement levels and ensure that such a philosophy is kept high on a PICU's agenda.

De-escalation

De-escalation is a technique that aims to prevent and/or diminish levels of hostility within human interaction. A number of models have been proposed for use in mental health and a specific one has been proposed for use within the psychiatric intensive care or low secure unit. It is important to recognise that as well as being a skill-set, de-escalation is a philosophy, and those responsible for the environment and regimes within in-patient services are required to take careful account of the ways in which characteristics of the institution itself might be modified to help prevent hostile responses.

Dix & Page (2008b) proposed a three-component cyclical model of successful de-escalation specifically for use in a PICU – the ACT (assessment, communication, tactics) model (Fig. 8.3). Using this model, assessment should be applied at all levels within the operational framework of the PICU, as well as in the context of specific interactions between people. There are a variety of communication techniques that aim to de-escalate situations that might be progressing towards hostility.

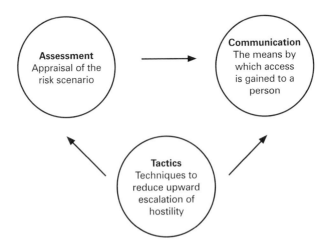

Fig 8.3 The ACT (assessment, communication, tactics) model (Dix & Page, 2008b).

Physical restraint

The nature of aggression, and thus also containment strategies such as restraint, will always contain elements of unpredictability. When examining staff strategies for applying emergency procedures with violent or threatening patients, Wynn (2002) found that physical restraint was a more common strategy in patients who were male, younger and non-psychotic. In contrast, seclusion was more likely with older male patients with an organic psychotic disorder. Although the Mental Health Act 1983 does not specifically deal with the legal authority to restrain, detailed guidance is given within the associated Code of Practice (Department of Health, 2008) and practitioners should consider this (or similar appropriate legislative guides) in all episodes of restraint (Box 8.1).

Following growing concern over the ability (and training) of staff to manage violence within psychiatric hospitals in a safe manner (Brailsford & Stevenson, 1973; Bridges *et al*, 1981), more systematised methods of physical restraint were developed (Lee *et al*, 2001). In 2014, much heterogeneity still exists in the restraint techniques being taught to clinical staff, and this has led to concerns about the generalisability, reliability and validity of such interventions.

Several authors have offered perspectives on maximising restraint safety (Parkes, 2002; Paterson & Leadbetter, 2004; Macpherson *et al*, 2005; Metherall *et al*, 2006). Factors either relate to the individual (e.g. pre-existing medical conditions, obesity, high doses of medication) or to the restraint process itself (e.g. length of restraint, restraint in prone position, pressure applied to thorax causing positional asphyxia). One important factor is the duration of restraint in the prone position. The independent inquiry following the death of David Bennett recommended that under no circumstances should any patient be restrained in a prone position for a period longer than 3 min (Norfolk, Suffolk and Cambridgeshire SHA, 2003). National Institute for Health and Care Excellence (NICE) guidance states that physical intervention must be 'appropriate, reasonable and proportionate to a specific situation and should be applied for the minimum possible amount of time' (NICE, 2005). In the event of a prolonged episode of restraint, careful consideration must be given to the risk to the patient of continuing restraint and the risk of further assault to others if restraint is discontinued.

It is good practice to measure length of time, but unless an individual is specifically monitoring the patient's physical well-being when subject to these interventions, timings are subject to errors. Metherall *et al* (2006) reported on the creation of medical emergency response teams available to respond quickly to episodes of restraint. These teams included an independent assessor trained to intermediate life-support standards whose sole role was to monitor the physical condition of the patient being restrained and alert staff to the physical healthcare risks described above.

Box 8.1 Summary of Code of Practice restraint guidance

- Clear written policy that includes provision for post incident review.
- Each episode is documented and reviewed.
- Any restraint is:
  - to be used as a last resort in an emergency, when there is a real possibility of harm if no intervention made
  - to be reasonable, justifiable and proportionate to risk
  - to be used only as long as absolutely necessary
  - to involve recognised restraint techniques
  - not to involve deliberate application of pain
  - to be carried out by those with appropriate training
  - to use mechanical restraint only in 'exceptional' circumstances, with a clear governing policy
- Non physical interventions to be used initially
- Individual member of staff to take control of incident
- Individual member of staff to take lead in caring for other patients
- Take into consideration special needs of patients with sensory impairments
- Continue with verbal de-escalation throughout
- Doctor should be quickly available to attend an alert by staff
- Patient's physical and psychological well-being should be monitored
- Emergency resuscitation devices should be readily available
- Post-incident support should be given that caters for the needs of patient, staff, carers and visitors who witnessed the incident and allows organisational learning
- The patient's care plan should be re-assessed and the patient given the opportunity to write an account of episode
- Restraint may not be used to treat an informal patient who has the capacity to refuse treatment
- If a patient is not detained, but restraint has been deemed necessary, consideration should be given to appropriateness of formal detention

Source: Department of Health (2008)

Zoning and time-out

Zoning and time-out interventions are examples of the restriction of free movement of patients within a PICU. Some would see such interventions as being on a non-linear continuum with other clinical interventions such as physical restraint and seclusion.

Zoning within the PICU unit involves the restriction of the patient's movements to within a certain area (or zone) within the PICU. The zone should not be a single room from which exit is barred as this would meet the definition for seclusion. The rationale for zoning must be based on a clinical or risk management need for the patient, which requires intensive care apart from the other patients on the ward. The majority of zoning occurs in the context of an otherwise unmanageable level of risk to others within the PICU ward. There is an idea that zoning is less restrictive than alternatives such as seclusion, but extended zoning might, to the patient, be little different to seclusion if used inappropriately, especially if it is used for long periods.

An underlying assumption is that it is possible to maintain the zone as an intensive care environment in itself, with all the aspects of care, treatment, safety and dignity that would normally be available to the patient in the main PICU. Maintaining these standards in a zone is clearly a challenge in most PICU environments, and probably one of the major reasons why zoning is not commonly used. Most PICUs ensure that a patient being zoned is at least subject to continuous enhanced observations for the duration of the zoning intervention.

Zoning (or something similar by another name) probably occurs in units that do not have a purposely designed extra care area. In certain circumstances (e.g. if the patient is physically prevented from leaving a specified area within the unit), the definition of extended segregation (as per the Mental Health Act) is met and the appropriate guidelines should be followed.

Time-out is a behavioural approach characterised by the removal of positive reinforcement from a patient for a short period of time, usually a maximum of 15 min. The trigger for time-out is usually the occurrence of repetitive, disruptive behaviour of a serious nature. The approach should be part of the pre-designed care plan for the patient, which clearly outlines the behaviours that would lead to the initiation of time-out. Most PICUs would ensure that a patient on time-out would be subject to continuous enhanced observations for the duration of the time-out intervention.

Time-out should take place on the basis of a negotiated, agreed care plan with a capacitous patient. Time-out should not take place in a locked environment. The defining factor for time-out is that the patient can choose to discontinue it at any time and is not physically restricted to an area within the unit or room. If a designated area for time-out is locked, or the person is taken to a room that is locked, then the procedure would meet the criteria for an extra care area or seclusion.

Extra care area

To take the idea of zoning one step further, specific areas of in-patient units have been used to separate a patient who is acutely disturbed or physically aggressive from the main body of the unit. Often known as an extra care area, it is supervised and specified accommodation in which an acutely disturbed patient might be engaged away from the main unit population (Kinsella & Brosnan, 1993; Dix & Williams, 1996). It could be argued that this is little more than formalised zoning, but that in itself affords better procedural safeguards as this might be more clearly identified as extended segregation within the meaning of the Mental Health Act Code of Practice (Department of Health, 2008).

The advantage of the extra care area over seclusion is that patients and staff are kept in close proximity to each other during the entire episode of disturbance. The skills required to manage an acutely disturbed episode can be developed and enhanced through the use of an extra care area.

The Mental Health Act Code of Practice (Department of Health, 2008) defines procedures required for administering extended segregation (segregation is another generic term often used interchangeably with zoning and extra care area). These procedures are similar to those that apply to seclusion. They specify regular assessment and reconsideration at intervals throughout the process of segregation.

While the use of an extra care area can have significant benefits in managing acutely disturbed episodes and might offer significant advantages over seclusion, there is the possibility of secondary behavioural disturbance resulting from the close contact and attention that arises within the extra care area (Shugar & Rehaluk, 1990; Kinsella & Brosnan, 1993; Dix & Page, 2008b). Generally speaking, the extra care area should be used for the minimum amount of time possible and determined efforts should be made to ensure this does not exceed 72 h. Extended use can result in it becoming difficult to create the conditions to return the patient to the main ward. There are also significant resource issues to consider, given that operation of the extra care area will require a significant proportion of the staff who would ordinarily be required to staff the main unit.

Use of an extra care area should follow clear policies and procedures above those required by the Code of Practice. These should include a specified level of accommodation within the extra care area (Curran et al, 2005) and specific guidance as to the sorts of interventions that can be employed (e.g. access to television and music), as well as a clear process for exiting the extra care area.

Seclusion

In England, seclusion is defined as 'the supervised confinement of a patient in a room, which may be locked. Its sole aim is to contain severely disturbed behaviour which is likely to cause harm to others' (Department of Health, 2008).

Given the nature of disturbed behaviour, the use of seclusion in clinical treatment will always produce variation in practice. Even so, it is indefensible not to have clear, agreed and well-thought-out policies to guide practice. Policies should ensure the safety of the secluded individual in a designated room meeting the Mental Health Act Commission's standards for seclusion (further guidance is given by Curran et al, 2005) and accord with the Code of Practice (Department of Health, 2008) and NICE (2005) guidelines. Seclusion should be used for the shortest amount of time possible. To enable this, regular multidisciplinary reviews should be conducted at predetermined intervals to establish the need (or not) for continued seclusion, the steps needed to bring it to an end as quickly as possible and the individual care needs of that patient.

Records of patient behaviour and ward factors that preceded seclusion should be identified and regularly reviewed. The input of professionals from outside the PICU should be sought both in policy development and in the practice of seclusion, to gain an independent perspective. Differences between time-out and seclusion, as described above, must be emphasised unambiguously to staff and patients and the implementation of seclusion for an informal patient must be viewed as an indication of a need for formal detention under the Mental Health Act.

Some acute psychiatric wards and even PICUs do not use seclusion. A report on mental health trusts revealed that 50/68 trusts operated seclusion within their acute service (Healthcare Commission, 2008) and in a survey of PICUs and low secure units, only 53% stated that seclusion was used (Pereira *et al*, 2006b). In a survey of seven PICUs, those that used seclusion did not differ significantly from those that did not use seclusion in rate of restraint use or duration of individual restraint episodes (Dye *et al*, 2009). However, physical intervention is usually needed to place someone in seclusion and the study does little to clarify whether the presence of seclusion facilities means that they are used to manage behaviour that could be managed in a less restrictive manner. It has been suggested that when a patient cannot co-operate and is at risk of being dangerous to self or others, seclusion might be the safest and most dignified intervention, especially if there are concerns arising from the patient's medical or psychiatric history (Farnham & Kennedy, 1997).

More recently, the development of comfort rooms or 'snoezelen' multisensory environments have been advocated as an alternative to traditional seclusion facilities (Cummings *et al*, 2010). These are multisensory, high-technology environments that can include music, fibre-optic light strands, calming image projections, vibrations of bubble tubes and soothing smells. There is emerging evidence that improving physical environments is associated with decreased levels of disturbance (Van der Schaaf *et al*, 2013; Jenkins *et al*, 2014; Papoulias *et al*, 2014) and some PICUs have done this in an attempt to decrease the use of seclusion.

Rapid tranquillisation

Where psychological and behavioural approaches have failed to de-escalate acutely disturbed behaviour, the treatment of last resort is rapid tranquillisation. In essence, rapid tranquillisation is the use of psychotropic medication to calm the severely aggressive or agitated patient. This area of clinical practice continues to be underpinned by a poor but improving evidence base and local clinical practice guidelines across the UK show considerable variation. A rapid tranquillisation pathway is shown in Fig. 8.4.

Box 8.2 lists the medications that can currently be used at different stages in the rapid tranquillisation pathway. The rationale for the practice of rapid tranquillisation is derived from NICE guidance (NICE, 2005), the

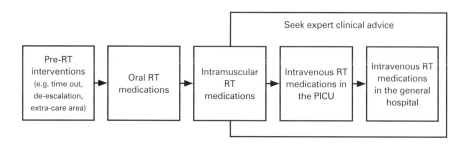

Fig. 8.4 Generalised rapid tranquillisation (RT) pathway.

influential TREC studies (TREC Collaborative Group, 2003; Alexander et al, 2004; Huf *et al*, 2007; Raveendran *et al*, 2007) and a raft of other academic publications in this area (Battaglia, 2005; Pereira *et al*, 2005c; Pratt *et al*, 2008; Huf *et al*, 2009). Along with the pragmatism derived from on-the-ground clinical practice, these documents have informed the majority of hospital rapid tranquillisation policies and protocols.

Depending on the stage arrived at in the rapid tranquillisation pathway, the choice of one medication over another is influenced by a number of factors: current and recent medication history, past history of side-effects, the clinical differential diagnosis, a comorbid acute influence of illicit drugs/ alcohol, medical concerns (e.g. cardiovascular risk, respiratory depression, susceptibility to neuroleptic malignant syndrome), neuroleptic naivety, and static patient factors such as age and gender (Innes & Sethi, 2012).

There are all manner of clinical and prescribing nuances, given the wide variety of clinical scenarios leading to rapid tranquillisation, and the heterogeneous group of medications that comprise the rapid tranquillisation family. The PICU medical team, supported by a pharmacist, should have special expertise in rapid tranquillisation scenarios, whether common or uncommon. Some examples of challenging rapid tranquillisation scenarios

---

Box 8.2 Medications used in rapid tranquilisation

Oral

- Diazepam
- Lorazepam
- Aripiprazole
- Haloperidol
- Olanzapine
- Quetiapine
- Risperidone
- Promethazine
- Buccal midazolam

Intramuscular

- Lorazepam
- Midazolam
- Aripiprazole
- Haloperidol
- Olanzapine
- Promethazine

Intravenous

- Diazepam
- Lorazepam
- Haloperidol

---

include pregnant women, the pharmacological treatment of patients with significant acute cardiovascular risk, ongoing concerns around neuroleptic malignant syndrome, and patients for whom the initial sequence of intramuscular medications has proven ineffective. This last, often termed end-stage rapid tranquillisation, will require senior psychiatrist support in association with pharmacy input. End-stage rapid tranquillisation can involve joint working between psychiatrists and physician colleagues (e.g. in the medical assessment unit, accident and emergency, or even medical intensive care).

Following rapid tranquillisation, there is usually a mandatory physical monitoring protocol (temperature, pulse, blood pressure and respiratory rate). Most such monitoring protocols focus on the requirements following parenteral medication administration. Examples of such a protocol can be found in the Maudsley Prescribing Guidelines (Taylor *et al*, 2012) and a recent review of post-rapid-tranquillisation monitoring practice in the UK (Innes & Iyeke, 2011). Psychiatric doctors in the PICU should obviously be well versed in the management of acute psychotropic medication side-effects, the management of common medical emergencies and resuscitation.

Management of acute medications

PICUs treat some of the most acutely disturbed patients in the in-patient mental health setting. In this respect, they have come to be considered the in-patient psychiatry 'emergency response'. This role requires a different approach to medication management and a healthy and dynamic relationship between medical, nursing and pharmacy professionals.

PICU teams review pharmacological treatment plans on regular basis, usually daily. This requires expert knowledge of the pharmacodynamics, pharmacokinetics, side-effect profiles, interactions and efficacy signatures of psychotropic medications. High-dose prescribing (in spite of recent cautionary statements against such practice), interactions with non-psychotropic medications (because of the high prevalence of associated physical health concerns in PICU patients), treatment-resistance prescribing scenarios, and medications given in a manner to maximise time to efficacy (e.g. loading dosages of sodium valproate in acute mania) are all examples of common scenarios faced by the average PICU clinician.

The challenge is often to make prescribing decisions under pressure and sometimes with little collateral information. Informed capacitous consent is not commonly present in the early phase of PICU admission, and this means that doctors and pharmacists are often acting somewhat blind, balancing patient choice and the impetus for risk reduction against the various safety mechanisms present to ensure that prescribing does not lead to unreasonable harm. Complex risk–benefit decisions are commonplace, with little luxury of time. Capacity issues aside, patients will frequently not consent to oral medications when acutely disturbed, which brings into play all sorts of legal and ethical dilemmas. Managing parenteral psychotropic medications in the PICU requires a high level of technical skill and the ability to make decisive treatment plans, often in the face of considerable clinical uncertainty. The input of non-medical and non-pharmacy PICU clinicians can play a significant role in medication planning on a PICU, because of the amount of mental state and behavioural information that is accumulated over short time-frames by the whole multidisciplinary team.

Acute psychological interventions

When patients arrive at a PICU, they are in crisis, and as such are often unable to engage in direct therapeutic interventions. The key priorities on arrival are to stabilise the patient and provide a protective environment. However, once the patient is stabilised, they are likely to be transferred back to an open ward. Hence, the opportunity for traditional one-to-one interventions is limited. The challenge for a clinical psychologist is to know how to intervene with and on behalf of someone who is in crisis.

From a psychological viewpoint, there are four general areas of intervention.

- Assessment of the psychological and social factors that have led up to and immediately triggered a patient's admission.
- Identifying, planning and delivering psychological therapy individually and/or in groups on the ward to address the immediate recovery needs, to improve social and psychological functioning and to instil hope in recovery.
- If appropriate, engaging patients in thinking psychologically about their problems and motivating them to attend psychological therapy after discharge.
- Helping PICU staff to create an optimal therapeutic environment to engage patients in their treatment and assist recovery.

Clinical psychologists aim to reduce psychological distress and to enhance psychological well-being. In PICU settings, they can offer specialised assessment of patients' needs, abilities and behaviour via a variety of methods, including cognitive assessment, psychometric testing, interviews and direct observation of behaviour on the ward. Psychologists can assist with the behavioural management of patients on in-patient units, for example, by helping the nursing team carry out a detailed functional analysis. This analysis can identify what might be triggering and reinforcing particular behaviours, and a behavioural management programme can then be devised. Cognitive assessments and psychometric testing can assist in detecting organic impairment, aid diagnosis, assess current level of functioning and help in monitoring progress. However, using objective and standardised assessment tools can be problematic in a PICU. This difficulty is mainly because of their lack of validity when a person is in acute distress and as such should only be administered if the patient is considered mentally stable.

Following assessment, psychologists work to produce shared formulations to help understand the client's problems better. Formulations integrate the information obtained during the assessment to clarify the probable development and maintenance of problems. This helps patients to make sense of their experiences and guides clinicians towards the appropriate interventions. Assessment and formulation are only the beginning of the process of working directly with patients. However, in PICUs it might be all that time allows. The next phase would be to develop goals and care plans that can build on the formulation, ideally in collaboration with the patient. Psychologists can also work closely with families to provide psycho-education, offer support and advice on managing their relative's difficulties, and work with the family more systemically.

The presence of a clinical psychologist in multidisciplinary team meetings and/or case discussion groups can be beneficial in a number of ways, for example by offering a psychological perspective or formulation of clients' difficulties. This can serve to broaden the team's understanding of the client, help select appropriate lines of treatment or modify treatment in progress. During multidisciplinary team discussions, psychologists can help the team to think creatively about managing aggression and risk. In addition, by being present in multidisciplinary team meetings, psychologists can identify which patients are presenting the biggest treatment problems or stress to the team. They can then offer appropriate support to the team, for example by offering debriefing following difficult incidents.

Working in a PICU is often stressful, with frequent high-risk patient behaviour, aggression, violence, and a sense of hopelessness when frequently re-presented with 'revolving door' patients. This results in high levels of staff turnover, burnout and lack of motivation. In order to cope with high levels of distress and extreme crisis, staff become task driven and rely heavily on medication and symptom management. To change to a therapeutic milieu, staff need to have time to reflect, so that the anxiety of working with high-risk patients in extreme distress can be comprehended and contained. Reflective practice groups facilitated by a psychologist provide an opportunity for debriefing and reviewing difficult situations in a non-judgemental setting, and they are helpful in making staff feel valued and consulted. Working with staff directly to support and empower them can help the team develop and grow so that it can deliver excellence in care. A number of PICUs have enlarged on this theme by integrating the role of a psychotherapist to provide more psychodynamics-based staff-support groups in the tradition of Balint groups.

Occupational therapy interventions

A common misconception is that the role of the occupational therapist is as an activity provider, appointed to keep patients engaged so as to reduce levels of violence and aggression. At a most basic level, occupational therapists are involved in developing and overseeing activity programmes and evidence suggests that keeping patients busy has an effect on violence and aggression (Davidson, 2005; Department of Health, 2002). However, the core skills of occupational therapists are using meaningful activity as a therapeutic tool, assessment of functioning and how this is affected by illness, activity analysis, grading of therapeutic activities and manipulation of the environment (Creek, 2003; Finlay, 2004). An intervention that embraces core principles of occupational therapy is remotivation (De las Heras *et al*, 2003a).

In the PICU environment, occupational therapists can start addressing the severe volitional difficulties that patients tend to present with. Helping patients to improve their ability to perform meaningful activities and address their motivational needs is necessary to bring about long-standing change and support mental well-being (Kielhofner, 2008). Volition is understood as an innate motivation to 'do', to act upon the world – a drive that guides actions and choices and is informed by a person's values. This in turn affects a person's self-image and how they organise themselves (De las Heras *et al*, 2003a). Patients in PICU settings have difficulties with components of motivation, such as their ability to appraise their strengths and limitations, their expectation of success and their belief in their ability to be effective. Whether over- or under-inflated, and masking underlying insecurities and fears, patients' unrealistic expectations and beliefs influence their sense of confidence and optimism and affect occupational performance (doing) and participation (doing with others). Additional volitional difficulties observed concern the ability to make choices that support mental well-being, difficulties identifying interests and sometimes holding antisocial values.

Occupational therapists in a PICU setting can support patients in the early stages of their recovery through early remotivation work, which could be group work and/or one-to-one sessions. Assessments such as the Model of Human Occupation Screening Tool (Parkinson *et al*, 2004) and the Volitional Questionnaire (De las Heras *et al*, 2003b) enable identification of a person's strengths and needs, including within the areas of motivation. The remotivation process supports the development of graded interventions designed to promote improvement in various aspects of motivation, and is divided into three stages (De las Heras *et al*, 2003a). For example, the first stage, 'exploration', focuses on early engagement, exploration of how and when someone participates, promotion of independent choice, expression of curiosity, forming of trust in the therapeutic relationship, acceptance and containment of chaotic behaviours, opportunities for self-evaluation, and manipulation of the environment to enable patients to experience success and maximise independence. Activity is purely the medium through which the process is applied. Interventions are developed and supervised by occupational therapists, but sessions can be implemented by other members of the clinical team.

The other two stages of the remotivation process are 'competency' and 'achievement'. It might be premature to address such stages within a

PICU. However, the remotivation process is widely used in acute settings and is appropriate to community treatment. The early remotivation work carried out in PICUs offers the opportunity for a streamlined approach to occupational therapy mental healthcare across in-patient and out-patient pathways.

Conclusions

PICUs have featured on the spectrum of acute mental health services in the UK for at least 25 years. During that time, they have continued to evolve and are now considered essential facilities within which acute and emergency situations can be effectively engaged.

The professional literature and forums within the psychiatric intensive care clinical community have recorded and disseminated a comprehensive skill set required for responding to acute situations in the specialist PICU environment. This chapter has outlined the core elements considered to be an essential part of PICU infrastructure: the PICU security matrix, acute and dynamic risk assessment and management, and a wide range of clinical interventions. These interventions include engagement, observation, de-escalation, physical restraint in a controlled manner, time-out, zoning, extra care area practice, seclusion, rapid tranquillisation, acute medication management, acute psychological intervention and acute occupational therapy.

It is important that too great an emphasis is not placed on any one of the domains within which intervention can be framed. A successful PICU approach will be multifaceted, and involve well-developed strategies for pharmaceutical, psychological, engagement and security interventions. PICU clinicians need to be complete clinicians, in that their expertise needs to be broad. They will necessarily need some expertise in the biological, psychological, psychodynamic and socio-cultural factors associated with acute disturbance. Irrespective of their primary health discipline, PICU clinicians must have the ability to work across health disciplines and interface with a range of non-health agencies. They need to be operationally astute and emotionally intelligent and simultaneously excel at being team-players and leaders, all in a truly multidisciplinary environment.

The key to the most successful PICU response is the underpinning philosophy of the unit's clinical leadership and operational management. The attitude and philosophy of the clinical team and clinical approaches should be aligned to the notion of therapeutic intervention, rather than one of containment. PICUs can be challenging environments in which a clinical team's positive attitude, self-awareness and resilience are crucial in enabling a consistent focus on therapeutic intervention. Treatment approaches to acute disturbance are continually developed on the basis of previous experience, research and dissemination of best practice. A sense of innovation is a key attribute of any clinical team that routinely deals with psychiatric emergencies.

References

Alexander J, Tharyan P, Adams C, *et al* (2004) Rapid tranquillisation of violent or agitated patients in a psychiatric emergency setting: pragmatic randomised trial of intramuscular lorazepam v. haloperidol plus promethazine. *British Journal of Psychiatry*, **185**: 63–69.

Almvik R, Woods P (2003) Short-term risk prediction: the Bröset Violence Checklist. *Journal of Psychiatric and Mental Health Nursing*, **10**: 236–238.

Battaglia J (2005) Pharmacological management of acute agitation. *Drugs*, **65**: 1207–1222.

Beer MD, Paton C, Pereira S (1997) Hotbeds of general psychiatry: a national survey of psychiatric intensive care units. *Psychiatric Bulletin*, **21**: 142–144.

Bowers L, Simpson A, Alexander J (2003) Patient-staff conflict: results of a survey on acute psychiatric wards. *Social Psychiatry and Psychiatric Epidemiology*, **38**: 402–408.

Bowers L, Simpson A, Nijman H, *et al* (2008) Patient ethnicity and three psychiatric units compared: the Tompkins acute ward study. *Journal of Psychiatric and Mental Health Nursing*, **15**: 195–202.

Bowers L, Brennan G, Ransom S, *et al* (2011) The Nursing Observed Illness Intensity Scale (NOIIS). *Journal of Psychiatric and Mental Health Nursing*, **18**: 28–34.

Bowles N (2002) A solution-focused approach to engagement in acute psychiatry. *Nursing Times*, **98**: 26.

Brailsford D, Stevenson J (1973) Factors relating to violent and unpredictable behaviour in psychiatric hospitals. *Nursing Times*, **69** (Suppl): 9–11.

Bridges W, Dunane P, Speight I (1981) The provision of post basic education in psychiatric nursing. *Nursing Times*, **23**: 141–144.

Brown S, Bass N (2004) The psychiatric intensive care unit (PICU): patient characteristics, treatment and outcome. *Journal of Mental Health*, **13**: 601–609.

Brown S, Chhina N, Dye S (2008) The psychiatric intensive care unit: a prospective survey of patient demographics and outcomes at seven English PICUs. *Journal of Psychiatric Intensive Care*, **4**: 17–27.

Creek J (2003) *Occupational Therapy Defined as a Complex Intervention*. College of Occupational Therapists.

Cresswell J, Beavon M, Glover N (2009) *Accreditation for Inpatient Mental Health Services: Standards for Psychiatric Intensive Care Units (PICUs)* (CRTU078). Royal College of Psychiatrists.

Cummings KS, Grandfield SA, Coldwell CM, *et al* (2010) Caring with comfort rooms: reducing seclusion and restraint use in psychiatric facilities. *Journal of Psychosocial Nursing & Mental Health Services*, **48**: 26–30.

Curran C, Adnett C, Zigmond A (2005) Seclusion: factors to consider when designing and using a seclusion suite in a mental hospital. *Hospital Development*, **36**: 19–26.

Davidson SE (2005) The management of violence in general psychiatry. *Advances in Psychiatric Treatment*, **11**: 362–370.

De las Heras CG, Llerena V, Kielhofner G (2003a) *Remotivation Process: Progressive Intervention for Individuals with Severe Volitional Challenges* (Version 1.0). University of Illinois at Chicago

De las Heras CG, Geist R, Kielhofner G, *et al* (2003b) *The Volitional Questionnaire (VQ)* (Version 4.0). University of Illinois at Chicago.

Department of Health (2002) *Mental Health Policy Implementation Guide. National Minimum Standards for General Adult Services in Psychiatric Intensive Care Units (PICU) and Low Secure Environments*. The Stationery Office.

Department of Health (2008) *Code of Practice: Mental Health Act 1983*. The Stationery Office.

Department of Health (2010) *See, Think, Act: Your Guide to Relational Security*. The Stationery Office.

Department of Health (2013) *Mental Health Payment by Results Guidance for 2013–14*. Department of Health.

Dix R, Page M (2008a) Physical environment. In *Psychiatric Intensive Care* (2nd edn) (eds MD Beer, S Pereira, C Paton). Cambridge University Press.

Dix R, Page M (2008b) De-escalation. In *Psychiatric Intensive Care* (2nd edn) (eds MD Beer, S Pereira, C Paton). Cambridge University Press.

Dix R, Williams K (1996) Psychiatric intensive care units, a design for living. *Psychiatric Bulletin*, **20**: 527–529.

Dix R, Pereira SM, Chaudhry K, *et al* (2005) A PICU/LSU environment assessment inventory. *Journal of Psychiatric Intensive Care*, **1**: 65–69.

Dye S, Johnston A, Pereira S (2005) The national psychiatric intensive care governance network 2004–5. *Journal of Psychiatric Intensive Care*, **1**: 97–104.

Dye S, Brown S, Chhina N (2009) Seclusion and restraint usage in seven English psychiatric intensive care units (PICUs). *Journal of Psychiatric Intensive Care*, **5**: 69–79.

Farnham FR, Kennedy HG (1997) Acute excited states and sudden death. *British Medical Journal*, **315**: 1107–1108.

Feinstein A, Holloway F (2002) Evaluating the use of a psychiatric intensive care unit: is ethnicity a risk factor for admission? *International Journal of Social Psychiatry*, **48**: 38–46.

Finlay L (2004) *The Practice of Psychosocial Occupational Therapy* (3rd edn). Nelson Thornes.

Healthcare Commission (2008) *The Pathway to Recovery: A Review of NHS Acute Inpatient Mental Health Services*. Commission for Healthcare Audit and Inspection.

Huf G, Coutinho ESF, Adams CE, *et al* (2007) Rapid tranquillisation in psychiatric emergency settings in Brazil: pragmatic randomised controlled trial of intramuscular haloperidol versus intramuscular haloperidol and promethazine. *BMJ*, **335**: 869–872.

Huf G, Alexander J, Allen M, *et al* (2009) Haloperidol plus promethazine for psychosis-induced aggression. *Cochrane Library*, **3**: CD005146.

Innes J, Iyeke L (2011) A review of the practice and position of monitoring in today's rapid tranquilisation protocols. *Journal of Psychiatric Intensive Care*, **8**: 15–24.

Innes J, Sethi F (2012) Current rapid tranquillisation documents in the UK: a review of the drugs recommended, their routes of administration and clinical parameters influencing their use. *Journal of Psychiatric Intensive Care*, **9**: 110–118.

Jenkins O, Dye S, Foy C (2015) A study of agitation, conflict and containment in association with change in ward physical environment. *Journal of Psychiatric Intensive Care*, **11**: 27–35.

Kearney T, Dye S (2010) Lean thinking and more: development of patient needs types in psychiatric intensive care. *Journal of Psychiatric Intensive Care*, **6**: 57–63.

Kielhofner G (2008) *Model of Human Occupation: Theory and Application* (4th edn). Lippincott, Williams & Wilkins.

Kinsella C, Brosnan C (1993) An alternative to seclusion? *Nursing Times*, **89**: 62–64.

Lee S, Wright S, Sayer J, *et al* (2001) Physical restraint for nurses in English and Welsh psychiatric intensive care and regional secure units. *Journal of Mental Health*, **10**: 151–162.

Leucht S, Kane JM, Kissling W, *et al* (2005) Clinical implications of Brief Psychiatric Rating Scale scores. *British Journal of Psychiatry*, **187**: 366–371.

Macpherson R, Dix R, Morgan S (2005) A growing evidence base for management guidelines: revisiting … guidelines for the management of acutely disturbed psychiatric patients. *Advances in Psychiatric Treatment*, **11**: 404–415.

Metherall A, Worthington R, Keyte A (2006) Twenty four hour medical emergency response teams in a mental health in-patient facility – new approaches for safer restraint. *Journal of Psychiatric Intensive Care*, **1**: 21–29.

National Association of Psychiatric Intensive Care Units (2014) *National Minimum Standards for Psychiatric Intensive Care in General Adult Services: updated 2014*. NAPICU.

National Institute for Health and Clinical Excellence (2005) *Violence: The Short-Term Management of Disturbed/Violent Behaviour in Psychiatric In-Patient Settings and Emergency Departments (NICE Clinical Guideline 25)*. NICE.

Nijman H, Palmstierna T (2002) Measuring aggression with the staff observation aggression scale – revised. *Acta Psychiatrica Scandinavica*, **106** (suppl 412): 101–102.

Norfolk, Suffolk and Cambridgeshire SHA (2003) *Independent Inquiry into the Death of David Bennett*. Norfolk, Suffolk and Cambridgeshire SHA.

Papoulias C, Csipke E, Rose D, *et al* (2014) The psychiatric ward as a therapeutic space: systematic review. *British Journal of Psychiatry*, **205**: 171–176.

Parkes J (2002) A review of the literature on positional asphyxia as a possible cause of sudden death during restraint. *British Journal of Forensic Practice*, **4**: 24–27.

Parkinson S, Forsyth K, Kielhofner G (2004) *Model of Human Occupation Screening Tool (MOHOST)* (Version 2.0). University of Illinois at Chicago.

Paterson B, Leadbetter D (2004) Learning the right lessons. *Mental Health Practice*, **7**: 12–15.

Pereira S, Beer D, Paton C (1999) Good practice issues in psychiatric intensive-care units: findings from a national survey. *Psychiatric Bulletin*, **23**: 397–400.

Pereira S, Chaudhry K, Pietromartire S, *et al* (2005a) Design in Psychiatric Intensive Care Units: problems and issues. *Journal of Psychiatric Intensive Care*, **1**: 70–76.

Pereira S, Sarsam M, Bhu K, *et al* (2005b) The London Survey of Psychiatric Intensive Care Units: psychiatric intensive care; patient characteristics and pathways for admission and discharge. *Journal of Psychiatric Intensive Care*, **1**: 17–24.

Pereira S, Paton C, Walker L, *et al* (2005c) Treatment of acute behavioural disturbance: a UK national survey of rapid tranquillisation. *Journal of Psychiatric Intensive Care*, **1**: 1–5.

Pereira S, Dawson P, Sarsam M (2006a) The National Survey of PICU and low secure services: 1. Patient characteristics. *Journal of Psychiatric Intensive Care*, **2**: 7–12.

Pereira S, Dawson P, Sarsam M (2006b) The National Survey of PICU and low secure services: 2. Unit characteristics. *Journal of Psychiatric Intensive Care*, **2**: 13–19.

Pratt P, Chandler-Oatts J, Nelstrop L, *et al* (2008) Establishing gold standard approaches to rapid tranquillisation: a review and discussion of the evidence on the safety and efficacy of medications currently used. *Journal of Psychiatric Intensive Care*, **4**: 43–57.

Raveendran NS, Tharyan P, Alexander J, *et al* (2007) Rapid tranquillisation in psychiatric emergency settings in India: pragmatic randomised controlled trial of intramuscular olanzapine versus intramuscular haloperidol plus promethazine. *BMJ*, **335**: 865–869.

Shugar G, Rehaluk R (1990) Continuous observation for psychiatric inpatients: a critical evaluation. *Comprehensive Psychiatry*, **31**: 48–55.

Taylor D, Paton C, Kapur S (2012) *The Maudsley Prescribing Guidelines* (11th edn). Wiley–Blackwell.

TREC Collaborative Group (2003) Rapid tranquillisation for agitated patients in emergency psychiatric rooms: a randomised trial of midazolam versus haloperidol plus promethazine. *BMJ*, **327**: 708–713.

Van der Schaaf PS, Dusseldorp E, Keuning FM, *et al* (2013) Impact of the physical environment of psychiatric wards on the use of seclusion. *British Journal of Psychiatry*, **202**: 142–149.

Wynn R (2002) Medicate, restrain or seclude? Strategies for dealing with violent and threatening behaviour in a Norwegian university psychiatric hospital. *Scandinavian Journal of Caring Sciences*, **16**: 287–291.

Yudofsky SC, Silver JM, Jackson W, *et al* (1986) The Overt Aggression Scale for the objective rating of verbal and physical aggression. *American Journal of Psychiatry*, **143**: 35–39.

Zigmond A (1995) Special care wards: are they special? *Psychiatric Bulletin*, **19**: 310–312.

CHAPTER 9

Safeguarding

Jennifer Crisp

'All that is necessary for evil to triumph is for good men to do nothing.'
(attributed to Edmund Burke)

Safeguarding the welfare of vulnerable children and adults is increasingly a key strand in all comprehensive psychiatric and intellectual disability assessments. Safeguarding concerns can be part of an unfolding psychiatric emergency or constitute an emergency within otherwise routine care. Whatever the age of the patient, family circumstances, the impact of mental health problems, substance misuse and abusive behaviours now take centre stage in social assessments alongside the biological, medical and psychological aspects. This chapter will focus on safeguarding issues in emergency situations but the importance of recognising abuse as soon as possible, allowing early intervention to become part of the care offered in order to prevent, or protect from more serious harm occurring, is the aim.

This chapter will describe the nature of abuse and abusive behaviour, the harms caused, and the harmful impact of severe neglect and outline the legal framework relevant to safeguarding both children and vulnerable adults. A systematic approach to identifying, assessing and responding to abuse and neglect in routine care and as it presents in emergency situations will be proposed. Case studies will illustrate key issues for service providers and practitioners.

The 'toxic triad' of parental mental health problems, parental substance misuse and domestic violence is a particularly risk-laden environment for children to grow up in. Studies of serious case reviews consistently demonstrate the effects of these risk factors. Parental mental illness by itself does not necessarily mean parenting will be impaired and, with support and understanding, a child's vulnerability can be mitigated. However, the more difficulty a parent has in managing their own emotional distress or their use of drugs or alcohol, the more likely it is that the child will experience adverse consequences or actual harm. Where violence is also a feature, emotional harm is significantly increased. Studies suggest that more than 50% of children living in such households might also be physically abused (Hester & Pearson, 1998; Howe, 2005). The negative effects of growing up in chaotic and disturbed households are cumulative, potentially lifelong and, by virtue of the damaged attachment patterns created, can produce personality disturbances and future difficulties with parenting. Hence, for some families, abusive patterns repeat themselves down generations.

Such patterns of disturbed relationships and behaviour are well understood as important in mental health and intellectual disability services, but not always thoroughly assessed or even acknowledged by practitioners from medical, nursing or other professional backgrounds. Undue emphasis on the medical and biological aspects of assessment, without wider exploration of the context of the distress or symptoms, can mislead or result in the medicalisation of underlying social causes of emotional disturbance, compounding the practitioner's failure to understand and intervene appropriately.

Maltreatment of adults has similar detrimental effects, reducing well-being, causing harm and eroding choice, trust and confidence. As the foreword to the *No Secrets* guidance on multi-agency policies and procedures says, 'there can be no secrets and no hiding place when it comes to exposing the abuse of vulnerable adults' (Department of Health, 2000). Vulnerable adults require a different approach to that needed for children: one that acknowledges the adult's right to information, choice and involvement in decision making. The safeguarding processes should result in empowerment and justice, as well as protection from harm. Advocacy can play a key role in ensuring the patient's concerns are heard and understood. Providing robust but sensitive safeguarding in emergency situations for children and vulnerable adults is particularly challenging when opportunities to think calmly are compromised by the circumstances.

Legal framework and definitions

Children

A basic knowledge of the legal framework underpinning the safeguarding of children and adults is required to practice competently and safely. Abusive and neglectful behaviours, and the harms that are likely to result, are defined in respect of the legislation as it applies to children and 'Vulnerable Adults'.

Abuse of children is defined in the Children Act 1989 as 'neglect, physical injury, sexual abuse or emotional abuse inflicted or knowingly not prevented, which causes significant harm or death'. 'Knowingly not prevented' has been added into the definition, allowing the prosecution of perpetrators of child abuse when a number of individuals deny personal responsibility for the harm caused.

The Children Act 1989 (amended by the Adoption and Children Act 2002) defines harm as 'ill-treatment or the impairment of health or development, including, for example, impairment suffered from seeing or hearing the ill-treatment of another'. Health is physical or mental and development is physical, emotional, social or behavioural. These definitions are deliberately broad enough to include all forms of harm suffered by a child, whether done intentionally or not. The clause 'seeing or hearing the ill-treatment of another' was added to specifically identify the harm suffered by children living in households where domestic abuse and violence occurs between adults.

The Children Act 1989 introduced the concept of 'significant harm' as the threshold of harm that justifies a formal child protection enquiry. There are no set criteria for judging significant harm, as it depends on several factors (Department for Children, Schools and Families, 2010):

- the degree and extent of physical or mental harm
- the duration of abuse and neglect
- the extent of premeditation
- the presence of threat, coercion, sadism and bizarre or unusual elements
- the impact on the child's health and development
- special needs that affect the child's development and care
- the capacity of the parents to adequately meet the child's needs
- the wider family and community environment.

Adults

Adult protection legislation in the UK is not as concisely framed as the law safeguarding children. The Human Rights Act 1998 provided the basic precepts, and the *No Secrets* guidance (Department of Health, 2000) set out the key framework for the protection of vulnerable adults. An adult in English law is a person over the age of 18.

A vulnerable adult is defined in *No Secrets* as a person aged at least 18 years of age:

> 'who is or may be in need of community care services by reason of mental or other disability, age or illness; and who is or may be unable to take care of him or herself, or unable to protect him or herself against significant harm or exploitation.'

By this definition anyone accessing mental health or intellectual disability services, over the age of 18, potentially becomes a vulnerable adult if they are unable to take care of themselves or are unable to protect themselves from significant harm or exploitation. In all cases, the criteria include a test of vulnerability (by definition a child is vulnerable by reason of age) and of experience of significant harm or exploitation (or being at risk of significant harm).

Categories of adult abuse include the following:

- neglect, physical, emotional and sexual abuse
- financial abuse (common but under-reported)
- discriminatory abuse.

'Discriminatory abuse – including racist, sexist, that based on a person's disability and other forms of harassment, slurs or similar treatment. Any or all of these types of abuse may be perpetrated as the result of deliberate intent, negligence or ignorance.' (Department of Health, 2000)

Abuse of a vulnerable adult can consist of a single act or repeated acts. It can be physical, verbal, or psychological in nature, an act of neglect (an omission), or it might occur when a vulnerable person is persuaded to enter into a financial or sexual transaction to which he or she has not consented or cannot consent.

Abuse can occur in any relationship and the exploitation, deception, misuse of authority, intimidation or coercion that attends it can render a vulnerable adult incapable of communicating his or her concerns or wishes. Such behaviours accompanying abuse would be taken into account when judging the severity and significance of resulting harm.

Information sharing

Good information sharing is critical to effective safeguarding. Failures in communication are commonly cited in serious case reviews where significant harm or death has occurred. This communication challenges professionals, patients and carers, as safeguarding information is by its nature private and sensitive, often hard to elicit and can provoke defensive and even hostile responses from the adults and professionals involved.

Seven 'golden rules' for information sharing were set out by the government (Department for Education, 2008):

1   The Data Protection Act 1998 is not a barrier to information sharing.
2   Be open and honest.
3   Seek advice.
4   Share with consent where appropriate.
5   Consider safety and well-being.
6   Be sure it's necessary, proportionate, relevant, timely and secure, ensuring any information shared is necessary for the purpose and shared only with those who need to know.
7   Keep a record.

Consent

Obtaining consent from parents in responding to concerns about a child is good practice and is required using the common assessment framework or making a child in need referral to children's services. Consent, however, is not required if making a child protection or vulnerable adult referral if obtaining that consent would place a child at increased risk of significant harm or a vulnerable adult at risk of serious harm; or if obtaining it would prejudice the prevention or detection of a serious crime or lead to an unjustified delay in investigating the case.

Consent obtained or the reasons why consent has not been sought must be properly documented. Consent and assessment of capacity in adults are subject to the Mental Capacity Act 2005. All treatment and care decisions must have informed consent and, if mental capacity is impaired (temporarily or longer term), all decisions must be subject to a formal test of capacity.

Long-term impact of abuse

Abusers of children and adults are rarely strangers to their victim and abuse and neglect occur most frequently in domestic settings: in the person's home or in residential facilities. The most frequently identified groups of abusers are family and relatives, but professional staff and paid care workers also abuse vulnerable children and adults. Children with disabilities are two to three times more likely to be abused than non-disabled children and social isolation and challenging behaviours create greater risk. Children in care can experience abuse and run away. Children and young people who end up living on the streets are especially vulnerable to exploitation. The betrayal of trust tends to be repeated in recurring patterns throughout life, unless the vicious circle of abuse and victimhood can be broken.

The seriousness of abuse and the risk of resulting harm has to be assessed individually, taking into account the nature and extent of the abuse and length of time it has been occurring. The vulnerability of the victim and the risk of repeated or escalating abusive acts involving them or others also have to be considered. Resilience and protective factors must be evaluated so that a balanced view can emerge. Findings from serious case reviews of both adult and child cases emphasise that abuse, left unchecked, erodes a victim's trust and ability to disclose, and in the worst cases escalates dramatically into lethal violence.

Key cases of national influence

Case study 1

Victoria Climbié was 7 years old when she arrived with her great aunt in the UK in April 1999. Aunt and child were put into homeless accommodation for a few weeks before the aunt formed a liaison with a younger man from Ghana, who was already working in London. Victoria and her aunt had moved into his flat in Haringey by July 1999. Only 6 months later, Victoria was dead, having become known to four social services departments, three housing departments, two police forces, two hospitals and the NSPCC. She was starved and beaten because of her bed-wetting and spent the last 4 months of her life tied up in a bin liner in the bath. Victoria never went to school in the UK and, although she was considered to be a child at risk of non-accidental injury, no one spoke to her in the last few months of her life.

The horror of her life and her death in 2000 led to a public enquiry (House of Commons Health Committee, 2003). The enquiry led to a revision of the Children Act 1989 and the setting up of Local Safeguarding Children

Boards in each Local Authority in England and Wales. Victoria's terrible experience illustrates the risks to a vulnerable and isolated child living with non-biologically related adults who collude in ill-treatment. Both adults and all the services failed to safeguard Victoria's safety and her life.

Case study 2

Peter Connelly, known as 'Baby P', died in Haringey 7 years after Victoria. He was 17 months old when he died of injuries inflicted in his home. His mother and grandmother had alcohol-related problems and many social difficulties. Six months before his death, he was put on a child protection plan, but his mother's partner moved into the household and 4 months later his older brother also came to stay in the crowded house. Peter died of 68 separate injuries. The adults blamed one another, each denying responsibility: each has been convicted of failing to prevent his death.

In neither of these cases were mental health services involved, but they easily could have been. Many other services were involved and failed in their duty to protect. It is likely that mental health services would also have failed these children. The risk to vulnerable young children of living with non-biologically related adults, especially where personality disorder or substance misuse are involved, is repeatedly found in child protection cases. The potential for serious physical, emotional and sexual abuse has to be considered in medical assessments made in such circumstances.

The second serious case review of this death says: 'A man joining a single parent household, who is unrelated to the children, is well established in research as a potentially serious threat to the well-being of the children. He needs to be checked out and his involvement with and relationship to the children carefully assessed' (Haringey Local Safeguarding Children Board, 2010). The next two well-known cases feature mental health and intellectual disability services and illustrate multi-agency failures of information sharing and assessment of risk.

Case study 3

Kyra Ishaq was 7 years old when she died of starvation, pneumonia and septicaemia at her home in 2008. Her mother and her mother's partner were convicted of the manslaughter of the child and of cruelty to her siblings. Her mother had become depressed, hostile and defensive, withdrawing her daughter from school. Her mother's partner believed that she was possessed by evil spirits causing bed-wetting. He imposed beatings and food withdrawal as punishment. He had mental health problems and had received treatment previously for psychosis. In his own early childhood he had lost two siblings, one from cot death and one, a 3-year-old sister, killed by his violent father (who served 7 years in prison for her manslaughter). The children missed 129 professional appointments in the 10 years leading up to Kyra's death. Her mother prevented a wide range of professionals from seeing or speaking to her daughter. All the children suffered in the household, but Kyra was particularly targeted.

The adults were defensive and disturbed in their relationships with professionals and developed a belief that the child was possessed by evil.

The non-related male in the household was allowed to dominate. History repeated itself with the manslaughter of a child in a second generation.

Case study 4

> Steven Hoskin was a 39-year-old man with an intellectual disability, who was killed by two younger 'friends' after months of abuse and being terrorised in his bedsit in 2006. He was the only son of a single mother who herself had intellectual disabilities and grew up with his mother and maternal grandmother in rural Devon. He attended a residential school from 12 to 16 years of age and was assessed as having a reading age of 6 years. On leaving school, he was unemployed and was later admitted to an assessment and treatment unit for 14 months. He was victimised in youth training activities while resident there. On discharge, he returned to live with his mother and grandmother. He was described as 'a kind hearted, generous and understanding young man, who was fond of music'.
>
> His relationship with his mother deteriorated during his 20s, exacerbated by his alcohol use and the death of his grandmother. Aged 26, he had a community assessment after he assaulted his mother; he was put on probation and re-housed in a nearby town. His mother was provided with sheltered accommodation.
>
> A number of young people subsequently 'befriended' Steven while staying at his bedsit. Steven ended his adult social care plan in 2005, saying he now had friends providing company. In reality, his life was dominated by drug dealing, alcohol, 999 calls and police visits. Steven had an in-patient admission in 1983, a reassessment by Community Services in 1993 and a further reassessment in 2003. His abusers were a local drug dealer, the dealer's underage girlfriend and three other youths. They increasingly intimidated and humiliated Steven, named him as a paedophile and tormented him. They put a dog lead on him and fed him out of a dog bowl. On the day of his murder, he was forced to take an overdose of paracetamol, then taken to a viaduct and eventually pushed over.

Five young people were tried for his murder. Two were convicted of murder and a third of manslaughter. His principal assailant had been a runaway himself and viewed as high risk since the age of 16. He had convictions for assault, arson, street robbery and domestic violence. His children were known to child protection services. He was well known for violence, alcohol use and drug dealing, and had a diagnosis of borderline personality disorder. He had numerous contacts with mental health services, including multi-agency working by a specialist forensic team. He had been detained under the Mental Health Act. His young girlfriend was his fifth underage partner. She had dropped out of college and run away with him and miscarried shortly before the murder. Her family had reported her missing to the police, social care and housing departments. Her midwife had reported her vulnerability following her miscarriage.

The serious case review cited poor communication and information sharing and serial failures to recognise Steven as a vulnerable adult. 'He was regarded as a public nuisance because of the antisocial behaviour, rather than as a vulnerable adult needing protection from abuse and neglect' (Cornwall Adult Protection Committee, 2007).

These case studies illustrate the cumulative impact of disturbed behaviour, mood and beliefs, compounded by alcohol and drug misuse, that resulted in an escalation of violence and the death of a vulnerable individual. They also convey the difficulties of working with such people and the reluctance of professionals to face the nature and extent of such abuse, skilfully concealed by the perpetrator and not disclosed by the victim. A common professional failing is to not keep the possibility of abuse in mind and to fail to make direct enquiries.

Other safeguarding situations in acute psychiatry in which parental mental health problems and abuse are a contributory factor, are now illustrated by two narratives less well known than those above. The story of Daksha and Freya Emson is of particular relevance to psychiatrists (North East London Strategic Health Authority (2003).

Case study 5

Daksha Emson was a high-flying senior registrar in psychiatry in 2000 when she had her daughter Freya. She became depressed after the birth but was reticent with both her physicians and family about the depth of her despair and her suicidal thoughts. When her daughter was 3 months old, Daksha killed herself and her child. Her case reminds us of the risks to both mother and baby when a mother has puerpural psychosis. She knew the risks. The stigma she felt clearly made it harder for her and others to manage her illness. There was no care plan or risk assessment, and the risks to her child were not fully considered. The serious case review printed her suicide note as a poignant foreword, and specifically highlighted the difficulties of providing robust care for medical colleagues, describing the 'grey market' in the treatment of doctors.

In 2007, a mother with severe mental health problems killed both her children while they were on an overnight visit with her. Their story is told in a serious case review (City and Hackney Local Safeguarding Children Board, 2008), and summarised below.

Case study 6

The mother of two children had become increasingly unwell with an acute delusional disorder after separating from their father. She was eventually admitted to hospital under Section 2 of the Mental Health Act 2007 with delusional ideas that both children had been substituted at birth and were not her biological children. She was treated with antipsychotic medication and seemed to have made good progress. Staff believed that her delusional ideation had responded to treatment and she was discharged with an enhanced care package and follow-up. The children, meanwhile, went to live with their father and paternal grandparents.

The children were separately the subject of a referral to children's social care and access visits by their mother, which were subject to formal supervision. The first supervised contact went well, but when the social worker went on leave, further visits from the mother occurred without supervision. The adult mental health team looking after the mother believed that she was recovering and that the children were safeguarded by residence with their father and grandparents. Three months later, after two overnight visits to their mother, she killed both children. The subsequent forensic investigation revealed that her delusional ideas were unmodified and there was no evidence of psychotropic medication in her system.

The serious case review praised the care offered to the mother, and acknowledged that it can be difficult to know when a patient is deliberately concealing their symptoms. However, the care provided for the children was criticised. The review concluded that the adult mental health practitioners and children's social care failed to safeguard the children by assuming they were safe in the care of their father. Urgent National Patient Safety Agency guidance (2009) stated that any children who are the subject of a parent's delusional ideas or suicidal plans require a mandatory child protection referral, and that a consultant psychiatrist must have formal charge of the care of the adult patients, with an additional remit ot keep the welfare of the children in view.

Drug and alcohol misuse and dependence

Drug and alcohol misuse and dependence increases vulnerability in multiple ways for individuals and their families. Drug and alcohol workers have to be constantly alert for safeguarding emergencies on the street and in the home. Adults and children who use substances are more likely to experience abusive and exploitative situations and to behave antisocially and abusively to fund their drug habits. The chaos of the lives led by some substance users is imported into the lives of their families. This has been described as 'hidden harm' in the literature. Risks to the unborn children of drug- and alcohol-using pregnant mothers, risky storage of substances resulting in young children overdosing on parental drugs, and exposure to the chronic social chaos of dependent drug use is harmful to children in many ways. Safeguarding is a routine part of offering care to such families and often has to be done in distressing and challenging emergency situations.

Three other categories of abusive behaviour are particularly hidden and difficult to disclose or discern, and might lead directly to acute mental health crises or contribute significantly to psychiatric emergencies: sexual abuse and exploitation, cyber abuse, and domestic violence. Studies of all these phenomena suggest they occur more commonly than realised and cause emotional turmoil that might be attributed to other causes or go unrecognised.

Sexual abuse

Sexual abuse is probably the most under-detected form of abuse. It is especially difficult for children being sexually abused by a parent or other relative to speak openly about the abuse. A case from 1999 demonstrates

159

how difficult it can be to understand a coded disclosure from a child when the truth could not be spoken.

Case study 7

> 'A', a 7-year-old boy, had presented to child and adolescent mental health services in 1997 with an obsession about death. He had been born prematurely at 31 weeks gestation and spent 8 weeks in a special care baby unit. He was put on the child protection register when he was 2 years old because of a non-accidental injury. A half-sibling born 5 years later was also put on the register as an infant. In 1998, a further child protection investigation was undertaken because of A's disturbed behaviour, but attention was directed at his mother's new partner, who was known to be a schedule I sex offender. His mother and maternal grandmother expressed concerns about his biological father but were ignored in the investigation. 'A' was subsequently killed by his father, just as the local authority was pursuing care proceedings. The police investigation strongly suggested his father was involved with a local paedophile ring abusing the boy, but that evidence never came to court. Child A's obsession with death was not understood as an attempt to disclose the severe abuse he was subject to or his fears for his life; neither were the concerns of the two women in the family heard.

Paedophilia, sexual exploitation, grooming and trafficking are situations that cause severe and enduring harm to some of society's most vulnerable and hidden young people. Many wil be 'looked after' children or have previously been in care. Drug and alcohol use, grooming and forced prostitution (boys and girls) mean some of these victims are known to substance misuse and mental health services. Engaging with and winning the trust of such victims in order to plan effective interventions takes great skill and perseverance. It is unlikely that formal procedures for protection will succeed for this client group, because most victims will simply disappear if they feel pursued or coerced by services.

Cyber abuse

This is a rapidly growing problem that is likely to become important in mental health and intellectual disability services because of the ubiquity and increasing sophistication of electronic media and the naivety of many users. It is already a major agenda for schools and the police, and will be a hidden stressor in some psychiatric assessments. This chapter only has space to acknowledge the issue and its emerging importance in safeguarding work. Virtual reality has created a separate world available to bullies and abusers and has changed the landscape of bullying, spawning new forms. The advent of mobile electronic devices, carried on the person and set up in bedrooms, permanently switched on and giving an illusion of privacy, enables abuse of various forms from abusers who would not usually be perpetrators in everyday, physical reality.

Whether casual and random, or targeted and systematic, cyber bullies bring distress and danger to vulnerable audiences who are often young (some very young indeed). Grooming, paedophilia, incitement to hatred, the posting of indecent images and videos, 'happy slapping', 'trolling' and websites encouraging eating disorders, suicide, self-harm and radicalization are a few of the ways digital technology is deliberately used to upset another in their private, personal space. This emerging use of digital technology to bully, record abuse and coerce or exploit vulnerable young people and adults might require child and adult protection policies and procedures to be used when cyber abuse is suspected. Specialist police units investigate, target serious perpetrators and rescue victims around the world.

Domestic abuse and violence

Domestic abuse and violence in all its forms is as old as human society. A determined cross-government campaign has been underway in the UK over the past decade, raising awareness of the nature and extent of the problem, creating victim and perpetrator programmes and school- and university-based educational programmes. The National Health Service (NHS) actively campaigned throughout 2010 to improve services for victims of domestic violence. Studies suggest a high percentage of female mental health admissions have current or past histories of domestic and sexual abuse (Morgan *et al*, 2010). Midwifery studies reveal women typically endure 35 assaults before they disclose the abuse (Yearnshaw, 1997). Sexual control and violence is a common accompaniment of domestic abuse. Two women each year die in England and Wales at the hands of an abusive partner or ex-partner (Department of Health, 2005). Less frequently, women kill their partners. The relationships in which violent behaviours occur are often long-standing and repeatedly abusive. Recent research demonstrates the young age of many perpetrators and victims and new legislation proposed will recognise this vulnerability (Department of Health, 2009).

The Domestic Crime and Violence Act 2003 provided legal powers for intervening and prosecuting offenders. Multi-agency risk assessment conferences are led by the police and hold regular information-sharing meetings for the most serious cases, which health providers attend. Although domestic abuse remains a major social problem, often aggravated by alcohol consumption, it should no longer be cause for therapeutic despair. In most areas, an increasing range of support systems and education programmes exist and refuge places are available for those most at risk. Formal processes should be invoked where harm is demonstrated, including child protection referrals, vulnerable adult referrals and, in emergencies, police powers. The police have specialist domestic violence teams that can be called out and have the power to remove children to a place of safety. Independent domestic violence advisors are available to support and inform victims, and independent sexual violence advisors perform a similar role for sexual violence, often working closely with their domestic violence colleagues.

Emotional neglect

This is a particularly difficult cause of harm to recognise or prove, as it leaves only indirect signs of the lack of due regard or care. The impact of severe emotional neglect, however, can be profound if undetected and the younger the child, the greater the developmental delays that can result. Severe depression or psychosis can result in a parent being unable to respond intuitively and appropriately to a child's emotional needs and additional help should be sought from family or friends to mitigate the impact of that parent's impaired emotional responsiveness. If family members are not available, nursery placements or extended school hours and pre- and after-school clubs can help some children. Children who are carers are another group who might need additional support, as they have to support adults or siblings who rely on their help in everyday life. Quiet emergencies occur behind the scenes if those carers' needs are not recognised and responded to. Lesser degrees of emotional deprivation for children can accompany parental mental distress of many kinds, sewing their own problems for the future, but recognition and understanding with support can help significantly.

Elder abuse

Elderly people are one of the most vulnerable groups by reason of age, infirmity, cognitive decline and need for care. Although older age does not necessarily bring loss of autonomy and mental incapacity, Western societies have increasing numbers of octogenarian and older citizens. Multiple disadvantages become more common with increasing age and include loneliness, poverty, disability and ill-health. Emergencies in this patient group are often caused by a combination of disability and vulnerability, as coping abilities are overwhelmed. Elderly patients often have little voice and limited choices, and opportunities for neglect and abuse are therefore increased. Public outcry seems to achieve little improvement in the quality of care offered to this group of older citizens. Reports regularly cite elderly patients being poorly fed in hospital (and sometimes at home), as support for feeding and nutrition is overlooked. Standards of care for older people in hospital are not always safeguarded and protection of dignity, privacy and choice not always prioritised. Elderly people are sometimes physically and emotionally abused by family members or carers and occasionally killed. It is thought likely that financial abuse often goes unrecognised as part of the picture. It is rare that such events are attended by warning signs or can be easily prevented.

The Care Quality Commission is charged with registration and inspection regimes for quality assurance of public and private care provided in hospitals and care homes. Commissioners of NHS services now require evidence of quality standards being achieved for the more vulnerable users of services. Mental health services for older people have to be particularly proactive in in-patient, day and out-patient settings. Out-of-hours emergency assessments for older people are often complex and challenging, associated with carers no longer being able or willing to cope. Being vigilant about the possibility of neglect and abuse is necessary if assessment is to identify any maltreatment present.

Intellectual disability services

A similar argument applies to intellectual disability services in the public and private sector, as a recent scandal at a privately run care unit exposed by a 2011 *Panorama* programme in revealed. A closed community of vulnerable individuals, out of sight of families and friends, were tormented by a staff group of mainly unqualified and unsupervised individuals. At its worst, humiliating, degrading and physically abusive care was inflicted on the clients. Encountering any instance of severe institutional neglect or abuse is an emergency and needs immediate reporting to the relevant authorities, through local children or adult protection procedures.

Institutional neglect and abuse

A safeguarding chapter in a book on psychiatric emergencies must acknowledge the issue of institutional neglect and abuse, which has already been referred to several times. The Winterbourne View and Stafford Hospital scandals, the child sexual exploitation trials in Oxford, Rotherham, Derby and Rochdale, and the investigation into Jimmy Savile and the abuse he perpetrated in many institutions over decades illustrate the widespread and pervasive nature of such occurrences. Such abuse and neglect is incremental in its repetition until finally exposed. Celebrity status can be an significant barrier to the recognition of abusive behaviour, as is the silence of the average victim of abuse; that is, until publicity begins to break down the taboo of speaking out. Gradually our social culture is changing with so many recent high-profile exposures, and new victims are emerging as old crimes, previously unreported, are now investigated.

The institutional settings in which neglect and abuse surface (e.g. hospitals, care homes, nursing homes, educational and religious institutions, prisons and domiciliary care services) are ones in which the ordinary human needs of patients, and their entitlement to respect and dignity, have been lost sight of, resulting in harm. If this harm becomes significant, it requires immediate action. All such concerns should be reported using established national safeguarding policies and procedures. Serious incidents in healthcare establishments and services must be reported to the Care Quality Commission, although this itself came under the scrutiny of the Francis Inquiry into neglect at Stafford Hospital (Francis, 2013). All NHS trusts have policies and procedures in place that mirror national directives and protocols.

A new focus on social and institutional factors that predispose to or contribute to neglect and abuse is now being taken up by commissioning processes for service quality, as well as by national registration and inspection regimes. Factors that protect against neglect and abuse in institutions include the following:

- a zero-tolerance professional and managerial culture
- the explicit attention of directors of NHS trust boards, their chairmen and chief executives
- priority being given to specialist training and supervision for staff
- a proactive organisational stance on reporting, monitoring and the learning of lessons.

The forthcoming independent inquiry into child sexual abuse, commissioned by the Home Secretary, should take public concern to the highest levels of Government and the Establishment. The outcome of this inquiry remains to be seen!

Taking appropriate action when neglect or abuse is suspected

Some general principles can be stated, but local policies and procedures must be followed in all instances, as these should be up to date and in line with local systems and national guidance. They will guide the practitioner to their local safeguarding children board or adult protection partnership. At the time of writing, the national guidance for the safeguarding of children is *Working Together to Safeguard Children* (Department of Education, 2013).

Disclosure of abuse or suspicion of harm requires reporting through local referral mechanisms and investigations will be governed by the local procedures, as set out in *Working Together to Safeguard Children* (or in local adult protection partnership procedures for a vulnerable adult).

There are some key principles when making a referral or expressing concerns, which should provide the practitioner with professional protection if followed.

- The reasons for concern, and actions taken or not taken, must be fully documented, dated and signed in case notes.
- Safeguarding concerns and actions should be recorded in, and followed up through, the relevant care documentation, including concerns for any children in the family in an adult's notes.
- Remember the seven golden rules of information sharing.
- Seek advice from senior colleagues, or the local safeguarding team. Never feel alone with a safeguarding concern – talk to another person in the 'best interest' of the patient or vulnerable individual.
- Access appropriate safeguarding training and keep up to date as part of your continuing professional development.
- Be sure to access safeguarding supervision for any concerns.

References

City and Hackney Local Safeguarding Children Board (2008) *Serious Case Review into the Deaths of Child A and Child B*. City and Hackney Local Safeguarding Children Board.

Cornwall Adult Protection Committee (2007) *The Murder of Steven Hoskin. A Serious Case Review. Executive Summary*. Adult Protection Cornwall.

Department for Children, Schools and Families (2010) *Working Together to Safeguard Children: A Guide to Inter-Agency Working to Safeguard and Promote the Welfare of Children*. HM Government.

Department for Education (2008) *Information Sharing: Guidance for Practitioners and Managers*. Department for Children, Schools and Families, and Communities and Local Government.

Department for Education (2013) *Working Together to Safeguard Children: A Guide to Inter-Agency Working to Safeguard and Promote the Welfare of Children*. HM Government.

Department of Health (2000) *No Secrets: Guidance on Developing and Implementing Multi-Agency Policies and Procedures to Protect Vulnerable Adults from Abuse*. Department of Health.

Department of Health (2005) *Responding to Domestic Abuse: A Handbook for Health Professionals*. Department of Health.

Department of Health (2009) *Improving Safety, Reducing Harm: Children, Young People and Domestic Violence*. Department of Health.

Francis R (2013) *Report of the Mid Staffordshire NHS Foundation Trust Public Inquiry. Executive Summary*. The Stationery Office.

Haringey Local Safeguarding Children Board (2010) *Serious Case Review: Child 'A'*. Department of Education.

Hester M, Pearson C (1998) *From Periphery to Centre: Domestic Violence in Work with Abused Children*. Policy Press.

House of Commons Health Committee (2003) *The Victoria Climbié Inquiry Report*. The Stationery Office.

Howe D (2005) *Child Abuse and Neglect: Attachment, Development and Intervention*. Palgrave Macmillan.

Morgan JF, Zolese G, McNulty J, *et al* (2010) Domestic violence among female psychiatric patients: cross sectional survey. *Psychiatric Bulletin*, **34**: 461–464.

National Patient Safety Agency (2009) *Preventing Harm to Children from Parents with Mental Health Needs. NPSA/RRR/003*. NPSA.

North East London Strategic Health Authority (2003) *Report of an Independent Inquiry into the Care and Treatment of Daksha Emson MBBS, MRCPsych, MSc and her Daughter Freya*. North East London Strategic Health Authority.

Yearnshaw S (1997) Analysis of cohort. In *Violence Against Women* (eds S Bewley, J Friend, G Mezey). Royal College of Obstetricians and Gynaecologists.

CHAPTER 10

Emergency electroconvulsive therapy

Kevin Nicholls

Convulsive therapies have been used for at least 200 years, particularly for psychiatric disorder. Following the discovery that electrical stimulation can reliably induce seizures, the clinical applications were soon exploited. Techniques have improved significantly over the years and modern electroconvulsive therapy (ECT) has proved to be the most effective treatment for severe or unremitting depression, and for certain other conditions (Prudic *et al*, 1990, 1996; UK ECT Review Group, 2003; Dombrovski *et al*, 2005; Fink, 2009).

ECT is viewed with suspicion by some people and with outright hostility by others. Much of this is due to a perception that the therapy is dangerous or, more misguidedly, a form of punishment. Mainstream UK consultant psychiatrists' opinion is that ECT is a humane, ethical and effective treatment, underpinned by a solid research base that confirms its efficacy. An authoritative review from the US National Network of Depression Centers has recently endorsed ECT as a 'substantially underestimated' means of 'produc[ing] large clinical improvements for individuals suffering from severe major depressive disorders' (Weiner *et al*, 2013). There is more clarity in contemporary practice around which conditions respond to ECT and how to most effectively administer the treatment, resulting in successful response rates of up to 90% in severe depression (Abrams, 2002).

History

The Romans used current generated by electric eels for the treatment of headaches and gout and to assist in obstetric procedures. Coin-operated, non-seizure-inducing, electrical stimulation of the head was common in late Victorian chemist shops and advocated for a wide range of ailments, including 'nervous debility'. But ECT benefits are, crucially, a function of the seizures involved, not electric current *per se*. The first description of the therapeutic effect of convulsions on psychiatric disorders has been credited to Paracelsus in the 16th century, and in 1785 the therapeutic use of drug-induced seizures was described in the *London Medical Journal* (Abrams, 2002). A Viennese textbook of 1798 described the treatment of mania by camphor-induced seizures by Weickhardt of the Imperial Russian College (Mowbray, 1959).

Chemically induced convulsive treatment was re-invented in the 1930s by Ladislaus Meduna. Camphor was initally used to produce seizures, but was quickly superseded by more potent pro-convulsive drugs (such as pentylenetetrazol), favoured for their solubility and consequentially rapid seizure induction. Bini and Cerletti, working in Rome, developed the safer and more reliable method of initiating seizures with electricity. Cerletti induced *grand mal* seizures in psychotic, depressed and otherwise disturbed or mute patients with positive effects from 1938. This encouraged further developments in the procedure, leading to the advent of recognisably modern ECT and its rapid widespread use in the UK and USA in the post-war period.

In the early years, ECT caused serious injury, including fractured bones and joint dislocations following violent seizure-induced muscular contraction. The introduction of general anaesthesia and muscle relaxants effectively prevents these serious complications and there should be no place for unmodified ECT nowadays, although it is still relied on in some low-income health systems.

How does ECT work?

The practice of ECT is often criticised because its mechanism of action is poorly understood. But its use has been likened to the giving of citrus fruits to prevent scurvy before people had knowledge of vitamin C. Although the complex effects of ECT are not fully understood, its clinical benefits are well recognised. Early observation linked amnesia to efficacy, but research rapidly discredited this hypothesis. Gliosis was also put forward in early days as the mechanism of action, on the basis of a theory that glial cell proliferation interrupted normal brain function and that ECT rectified this. Enhanced dendritic function is a probable benefit of ECT; however, this is mediated by increased spine density, a reversal of dendritic-atrophy-causing factors or a combination of both of these. This dendritic potentiation is in line with changes seen after antidepressant drug treatment. A detailed review of this and other candidate mechanisms believed to be synergistically implicated has recently been published (Rotheneichner *et al*, 2014). Normalisation of the hypothalamic–pituitary–adrenal axis and increased ECT-induced cell plasticity with hippocampal neurones sprouting mossy fibres but lacking abnormal connectivity seen after epileptic seizures are described.

Certain myths surrounding ECT can be dispelled. The notion that it is merely a 'shock' effect can be dismissed. The patient is, after all, under general anaesthetic and the fact that seizure duration is linked to efficacy also implicates this as an effective therapeutic event. This has been confirmed by sham ECT studies, in which general anaesthetic drugs given in modified ECT (plus adjunctive drugs like atropine and suxemethonium), but administered without electrical stimulation, proved significantly less effective in treating depression than real ECT (West, 1981; Brandon *et al*, 1984; Johnstone *et al*, 1985). The UK ECT Review Group (2003) pooled data from a total of 256 patients from six trials comparing sham with real ECT. A mean difference in Hamilton Rating Scale for Depression score of 9.67 was found in favour of ECT (95% CI 5.72–13.53). This is, of course, consistent with ECT being effective prior to the introduction of the modified procedure.

Contrary to early speculation, post-treatment amnesia is not an indicator of the therapeutic effectiveness of ECT, but some cognitive side-effects have been correlated with efficacy (McCall *et al*, 2000). This correlation might indicate a shared pathway (Perrin *et al*, 2012). Defining the underlying mechanisms of action has proved difficult. Inconclusive or contradictory research results are not uncommon and reflect the profound complexity of interacting brain systems. These intricacies can include synaptic transmitter concentration effects, differential receptor population densities and sensitivities, agonist/antagonist balance changes, enzyme functions, feedback mechanisms and second messengers, plus disparate transmitters in inter-dependent neuronal circuits (e.g. Blier & Abbott, 2001). Neurogenesis and synaptic plasticity mediated by neurotransmission-system-regulating proteins have been put forward as common mediators of beneficial ECT and antidepressant drug actions in depression (Racagni & Popoli, 2008).

Altered function in limbic and other nervous-system structures have been implicated in mood disorders, including the amygdala, hippocampus and cingulate cortex. Several reviews have given detailed information on current thinking on how ECT mediates its therapeutic effects (Nobler & Sackheim, 2008; Kato, 2009; Merkl *et al*, 2009; Scott, 2011).

Studies of ECT have identified electroencephalogram (EEG) changes and cerebrospinal fluid and serum neurotransmitter effects. Typically, the post-convulsion EEG shows high-frequency poly-spike activity followed by a slowing of brain waves compared with normal α and β activity. Trains of spike activity can occur in runs and post-ictal suppression is usually seen afterwards, with flattening of the EEG prior to a gradual return of normal activity. Slowing of the EEG is correlated with a positive response and frontal delta activity is particularly predictive of this. Slowing is more protracted after consecutive treatments and these EEG-induced changes can be detectable several weeks after treatment. A counter-kindling effect has been postulated, and this is perhaps consistent with anticonvulsive elevation of the seizure threshold with successive treatments. There are several physiological changes that are thought to mediate these changes, explained below.

Effects on neurotransmitters

Noradrenaline, adrenaline, serotonin, acetylcholine and dopamine can all be released by seizures. However, simplistic modelling founded on this and in line with the traditional monoamine theory of depression is outmoded. Recent work indicates that effects on transmitters can (unsurprisingly) be extraordinarily subtle and the benefits of ECT are not merely reflected in increased monoamine transmitter concentration (Cassidy *et al*, 1997, 2009). Variable changes to receptor subtypes and altered sensitivity for different transmitters indicates ever more complex and flexibly interactive neuronal circuits than previously postulated. For example, changes to dopamine receptor D_2 post-synaptic effects and catechol-o-methyltransferase gene expression (affecting COMT, the enzyme that catabolises catecholamines, including noradrenaline and dopamine) have been linked to ECT response (Merkl *et al*, 2009).

Changes in brain structure

Early theories on ECT's beneficial effects implicated glial cells, and more recent work perpetuates the possibility that the pro-neurogenic effects of ECT might be mediated by this means (Ongur & Heckers, 2004). As noted already, depressive illness seems linked with hippocampal neurone loss and successful treatment with ECT or antidepressant drugs can increase hippocampal volume. Memory disturbance caused by depression and ECT would also be consistent with hippocampal dysfunction (e.g. Gregory-Roberts *et al*, 2010). There is inconclusive evidence that ECT has specific effects on some areas of the brain, such as the fronto-temporal cortex, and a moderaton of hyper-connectivity in the dorsolateral prefrontal cortex has been implicated as a significant effect of ECT (Perrin *et al*, 2012).

Endocrine effects

It has long been recognised that endocrine systems are disturbed in mental disorders, and an underlying endocrine basis for brain dysfunction in depressive illness is seen as most likely by some (e.g. Bolwig, 2011). The effects of depression on the hypothalamic–pituitary axis are well established (e.g. de Kloet *et al*, 2007) and might substantially account for cognitive defects caused by depressive illness. The ability of ECT to restore normal dexamethasone suppression in depressed people with dysfunctional cortisol control is well established (Merkl *et al*, 2009). The hippocampus is also a possible site for beneficial corticosteroid effects. Whatever the predominant mode of action of ECT, it has to explain the rapid and often marked therapeutic improvements frequently experienced and appreciated by patients.

Contemporary ECT practice

In the UK, the National Institute for Health and Care Excellence (NICE) recognises ECT as a rapid and effective treatment for severe depressive illness, catatonia and prolonged or severe mania (NICE, 2003). However, there was concern within the Royal College of Psychiatrists that these guidelines were too restrictive. The Special Committee on ECT within the College convened to define areas of divergence in expert advice, and these were published in the second edition of *The ECT Handbook* (Scott, 2005). A slightly wider remit for ECT was sanctioned in depressive illness, including use following attempted suicide, strong suicidal ideation or life-threatening starvation or dehydration caused by depression. Use of ECT in severe depressive illness with associated stupor, psychomotor retardation or marked delusions or hallucinations was also deemed appropriate for some individuals. Additionally, ECT as a second- or third-line treatment where recovery from depression could not be fully achieved by other therapies was stated as an option in certain circumstances. The importance of patients, especially those who had previously been successfully treated with ECT, being offered the option of ECT was noted.

ECT as a second-line treatment for mania where treatment resistance or potentially fatal exhaustion is encountered was also sanctioned, as was its use in acute schizophrenia as a fourth-line measure where unremitting psychosis persists and is resistant to clozapine (or clozapine cannot be tolerated). A comprehensive analysis of the NICE guidance and supplementary advice to assist psychiatrists in areas where the NICE recommendations were silent or insufficient was helpfully provided in the second edition of *The ECT Handbook* (Scott, 2005).

NICE has not revisited its guidance directly to date, but has very helpfully provided supplementary guidance in the clinical guideline *Depression in Adults* (NICE, 2009). ECT was recognised in this revision as a valuable treatment option where depression is life-threatening, a rapid improvement is necessary or other treatments and therapies have failed. Failed response to previous treatment also indicates treatment with ECT in moderate as well as severe depression. ECT should not be used as a long-term treatment to prevent recurrent depression (i.e. maintenance ECT), or as a treatment for schizophrenia under normal circumstances. Following this clarification, there is no significant divergence of opinion now between NICE and the Royal College of Psychiatrists' third edition of *The ECT Handbook* (Waite & Easton, 2013). Their concurrence is also consistent with guidance from the British Association for Psychopharmacology (Anderson *et al*, 2008).

Further advice was also given that should be regarded as mandatory in contemporary practice and for good medico-legal reasons (NICE, 2003).

- Individual risk–benefit appraisal for each patient, which is carefully documented.

- Particular caution with pregnant women and patients who are young or older, with awareness of all special considerations in these groups.
- Careful reassessment after every treatment.

Notwithstanding the consensus regarding current indications for ECT, review of Royal College of Psychiatrists' advice is scheduled for 2017. Although funding for ECT research is insufficient (Versiani *et al*, 2011), it is not inconceivable that the use of ECT might be more widely indicated in better-defined circumstances for the treatment of psychosis, once we have a better understanding of its interactions with psychotropics (particularly antipsychotics).

ECT has been shown to be effective in the treatment of both unipolar and bipolar depressive states, without precipitating mania in depressed bipolar patients (Dierckx *et al*, 2012; Medda *et al*, 2013). Difficult-to-treat mixed bipolar states can also respond positively to ECT, which is relatively safe in comparison to high-dose polypharmacy and is probably under-used in these cases (Valenti *et al*, 2008). As noted already, ECT is also an effective means of managing drug-resistant mania.

ECT might be superior in the treatment of mania to lithium alone or combined therapy with lithium and haloperidol (Versiani *et al*, 2011). Evaluating the efficacy of ECT in treating bipolar disorder from this meta-analysis of 51 articles was frustrating, however, because of poor methodology and small participant numbers in many of the studies. The meta-analysis conclusions could not reflect the positive but still largely anecdotal clinical experience of successful ECT use in this disorder (Versiani *et al*, 2011).

ECT in schizophrenia might be undervalued, as adequate research in this area is probably being held back by negative attitudes and limited (non-industry-sponsored) research resources. It can be an effective treatment for people suffering schizophrenia, especially where catatonia, aggression, extreme depression or suicidality or other affective symptoms are a feature. Paranoid delusions can be ameliorated and improvement can be rapid. Such improvement might offer the patient a window of insight and allow co-operation with the commencement of clozapine where this has previously proved impossible. Furthermore, ECT might be useful in patients who have shown treatment resistance, by potentiating sensitivity to risperidone and clozapine and improving response to lower medication doses (Zervas *et al*, 2012; Pompili *et al*, 2013). Further research is needed in this area.

The Royal College of Psychiatrists recommends the use of ECT in schizophrenia as a fourth-line treatment (after clozapine therapy has failed) and for the treatment of catatonia that is resistant to lorazepam therapy (Fear *et al*, 2013).

A high relapse rate when ECT is used alone is a recognised problem. This rate might in part be due to a 'too soon' cessation of ECT as the patient responds, but also because this group of patients is often medication resistant (McCall, 2001; Tharyan & Adams, 2005). The use of maintenance

171

ECT to keep well patients who suffer severe and frequently relapsing affective disorders might reduce the exposure of these patients to high doses of atypical antipsychotic/mood-stabilising drugs. Adverse effects, including obesity, insulin resistance and other related features of metabolic syndrome, with the associated increased risk of hypertension, cardiovascular disease and type 2 diabetes, might be reduced (Moss & Vaidya, 2006). But maintenance ECT, as has already been noted, is not recommended by NICE.

Although doctors necessarily weigh guidelines with all due gravity, they do not necessarily rule out options that might need to be considered for an individual patient. As already noted, full appraisal of the risk–benefit formulation is essential. Obtaining an expert second opinion is wise if not mandatory (Mental Health Act 1983, 2007); indeed, a third opinion might be necessary. The patient should be kept fully informed of the situation and consulted as completely as possible.

The roles of independent advocates and carers must be properly emphasised and their views taken fully into account when the patient is too unwell to make a decision regarding treatment. In the event that the patient has made an advance directive against the use of ECT, this will normally be legally valid and alternative treatment strategies will need to be devised, even where the resulting treatment plan is suboptimal compared with ECT. In the small number of cases where the situation is so dire that ECT is imperative (e.g. actively suicidal behaviour or physiological collapse), the responsible clinician would be wise to seek judicial oversight to reinforce a decision to treat in any case where there is any legal uncertainty (e.g. over the validity of an advance directive). Review by hospital or trust solicitors and urgent application to the Court of Protection for explicit sanctioning of ECT treatment (or not) is strongly recommended in such circumstances.

A definitive review of the legal issues surrounding the administration of ECT defies abbreviation to the extent necessary to be accommodated in this chapter. Readers are instead referred to *The ECT Handbook* (Waite & Easton, 2013) for an authoritative reference on the subject.

Procedure

Typically, 6–12 ECT sessions are administered in a twice-weekly course of therapy (thrice weekly in some centres). There is convincing evidence that twice-weekly treatment is best, achieving the same antidepressant effect with fewer treatments (McAllister *et al*, 1987; Lerer *et al*, 1995; Shapira *et al*, 1998), but overall treatment duration can be longer (Charlson *et al*, 2012). On the morning of treatment, the patient, who has avoided food and drinks overnight, attends a dedicated ECT suite. Certain medications such as lithium and insulin can be omitted the night before and re-commenced after treatment.

A plastic cannula is placed in one arm to give drugs intravenously. A dental assessment will have been part of the work-up and during the procedure teeth are protected by a soft rubber guard. A senior anaesthetist administers the anaesthetic and is present throughout the procedure. Blood oxygen saturation is achieved by brief hyperventilation with oxygen when under anaesthetic and prior to treatment. This is done to reduce blood carbon dioxide concentration before treatment, but can also usefully lower the seizure threshold. For patients whose seizure threshold has been high in previous treatments, caffeine can also be prescribed before the next treatment to reduce this. Monitoring of the anaesthetised patient is essentially the same as for any other minor operation. The short-acting anaesthetics thiopental or propofol are commonly used, these having useful pro-convulsive properties (some alternative anaesthetics have anticonvulsant tendencies). These preferred anaesthetics also tend to cause increased post-ictal suppression, a parameter of ECT effectiveness (Azuma *et al*, 2007; Eser *et al*, 2010).

Following the stimulus, the resulting seizure is monitored by a basic EEG, which is integral to modern ECT machines. It allows the psychiatrist to monitor and record the seizure, assess its probable effectiveness and inform the management of future treatments. Peripheral signs of seizure are typically absent because of the use of muscle-relaxing medication.

The patient does not consciously experience or remember the stimulus or subsequent seizure. Recovery is supervised in a designated area and routine analgesia, such as paracetamol, is offered if headache or muscle pain is experienced. The patient usually becomes fully conscious and recovered within 30–60 min post-treatment. Treatment as an out-patient can be appropriate in some circumstances, if post-treatment recovery is assured and other arrangements such as suitable transport organised.

Stimulus and seizure threshold

The electrical stimulus administered is measured in millicoulombs (mC) and is calculated by the formula:

Charge (Q) = current (I) × time (t)

Modern ECG machines calculate the resistance between electrodes prior to the stimulus being given, thus allowing an optimum dose of electricity to be administered. Other approaches are also adopted to reduce the stimulus to the lowest effective level. Mains-source alternating sine-wave current is modified to minimise the area under the curve (and hence energy delivered) by squaring the shoulders off the sine wave (Sackeim *et al*, 2007). As well as pulse amplitude, wave width, train frequency, polarity and duration are other variables that can be manipulated. Most machines have the ability to vary one or more of these settings, but the most commonly adjusted setting is the charge. There is an argument for a more detailed and individually calculated stimulus dosage, based on parameters like pulse amplitude and shape, train frequency, directionality and polarity; simple metrics based on charge and energy alone to define dosage are regarded as inadequate by some (Peterchev *et al*, 2010).

The seizure threshold for an individual is unique to them at a given time, but in most cases is less than 250 mC. Scott & Dykes (1999) state that 7% of patients have a seizure threshold of less than 50 mC and that seizure threshold can vary by as much as 40-fold between patients; however, a less than 6-fold variation is normally found in practice (Bennett *et al*, 2012). Seizure threshold is higher for bilateral electrode placement than unilateral administration. The seizure threshold is determined initially by stimulus titration. Successively incrementally increased stimuli are given until a seizure is produced (usually limited to a maximum of two re-stimulations per titration session, to ensure adequate blood oxygenation and because the anaesthetic and muscle relaxant are very short-acting). This process enables judicious management of total stimulus dosage over a course of ECT and minimises adverse cognitive effects while optimising therapeutic effect.

A range of factors can increase the seizure threshold:

- age – threshold rises with age
- gender – men tend to have higher thresholds than women
- psychotropic medication – anti-epileptic medications (sometimes used as mood stabilisers), benzodiazepines and certain other medications raise the threshold (some medications, such as chlorpromazine, risperidone, clozapine and venlafaxine, decrease it, although these effects are rarely of clinical significance)
- seizures increase the threshold (including ECT-induced seizures; the threshold increases over a course of treatments).

The length of seizure required for therapeutic effect was commonly believed to be about 25 s. However, it is now evident that seizures of 15 s will often be effective (and possibly shorter periods, especially in older people), if the stimulus dose is also adequate. The relationship between seizure duration and therapeutic effect is not as straightforward as once believed, and might even be inverse (Abrams, 2002).

Therapeutic efficacy also depends on the electrical stimulus dose being sufficiently greater than the seizure threshold. This means that a seizure *per se* and its duration alone does not necessarily correlate with efficacy. Stronger stimuli might induce shorter but more effective seizures. A stimulus 1.5–2.5 times the seizure threshold is usual for bilateral ECT and will produce an efficacious seizure. In the case of unilateral ECT, a stimulus several times higher than the seizure threshold is necessary (perhaps six times the seizure threshold). Higher doses do not yield any greater benefit but cause incrementally more severe cognitive impairment (Sackeim *et al*, 1993; UK ECT Review Group, 2003). Pulse width is typically 0.8–1.5 ms (greater width also correlating with increased risk of negative cognitive effects). For a more detailed overview of ECT, please see *The ECT Handbook* (Waite & Easton, 2013).

Box 10.1 Possible contraindications to ECT

Cardiovascular disease
- Recent myocardial infarction
- Severe heart valve disease
- Clinically significant cardiac dysrhythmias
- Unstable angina

Neurological conditions
- Space-occupying lesions (high risk unless assessed as otherwise). Pre-existing high CSF pressure deemed as the putative aggravating factor.
- Conditions that do not preclude ECT, but require thorough assessment:
  - Cerebrovascular disease
  - Parkinson's disease unresponsive to drugs
  - Tardive dyskinesia (evidence contradictory)
  - Epilepsy
  - Cerebral lupus
  - Cardiovascular accident
  - Other neurodegenerative disorders that manifest extrapyramidal/pyramidal, autonomic or cerebellar signs (may have temporary and unpredictable beneficial effects on neurological status)
- Other medical conditions
  - Bronchospasm – possibly exacerbated in asthmatics
  - Bone or joint disease – might require increased muscle relaxant/other special care
  - Glaucoma – ophthalmological advice needed, as ECT increases intra-ocular pressure

Adapted from Waite & Easton (2013)

Safety

There is no absolute contraindication to ECT, but there are risks associated with ECT, mainly related to conditions that carry higher anaesthetic risk, such as cardiac or pulmonary disease (Box 10.1). Individualised risk–benefit assessments will determine whether the treatment should be offered. Additional contraindications include recent cardiovascular accident and raised intracranial pressure. However, such risks are sometimes mitigated by the amelioration of extreme, life-threatening morbidity (for example, imminent physiological collapse caused by debilitating mania) or other crucial risks, including suicidality.

Importantly, pregnancy is not a contraindication where the risk–benefit formulation favours ECT, but specialist advice from obstetricians and anaesthetists is essential. Pelvic wedges and left-side positioning on the treatment table might be needed to safeguard against pelvic vessel compression and placental hypoxia.

Administration of ECT to patients with implanted cardiac pacemakers is usually safe, as such devices are electrically isolated. However, temporary pacing devices are not similarly insulated and ECT is contraindicated for patients with these devices. Expert advice should be sought in any event. Medical conditions must be stabilised and a full risk–benefit assessment conducted, taking into account suitably specialist senior physician and anaesthetist opinions.

Overall, contemporary ECT is fundamentally safe and its effective use has been reported in patients as old as 102 years of age (Fink, 2009). A review of ECT in Veterans Affairs hospitals in the USA revealed there were no fatalities over the period 1999–2010. It is estimated that less than one death occurs for every 73 440 treatments (Watts *et al*, 2011).

The main risk is associated with the general anaesthetic, with approximately two deaths for every 100 000 treatments (Kramer, 1985, 1999). ECT might be safer than antidepressants in cases where selective serotonin-reuptake inhibitor (SSRI)-resistant depression indicates alternative or additional pharmacotherapy (e.g. tricyclics or mood stabilisers with the potential for cardiac dysrhythmia).

Older people might already be cardio-physiologically compromised, and patients who show QTc prolongation are more at risk from psychotropic-associated sudden death (ventricular fibrillation secondary to 'R on T'-induced dysrhythmia). A review of 121 papers that addressed the use of ECT in the elderly concluded that ECT is a safe and effective treatment of depressive illness in this group, including those suffering from dementia or Parkinson's disease (van der Wurff *et al*, 2003).

Patients with chronic obstructive pulmonary disease can be treated safely with ECT. Pre-procedure prophylactic use of inhaled bronchodilators is usually indicated. ECT should be considered with caution for patients prescribed theophylline, as this can lead to prolonged seizures and status epilepticus (Schak *et al*, 2008).

ECT can be used in patients with heart failure caused by left ventricular systolic function. In a retrospective review of 35 patients in this category, with a median age of 77 years and receiving a median of 10 treatments each, there were no deaths or decompensated heart failure, myocardial ischaemia or infarction during or within 24 h of ECT treatment. Patients were carefully monitored during treatment and excessive hypertension during previous ECT treated with prophylactic intravenous beta-blockers (necessary in 26 patients). Three patients developed transient and non-life-threatening cardiac arrhythmias (Rivera *et al*, 2011).

Eight patients with abdominal aortic aneurism have also been treated safely with ECT for severe depressive illness. The median age was 78.5 years (range 63–83 years). Imaging in six of these patients 11–29 months after ECT showed that increased dilatation of aneurisms was actually less than that which would normally be expected (3.3–5.3 cm; median 4.65 cm; Mueller *et al*, 2009). The safe use of ECT in patients with intracranial aneurisms has been indicated by a review that identified 15 such patients who had received ECT. Careful monitoring of blood pressure is necessary and use of a pro-hypotensive general anaesthetic, and possibly an antihypertensive agent, should be considered (van Herck *et al*, 2009).

In general, when considering ECT evaluate and document the following factors:

- the risks associated with general anaesthetic
- current medical morbidities
- potential adverse effects, especially cognitive side-effects
- the risks associated with not having ECT.

Does ECT cause brain damage?

Animal studies indicate that brain architecture is unaffected by ECT (e.g. Dwork *et al*, 2009). Levels of physiological markers of neurone damage are not increased following ECT (e.g. Agelink *et al*, 2001; Giltay *et al*, 2008; Palmio *et al*, 2010) and magnetic resonance imaging post-ECT is normal (Coffey *et al*, 1991). A clinical anecdote reported that a 63-year-old woman who received 325 sessions over 4 years demonstrated no change on computerised tomography scans (Kendell & Pratt, 1983).

ECT could cause harm in only two ways: passage of the electrical stimulus (causing tissue burning) or the resulting convulsion. The former possibility is dismissed by calculations showing that the absolute maximum temperature increase at neurone level caused by a modern ECT machine is approximately 0.1 °C. ECT effects on the brain are thus many orders of magnitude lower than would be required to inflict damage. However, the possibility of convulsion-induced damage to the brain has to be considered. The hippocampus is sensitive to damage by anoxia, which can complicate ill-administered ECT. This damage might be expected to cause memory loss. But the seizure intensity required to inflict injury is that of a generalised seizure lasting more than 90 min (or alternatively, more than 26 modified recurrent seizures in an 8-h period; or continuous limbic seizures lasting more than 3–5 h). This protracted seizure duration is much longer than the typical modified and oxygenated seizure duration of less than a minute in an ECT treatment (Devanand *et al*, 1994).

Side-effects

Headache and nausea are the two most common side-effects, but are usually transient and treated symptomatically. There is a view that taking mirtazapine can attenuate these post-ECT symptoms, the benefit postulated as being due to mirtazapine's serotonergic actions on 5-HT_1, 5-HT_2 and 5-HT_3 receptors (Li *et al*, 2011). A summary of cognitive side-effects is presented in Box 10.2.

Box 10.2   Factors linked to cognitive side effects

- Stimulus intensity
- Number of treatments
- Frequency of treatments
- Age of patient – older patients are more at risk
- Electrode placement – bilateral placement is associated with a higher risk than uniliateral placement, although this has been questioned (Kellner et al, 2010)

A frequently reported side-effect from ECT treatment is memory loss. These effects are typically mild and short-lived. The most obvious impairments are seen in the first 3 days after treatment, resolving within around 15 days, with some patients performing better than baseline after this period following treatment-induced improvement in depressed mood (Semkovska & McLoughlin, 2010). Adverse effects on memory are probably dose-dependent; therefore, every effort should be made to use the lowest stimulus to initiate a therapeutic seizure. Use of ketamine as an anaesthetic for ECT has theoretical advantages as an N-methyl-D-aspartate antagonist for ameliorating retrograde amnesia (Gregory-Roberts *et al*, 2010), and better word recall with ketamine compared with etomidate has been reported (McDaniel *et al*, 2006). However, ketamine's use in ECT is limited by other factors, such as a long recovery time and tendency to cause hypertension (Rassmussen *et al*, 1996).

Some evidence suggests that ECT can cause relatively short-term autobiographical memory impairment (memories of events occurring within 6 months either side of treatment). However, worrying anecdotal reports by patients of amnesia that is more extensive have been made. Further research controlling for the confounding effects of the co-existing depressive state has been called for (Fraser *et al*, 2008). Visuospatial deficits might also occur for up to a month or occasionally longer (Falconer *et al*, 2010). Systemic reviews have lent some clarity to these complex questions (Freeman, 2013).

- There are significant decreases in cognitive performance at 0–3 days post-ECT.
- Improvement occurs from 4 days, resulting in no detectable deficit at day 15. Indeed, at 15 days, 60% of patients showed better performance than on pre-ECT tests (but the most sensitive measures were not used and long-term follow-up is poor in ECT studies generally).
- Bilateral ECT is associated with increased verbal and visual episodic memory deficits.
- Brief-pulse ECT causes less impairment of visual episodic memory than sine-wave ECT.
- No relationship was found between cognitive changes and age.
- No relationship was found between the total number of ECT treatments and cognitive changes.

- No relationship was found between mean electrical dosage and cognitive changes.
- ECT can cause autobiographical memory impairment.

However, caution is required in interpreting these results, as factors might interact in inflicting impairment.

Patients should be informed of the following factors (Freeman, 2013).

- ECT causes memory problems.
- Difficulty with everyday memory, learning and retaining new information will be short-lived.
- Autobiographical memory might be affected for a longer period (up to 6 months) and some people complain of gaps in their memory that last for much longer than this.
- Depression can have marked effects on cognitive functions, including memory, and the longer the depression continues, the more severe and persistent these effects will be. Active treatment of depression therefore has a positive effect on memory.

Evaluation of progress between treatments will include the weighing up of side-effects and benefits with the patient. All discussions should be documented in the patient's notes. Re-consent after every couple of treatments is usual in Scotland and is good practice that should be the normal standard. The right for consenting patients to stop treatment at any time should be emphasised repeatedly.

NICE guidelines (2009) include assessment of cognitive function before the first treatment. Folstein's mini-mental state examination (Folstein *et al*, 1975), although not ideal, is commonly used for this purpose (Scott & Waite 2013). Subsequent monitoring of progress after every treatment using a validated outcome measure, such as The Clinical Global Impression of Improvement (Guy, 1976), is also recommended by NICE, as is monitoring of cognitive function every three or four treatments (NICE, 2009). In addition, measurement of new learning, retrograde amnesia and subjective memory impairment carried out at least 24 h post-treatment is advised (Scott & Waite, 2013). Any significant deterioration in cognition will trigger a reassessment of whether ECT should continue or a switch made to unilateral ECT. The anaesthetist should consider whether changing to an alternative drug might reduce the risk of adverse cognitive effects. Careful assessment of cognitive effects after the initial ECT treatment is especially important However, it should be noted that exposing patients to repeated, poorly validated testing that does not affect management or treatment already given is unethical.

Standards of ECT practice in the UK

In 1981, ECT was the subject of a critical editorial in *The Lancet* that highlighted the lamentable variation in ECT practice in the UK. Old equipment, poor facilities and absence of set standards and regulation

179

were all common at the time. Further surveys in the early 1990s by the Royal College of Psychiatrists showed little progress and led to the formation of the College's Special Committee on ECT and the setting up of training courses in ECT, which have since been attended by thousands of psychiatrists.

The Scottish ECT Accreditation Network (SEAN) was established in 1996 as the first such service in the UK. All ECT units are able to collate integrated care-pathway data electronically, and this is submitted for central analysis. The system is run in parallel with a biennial accreditation assessment against established standards, together with appraisal of an ECT session. A trained, multidisciplinary team, including a senior anaesthetist, observes a real treatment session and evaluates it against predefined standards. Feedback is provided during the visit and a formal report document subsequently provided to senior managers. The SEAN group produces an annual report detailing the number of patients who have received ECT in Scotland and various clinical and legal characteristics of practice and outcome, including pre- and post- ECT scores on the Montgomery–Åsberg Depression Rating Scale. Such data collection can demonstrate the effectiveness of the treatment on a national basis in a comprehensive clinical sample. Comprehensive information can be obtained via the SEAN website (www.sean.org.uk).

In May 2003, the ECT Accreditation Service was launched in England and Wales by the College's Centre for Quality Improvement and, by 2011, some 78% of ECT clinics were participating in the scheme. Accreditation is achieved by compliance with stringent standards and lasts for 3 years, subject to an interim 18-month review. Clinics that have completed two cycles have demonstrated sequential improvement, with the average percentage of standards met increasing from 87% to 95%. Details of accredited clinics, current standards and reports can be found via the College's website (www.rcpsych.ac.uk/cru/ECTAS.htm).

References

Abrams R (2002) *Electroconvulsive Therapy (4th edn)*. Oxford University Press.

Agelink MW, Andrich J, Postert T, *et al* (2001) Relation between electroconvulsive therapy, cognitive side-effects, neuron specific enolase, and protein S-100. *Journal of Neurology, Neurosurgery & Psychiatry,* **71**: 394–396.

Anderson IM, Ferrier IN, Baldwin RC, *et al* (2008) Evidence based guidelines for treating depressive disorders with antidepressants: a revision of the 2000 British Association for Psychopharmacology guidelines. *Journal of Psychopharmacology,* **22**: 434–396.

Azuma H, Fujita A, Sato K, *et al* (2007) Postictal suppression correlates with therapeutic efficacy for depression in bilateral sine and pulse wave electroconvulsive therapy. *Psychiatry and Clinical Neurosciences,* **61**: 168–173.

Bennett DM, Perrin JS, Currie J, *et al* (2012) A comparison of ECT dosing methods using a clinical sample. *Journal of Affective Disorders,* **141**: 222–226.

Blier P, Abbott EV (2001) Putative mechanisms of action of antidepressant drugs in affective and anxiety disorders and pain. *Journal of Science and Neuroscience,* **26**: 37–43.

Bolwig TG (2011) How does electroconvulsive therapy work? Theories on its mechanism. *Canadian Journal of Psychiatry*, **56**: 13–18.

Brandon S, Cowley P, McDonald C, *et al* (1984) Electroconvulsive therapy: results in depressive illness from the Leicestershire trial. *BMJ*, **288**: 22–25.

Cassidy F, Murry E, Weiner RD, *et al* (1997) Lack of relapse with tryptophan depletion following successful treatment with ECT. *American Journal of Psychiatry*, **154**: 1151–1152.

Cassidy F, Murry E, Weiner RD, *et al* (2009) Antidepressant response to antidepressant therapy is sustained after catecholamine depletion. *Progress in Neuropsychopharmacology and Biological Psychiatry*, **33**: 872–874.

Charlson F, Siskind D, Doi S, *et al* (2012) ECT efficacy and treatment course: a systemic review and meta-analysis of twice vs thrice weekly schedules. *Journal of Affective Disorders*, **138**: 1–8.

Coffey CE, Weiner RD, Djang WT, *et al* (1991) Brain anatomic effects of electroconvulsive therapy. A prospective magnetic resonance imaging study. *Archives of General Psychiatry*, **48**: 1013–1021.

de Kloet ER, Derijk RH, Meijer OC (2007) Therapy insight: is there an imbalanced response of mineralocorticoid and glucocorticoid receptors in depression? *Nature Reviews Endocrinology*, **3**: 168–179.

Devanand DP, Dwork AJ, Hutchinson ER, *et al* (1994) Does ECT alter brain structure? *American Journal of Psychiatry*, **151**: 957–970.

Dierckx B, Heijnen WT, van den Broek WW, *et al* (2012) Efficacy of electroconvulsive therapy in bipolar versus unipolar major depression: a meta-analysis. *Bipolar Disorders*, **14**: 146–150.

Dombrovski AY, Mulsant BH, Hasket RF, *et al* (2005) Predictors of remission after electroconvulsive therapy in unipolar major depression. *Journal of Clinical Psychiatry*, **66**: 1043–1049.

Dwork AJ, Christensen JR, Larsen KB, *et al* (2009) Unaltered neuronal and glial counts in animal models of magnetic seizure therapy and electroconvulsive therapy. *Neuroscience*, **164**: 1557–1564.

Eser D, Northdurfter C, Schule C, *et al* (2010) The influence of anaesthetic medication on safety, tolerability, and clinical effectiveness of electroconvulsive therapy. *World Journal of Biological Psychiatry*, **11**: 447–456.

Falconer DW, Cleland J, Fielding S, *et al* (2010) Using the Cambridge Neuropsychological Test Automated Battery (CANTAB) to assess the cognitive impact of electroconvulsive therapy on visual and visuospatial memory. *Psychological Medicine*, **40**: 1017–1025.

Fear CF, Dunn RA, McLoughlin DM (2013) The use of ECT in the treatment of schizophrenia and catatonia. In *The ECT Handbook (3rd edn)* (eds J Waite, A Easton). Royal College of Psychiatrists.

Fink M (2009) *Electroconvulsive Therapy: A Guide for Professionals and Their Patients (2nd edn)*. Oxford University Press, New York.

Folstein M, Folstein S, McHugh PR (1975) 'Mini-mental state': A practical measure for grading the cognitive state of patients for the clinician. *Journal of Psychiatric Research*, **12**: 189–198.

Fraser LM, O'Carroll RE, Ebmeier KP (2008) The effect of electroconvulsive therapy on autobiographical memory; a systemic review. *Journal of ECT*, **24**: 10–17.

Freeman CP (2013) Cognitive adverse effects of ECT. In *The ECT Handbook (Council Report 176) (3rd edn)* (eds J Waite, A Easton). Royal College of Psychiatrists: 76–86.

Giltay EJ, Kho KH, Blansjaar BA (2008) Serum markers of brain-cell damage and C-reactive protein are unaffected by electroconvulsive therapy. *World Journal of Biological Psychiatry*, **9**: 231–235.

Gregory-Roberts EM, Naismith SL, Cullen KM, *et al* (2010) Electroconvulsive therapy-induced persistent retrograde amnesia: could it be minimised by ketamine or other pharmacological approaches? *Journal of Affective Disorders*, **126**: 39–45.

Guy W (1976) Clinical Global Assessment Impressions. In *ECDEU. Assessment Manual for Psychopharmacology* (revised edn). National Institute for Mental Health: 217–222.

Johnstone EC, Deakin JF, Lawler P, *et al* (1985) The Northwick Park electroconvulsive therapy trial. *Lancet*, **2**: 1317–1320.

Kato N (2009) Neurophysiological mechanisms of electroconvulsive therapy for depression. *Neuroscience Research*, **64**: 3–11.

Kellner CH, Knapp R, Husain MM, *et al* (2010) Bifrontal, bitemporal and right unilateral electrode placement in ECT: randomised trial. *British Journal of Psychiatry*, **196**: 226–234.

Kendell B, Pratt RTC (1983) Brain damage and ECT. *British Journal of Psychiatry*, **143**: 99–100.

Kramer BA (1985) Use of ECT in California, 1977–1983. *American Journal of Psychiatry*, **142**: 1190–1192.

Kramer BA (1999) Use of ECT in California, revisited 1984–1994. *Journal of ECT*, **15**: 245–251.

Lerer B, Shapira B, Calev A, *et al* (1995) Antidepressant and cognitive effects of twice-versus three-times weekly ECT. *American Journal of Psychiatry*, **152**: 564–570.

Li T-C, Shiah I-S, Sun C-J, *et al* (2011) Mirtazapine relieves post-electroconvulsive therapy headaches and nausea: a case series and review of the literature. *Journal of ECT*, **27**: 165–167.

McAllister DA, Perri MG, Jordan MC, *et al* (1987) Effects of ECT given two vs three times weekly. *Psychiatry Research*, **21**: 63–69.

McCall WV (2001) Electroconvulsive therapy in the era of modern psychopharmacology. *International Journal of Neuropsychopharmacology*, **4**: 315–324.

McCall WV, Reboussin DM, Weiner RD, *et al* (2000) Titrated moderately suprathreshold vs fixed high-dose right unilateral electroconvulsive therapy: acute antidepressant and cognitive effect. *Archives of General Psychiatry*, **57**: 438–444.

McDaniel WW, Sahota AK, Byas BV, *et al* (2006) Ketamine appears associated with better word recall than etomidate after a course of six electroconvulsive therapies. *Journal of ECT*, **22**: 103–106.

Medda P, Mauri M, Fratta S, *et al* (2013) Long-term naturalistic follow-up of patients with bipolar depression and mixed state treated with electroconvulsive therapy. *Journal of ECT*, **29**: 179–188.

Merkl A, Heuser I, Bajbouj M (2009) Antidepressant electroconvulsive therapy, mechanism of action, recent advances and limitations. *Experimental Neurology*, **219**: 20–26.

Moss LE, Vaidya NA (2006) Electroconvulsive therapy as an alternative treatment for obese patients with mood disorders. *Journal of ECT*, **22**: 223–225.

Mowbray RM (1959) Historical aspects of electric convulsive therapy. *Scottish Medical Journal*, **4**: 373–378.

Mueller PS, Albin SM, Barnes RD, *et al* (2009) Safety of electroconvulsive therapy in patients with unrepaired aortic aneurysm: report of 8 patients. *Journal of ECT*, **25**: 165–169.

National Institute for Health and Clinical Excellence (2003) *Guidance on the Use of Electroconvulsive Therapy (NICE Technology Appraisal 59)*. NICE.

National Institute for Health and Clinical Excellence (2009) *Depression in Adults: The Treatment and Management of Depression in Adults (NICE Clinical Guideline 90)*. NICE.

Nobler M, Sackheim H (2008) Neurobiological correlates of the cognitive side effects of electroconvulsive therapy. *Journal of ECT*, **24**: 40–45.

Ongur D, Heckers S (2004) A role for glia in the action of electroconvulsive therapy. *Harvard Reviews of Psychiatry*, **12**: 253–262.

Palmio J, Huuhka M, Laine S, *et al* (2010) Electroconvulsive therapy and biomarkers of neuronal injury and plasticity: serum levels of neuron-specific enolase and S-100b protein. *Psychiatry Research*, **177**: 97–100.

Perrin JS, Merz S, Bennett DM, *et al* (2012) Electroconvulsive therapy reduces frontal cortical connectivity in severe depressive disorder. *Proceedings of the National Academy of Sciences of the United States of America*, **109**: 5464–5468.

Peterchev AV, Rosa MA, Deng ZD, *et al* (2010) Electroconvulsive therapy stimulus parameters: rethinking dosage. *Journal of ECT*, **26**: 159–174.

Pompili M, Lester D, Dominici G, *et al* (2013) Indications for electroconvulsive treatment in schizophrenia: a systematic review. *Schizophrenia Research*, **146**: 1–9.

Prudic J, Sackeim HA, Devanand DP (1990) Medication resistance and clinical response to ECT. *Psychiatry Research*, **31**: 287–296.

Prudic J, Haskett RF, Mulsant B, *et al* (1996) Resistance to antidepressant medications and short-term response to ECT. *American Journal of Psychiatry*, **153**: 985–992.

Racagni G, Popoli M (2008) Cellular and molecular mechanisms in the long-term action of antidepressants. *Dialogues in Clinical Neuroscience*, **10**: 385–400.

Rassmussen KG, Jarvis MR, Zarumski CF (1996) Ketamine anesthesia in electroconvulsive therapy. *Convulsive Therapy*, **12**: 217–223.

Rivera FA, Lapid MI, Sampson S, *et al* (2011) Safety of electroconvulsive therapy in patients with a history of heart failure and decreased left ventricular systolic heart function. *Journal of ECT*, **27**: 207–213.

Rotheneichner P, Lange S, O'Sullivan A, *et al* (2014) Hippocampal neurogenesis and antidepressive therapy: shocking relations. *Neural Plasticity*, **2014**: doi 10.1155/2014/723915.

Sackeim HA, Prudic J, Devanand DP, *et al* (1993) Effects of stimulus intensity and electrode placement on the efficacy and cognitive effects of electroconvulsive therapy. *New England Journal of Medicine*, **328**: 839–846.

Sackeim HA, Prudic J, Fuller R, *et al* (2007) The cognitive effects of electroconvulsive therapy in community settings. *Neuropsychopharmacology*, **32**: 244–254.

Schak KM, Mueller PS, Barnes RD, *et al* (2008) The safety of ECT in patients with chronic obstructive pulmonary disease. *Psychosomatics*, **49**: 208–211.

Scott AIF (ed.) (2005) *The ECT Handbook (2nd edn)*. Royal College of Psychiatrists.

Scott AIF (2011) Mode of action of electroconvulsive therapy – an update. *Advances in Psychiatric Treatment*, **17**: 15–22.

Scott AI, Dykes S (1999) Initial seizure threshold in the clinical practice of bilateral electroconvulsive therapy in Edinburgh, Scotland. *Journal of ECT*, **15**: 118–124.

Scott AIF, Waite J (2013) Monitoring a course of ECT. In *The ECT Handbook (3rd edn)* (eds J Waite, A Easton). Royal College of Psychiatrists.

Semkovska M, McLoughlin DM (2010) Objective cognitive performance associated with electroconvulsive therapy for depression: a systematic review and meta-analysis. *Biological Psychiatry*, **68**: 568–577.

Shapira B, Tubi N, Drexler H, *et al* (1998) Cost and benefit in the choice of ECT schedule. Twice versus three times weekly ECT. *British Journal of Psychiatry*, **172**: 44–48.

Tharyan P, Adams CE (2005) Electroconvulsive therapy for schizophrenia. *Cochrane Database of Systemic Reviews*, **2**: CD000076.

UK ECT Review Group (2003) Efficacy and safety of electro-convulsive therapy in depressive disorders; a systematic review and meta-analysis. *Lancet*, **361**: 799–808.

Valenti M, Benabarre A, Garcia-Amador M, *et al* (2008) Electroconvulsive therapy in the treatment of mixed states in bipolar disorder. *European Psychiatry*, **23**: 53–56.

van Herck E, Sienhaert P, Hagon A (2009) Electroconvulsive therapy for patients with intra-cranial aneurysms: a case study and literature review [Dutch]. *Tijdschrift voor Psychiatrie*, **51**: 43–51.

van der Wurff FB, Stek ML, Hoogendijk WJ, *et al* (2003) The efficacy and safety of ECT in depressed older adults: a literature review. *International Journal of Geriatric Psychiatry*, **18**: 894–904.

Versiani M, Cheniaux E, Landeira-Fernandez J (2011) Efficacy and safety of electroconvulsive therapy in the treatment of bipolar disorder: a systematic review. *Journal of ECT*, **27**: 153–164.

Waite J, Easton A (eds) (2013) *The ECT Handbook (3rd edn)*. Royal College of Psychiatrists.

183

Watts BV, Geoff A, Bagian JP, *et al* (2011) An examination of mortality and other adverse events related to electroconvulsive therapy using a national adverse event report system. *Journal of ECT*, **27**: 105–108.

Weiner R, Lisanby SH, Husain MM, *et al* (2013) Electroconvulsive therapy device classification; response to FDA advisory panel hearings and recommendations. *Journal of Clinical Psychiatry*, **74**: 38–42.

West ED (1981) Electric convulsion therapy in depression: A double-blind controlled trial. *BMJ*, **282**: 355–357.

Zervas IM, Theleritis C, Soldatos CR (2012) Using ECT in schizophrenia: a review from a clinical perspective. *World Journal of Biological Psychiatry*, **13**: 96–105.

CHAPTER 11

Life-threatening medical emergencies in a mental health unit

Nicholas Swift

Life-threatening medical emergencies on mental health units are mistakenly perceived as infrequent. In a 2-year study examining the frequency of call-outs of a US medical emergency team in a mental health unit, Cheung *et al* (2012) recorded an emergency response rate of 14.2 per 1000 admissions. This compared with 14.7 per 1000 admissions at the co-located medical hospital. Although this result might not be generalisable, it raises a clear question: why should a similar emergency medical need exist among mental health in-patients and patients of a medical hospital?

One explanation is that medical comorbidity is common for people with acute mental health problems. Lyketsos *et al* (2002) reported that 15% of patients in adult psychiatric hospitals had serious medical comorbidity on admission. Similarly, in a study of elderly patients admitted to a psychiatric emergency unit, 19% of the patients presented with a previously unrecognised medical disorder either causing or contributing to the psychiatric symptoms and 93% of all the patients had at least one chronic medical disorder (Woo, 2011). For those with intellectual disabilities, the risks of some specific medical illnesses are greater. For instance, the prevalence of epilepsy in this patient group is up to 30% (Wilson & Haire, 1990). In the elderly, falls have the potential for immediate life-threatening complications. On the basis of an analysis of falls in UK mental health units, an average rate of 2.1 falls per 1000 bed days is seen, with this rising to 13–25 falls per 1000 bed days in units providing exclusive care for the elderly (National Reporting and Learning Service, 2007). This included 4 deaths from falls and 85 cases of severe harm (e.g. brain damage or fractured neck of femur.)

Unfortunately, medical emergencies are rarely easy to predict. The acute medical complications of problems such as anorexia (Sharp & Freeman, 1993), dementia (Mukadam & Sampson, 2011), substance misuse and acute intoxication, although well recognised, are hard to predict by way of individual risk. The importance of early recognition of a deteriorating patient presenting with progressively worsening physiological derangement is regarded as crucial in avoiding a cardiorespiratory arrest scenario (National Confidential Inquiry into Patient Outcomes and Death, 2012).

The UK National Patient Safety Agency examined recorded cardiac arrest, respiratory arrest and choking incidents between 2006 and 2008 in mental health and intellectual disability units (Wilkins, 2008). In total, 599 incidents resulted in moderate harm, severe harm or death. In 26 cases, a significant lack of staff knowledge, skills, or equipment was evident. Three patient deaths occurred after choking on food. Another 22 reports were of moderate or severe harm following choking where responding staff lacked basic first-aid skills. When reviewed, these incidents also showed evidence of considerable variability in resuscitation techniques, failures in acting on observed deteriorations in physical symptoms and missed physical symptoms. Similarly, in a study of sudden unexplained deaths of psychiatric in-patients, Windfuhr *et al* (2011) found that cardiopulmonary resuscitation (CPR) was undertaken in only just over half of the cardiac arrests. This was despite 90% of the staff being trained in CPR. Alarmingly, appropriate equipment was only present in a third of wards.

Given the infrequency of emergencies and the typical staff skill mix in mental health units, human factors (such as a lack of recognition of acute physical symptoms or signs of illness, little practical repetition in the use of emergency equipment and unrehearsed teamwork) might all act to impede an effective response. Recognising this, the UK Department of Health (2009) defined a number of core skills as universal for all staff in *Competencies for Recognising and Responding to Acutely Ill Patients in Hospital* (Department of Health, 2009). An important, tiered 'chain of prevention' is made, encompassing non-clinical staff, recorders of observations, those who recognise and interpret observations, primary and secondary responders. Importantly, the initial care of any acutely ill patient is observed as a matter for all staff, not just doctors and nurses.

Specific risks are associated with managing disturbed or violent behaviour in the mental health setting (National Institute of Health and Care Excellence (NICE), 2005). Rapid tranquillisation is associated with a number of serious risks, including the risk of respiratory depression, respiratory arrest and cardiac arrest. Restraint can also lead to crush injury and airway and breathing obstruction. More specialised resuscitation provision might also need to be anticipated in special circumstances, such as where electroconvulsive therapy is provided or where patient groups are particularly young, old or challenging in behaviour. There also remains a wide range of potential serious and life-threatening adverse drug reactions, allergies, dangerous side-effects and interactions with the medications routinely initiated within mental health units (Simpson *et al*, 1987; Mehtonen *et al*, 1991). Examples include serotonin syndrome, neuroleptic malignant syndrome, seizure, laryngospasm, dystonia, skin reactions such as toxic epidermal necrolysis, haematological problems such as neutropenia, and physiological electrolyte disturbances. Other risks, perhaps not routinely anticipated, exist, such as a 90-fold increase in the risk of choking in patients receiving neuroleptics (Ruschena *et al*, 2003).

As such, the types of life-threatening emergencies can be highly varied, and the experience, equipment and resources of the mental health staff responding could be seen as inadequate when compared with those available at an acute hospital. Thus, the key remains early identification of any deteriorating patient, the provision of immediate life support and arranging safe transfer for acute care. The release of specific resuscitation quality standards and equipment guidance in the UK for mental health in-patient units is a welcome and overdue development (Resuscitation Council (UK), 2014a,b). These core standards for providing CPR include provision within mental health units of a resuscitation service structure, resuscitation lead officer and training programme. Importantly standards are also provided for prevention strategies for cardiorespiratory arrest, the resuscitation team, resuscitating children, resuscitating in special circumstances, transferring patients, post-cardiac arrest care, resuscitation equipment, decisions around resuscitation, audit and research.

Rather than trying to encompass a small medical textbook or resuscitation training programme, the aim of this chapter is to provide an overview of the common approaches to a limited number of acute medical conditions relevant to first responders or a medical emergency response team in a mental health unit. The approaches are not comprehensive but are aimed at aligning the skills, equipment and staff competencies to a common minimum standard of pre-hospital emergency care.

Assessment and immediate scene management of a life-threatening clinical situation

Clear leadership, good communication and teamwork are all critical. If the cause of acute illness is not readily identifiable or treatable, the immediate aim must be life-support while more specialist urgent assessment is arranged. In the subsequent handover of care, the patient's new specialist team should have immediate access to all necessary clinical information. The SAFE response (Fig. 11.1) is a helpful aide memoire used in pre-hospital care (Weekes, 1999) in emergency situations.

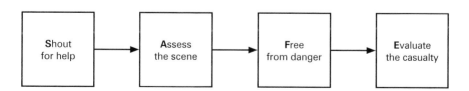

Fig. 11.1 The SAFE approach in pre-hospital care.

Help should be summoned, followed by an assessment of the situation and identification of any obvious hazards. Next, the scene must be cleared of immediate danger. This might require the removal of sharp items, unplugging electrical items or moving items for a safe approach. Further immediate life-threatening harm to the casualty must be eliminated. In some instances, this might merit moving the casualty to safety, cutting ligatures, or removing dangerous items where self-injury has occurred. A ligature knife should be stored safely but readily available to responding staff on all psychiatric wards.

In evaluating any casualty, it might also be necessary to initially triage a number of casualties. If the patient has been subject to mechanical trauma, potential cervical spine injury must be considered. If cervical injury is suspected, the cervical spine should be immobilised or the patient handled appropriately to avoid further injury. Cervical spine immobilisation should not hamper life-saving airway and breathing interventions. A patient might require immediate seclusion or separation from a situation of potential violence or aggression. An approach to emergency medical assessment is shown in Fig. 11.2.

The primary medical assessment (primary survey) and resuscitation

Rapid primary medical assessment in an emergency follows the key principles of simultaneously assessing, identifying and managing life-threatening problems. For any patient who is unconscious or has respiratory compromise, focal neurological problems, cardiovascular compromise, severe metabolic or endocrine abnormalities, trauma, sepsis or collapse in pregnancy, the ABCDE model should be followed, while also arranging for emergency ambulance transfer to an acute hospital:

- airway (and cervical spine control)
- breathing
- circulation (control bleeding and manage shock)
- disability of nervous system
- exposure and environmental control.

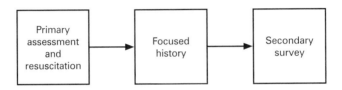

Fig. 11.2 An approach to emergency medical assessment.

This approach provides a priority of assessment and treatment. In some circumstances, for critically ill patients, nothing further than the primary medical assessment might be achieved. The priority here will be resuscitation and rapid transportation for definitive treatment. Constant re-evaluation should occur, with any deterioration in condition leading to a reassessment of the ABCDE. Basic physical monitoring, ideally using 'track and trigger' tools such as, for adults, the National Early Warning Score (NEWS) or, for children, the paediatric early warning score (PEWS) to record vital signs is recommended to identify early warning signs of deterioration (Royal College of Physicians, 2012). These scores help determine the frequency of observation needed and priority of medical response required.

All critically ill patients must be attached to a pulse oximeter, electrocardiogram (ECG) monitor and a non-invasive blood pressure monitor as soon as possible. An intravenous cannula should be sited and bloods taken for investigation.

(A) Airway

Look for signs of obstruction. The airway should be quickly checked and any obvious obstruction cleared. If the airway is compromised, it will have to be opened initially with a chin lift or jaw thrust. Airway adjuncts might be required (see below for airway management). If cervical spine injury is suspected, airway maintenance should still be carried out if breathing is compromised, but the spine should be protected from unnecessary movement. Anaphylaxis can cause obstruction through swelling, with early intubation often necessary, requiring expert help. This might be the stage to commence high-flow oxygen, if available.

(B) Breathing

Look, listen and feel for breathing for 10 s. A normal respiratory rate for an adult is 12–20 breaths per minute. If the patient is not breathing, CPR should be commenced (see below for resuscitation.) A fuller examination will be needed if breathing is difficult – to determine cause and treat accordingly. Listening to breath sounds and examining the chest will provide vital information in determining what treatment is needed. All critically ill patients should be given oxygen (O'Driscoll et al, 2011). Use of a pulse oximeter might help assessment at this stage. Initially the highest concentration of oxygen should be given with a mask with reservoir (aiming to keep the reservoir bag inflated during inspiration.) If using a pulse oximeter, the oxygen should be titrated to give a saturation of 94–98% (although, in the sickest patients, one might have to accept 90–92%). Some caution needs to be exercised with those with known chronic obstructive airway disease, aiming for a target saturation of 88–92% to avoid respiratory depression.

(C) Circulation

An examination focused on the signs of shock or haemorrhage should be performed. In almost all medical emergencies, assume hypovolaemia as the likeliest cause of shock until proven otherwise. Pulse rate, pulse volume, capillary refill, blood pressure, skin colour and skin moisture can all be useful indicators of shock. Any external major bleeding should be controlled with pressure or pressure bandaging until definitive treatment is obtained. Hypovolaemic shock should be treated initially by laying the patient down, leg raising, warmth and IV fluids. In pregnant women (over 20 weeks) a left lateral tilt should be used to avoid compression of the vena cava. Venous access should be undertaken early, given this can become more difficult as shock progresses. Consider anaphylaxis and treat at once if other signs exist (see below for anaphylaxis).

(D) Disability of nervous system

A brief assessment of consciousness can be done with the AVPU (alert, verbal, pain, unresponsive) scale:

- alert
- responds to verbal command
- responds to pain
- unresponsive.

The aim here is to check for gross neurological damage. The size and response to light of pupils should be determined, together with blood glucose level and any signs of neck stiffness (indicating meningism). A decreased level of consciousness is a sign of one of four possibilities: decreased cerebral oxygenation, central nervous system injury, drug or alcohol overdose, or metabolic derangement.

(E) Exposure and environmental control

In the case of traumatic injury, it is important to expose any injuries that could be hidden. This might require removal of clothing or moving the patient to see concealed areas of the body. Also, at this stage, consider preserving body temperature by covering the patient.

Rapid history and secondary survey

A well-performed primary medical assessment should have identified and stabilised life-endangering problems. At this stage a secondary assessment and history might well aid diagnosis. The rapid history should account for:

- events leading up to the illness or injury

- past medical history of serious medical illness (particularly cardiac or respiratory disease, diabetes or endocrine disease, epilepsy, drug or alcohol misuse and head injury)
- current medications used (with particular caution in all those using psychotropic medication for neuroleptic malignant syndrome, neutropenia serotonin syndrome and other adverse drug reactions)
- allergies.

The secondary survey involves a methodological physical examination of body systems and areas of the body to look for problems. It also allows for some reflection of all the information gained so far and the formulation of an initial management plan.

Communication and handover

In any emergency situation, good communication and appropriate clinical handover are paramount to clinical care. Communication errors account for a significant proportion of adverse events in healthcare. Human error is inevitable, particularly when managing an unfamiliar, medically complex or challenging situation that might only occur infrequently. Effective teamwork and good verbal and appropriate written communication can help prevent the inevitable human mistakes from becoming harmful events. Using standardised tools for communication can help foster a culture of appropriate, respectful assertion for professionals of varying competencies and backgrounds within a team.

The SBAR tool (Situation Background Assessment Recommendation) is recommended by the Resuscitation Council (UK) and is advocated as a means of standardising urgent clinical communication between clinicians in the UK National Health Service (Leonard, 2004). It is a situational briefing model originating in the airline industry and military which has been adapted for use in high-risk clinical environments. Such a tool might be of particular benefit when a staff member lacks confidence or is dealing with an unfamiliar or complex situation. Box 11.1 outlines the steps of this approach.

Key points

- Assessment and scene management for all acute clinical emergencies should follow the key principles of a SAFE ABCDE approach.
- A focused history and secondary survey should follow but, in the case of a critically ill patient, continuous resuscitation and stabilisation using the ABCDE method might be all that can be achieved pending specialist help or transfer.
- A culture of good teamwork, effective communication and diligent handover is crucial to patient safety in an emergency.

Box 11.1 Suggested SBAR (Situation Background Assessment Recommendation) template for handover of a medical emergency on a mental health unit

Situation (ideally in one sentence)
- Identify yourself, where you are and the patient
- Explain the reason for your call and your concern

Background (the details of the situation as you see it)
- Significant medical history
- Pertinent background information

Assessment
- Immediate clinical concerns
- Vital signs
- Clinical impression

Recommendation
- Explain what is needed
- Time-frame of action
- Make suggestions
- Clarify what you expect

Cardiac and respiratory arrest: CPR in mental health units

Survival in cardiac arrest is estimated at between 7.6% (for out-of-hospital cardiac arrest) and 18% (for in-hospital cardiac arrest); inference survival rates are improved by earlier provision of effective resuscitation (Nolan, 2011). For in-patients, where possible, advanced life support guidelines should be followed (Nolan *et al*, 2010). However, the reality is that not all responders in mental health units might have such competency and basic life support will be the default. In any eventuality, the initial care of any critically ill patient is an amalgamation of both basic and advanced life support and survival is optimised by early provision of effective CPR. Certain overriding principles for an in-patient are early recognition of an arrest, a standardised procedure for summoning help, and early provision of resuscitation (using airway adjuncts if necessary) with defibrillation within 3 min of arrest.

On a psychiatric ward, patients are often ambulatory and an arrest could occur in an area remote from the main ward. Wards must anticipate this with suitably portable resuscitation equipment and a common method of summoning help across the hospital. Any resuscitation team should be activated within 30 s of an arrest call. The common telephone number should be 2222 (National Patient Safety Agency, 2004), with a regularly tested and monitored continuity of emergency communication throughout all patient-accessible areas. Unless the mental health unit is part of an acute hospital, an ambulance should be called immediately for any patient who collapses.

Equipment to consider for an adult psychiatric resuscitation response kit is listed in Box 11.2. The equipment list must be tailored to the local needs (for instance the inclusion of size-appropriate equipment in a child and adolescent unit), standards of resuscitation (in co-located acute/mental health hospitals, the default standard might be advanced life support) and training. The equipment list and standards should ideally be determined by a hospital resuscitation committee on the basis of national standards of care, local needs and the specific clinical risks of their own units. Across any institution, the equipment, drugs and practices for CPR should be standardised (Resuscitation Council (UK), 2014*a*,*b*). CPR is a practical technique and the value of regular, hands-on training with simulated scenarios cannot be over-emphasised (Aggarwal *et al*, 2010). The knowledge and skills gained during training can deteriorate over 3 to 6 months (Soar *et al*, 2010*a*); thus, regular refresher training is needed to maintain skills.

The Resuscitation Council (UK) in-hospital adult resuscitation algorithm can be seen in Fig. 11.3. Paediatric basic life support is summarised in Fig. 11.4. The main aim of both is to ensure survival in cardiac arrest by the provision of early, effective chest compressions to restore the circulation of oxygen.

When a cardiac arrest is suspected, the first step following the scene safety check is to determine a response. If no trauma is evident, a shout of 'are you OK?' and shaking is usually sufficient (a gentle shake is enough if trauma is evident). In the event of unresponsiveness, aid should be summoned as quickly as possible. Assistance might be required not only in dealing with the casualty, but also elsewhere on the ward, given the sudden demands on staff in dealing with an emergency. Psychiatric units commonly employ an emergency response team, and this team should be quickly summoned.

CPR should begin with chest compressions while airway equipment arrives, repositioning the body if necessary. Airway management and ventilation are key steps. In the event of airway obstruction, the basic head tilt and chin lift procedure can move the tongue off the airway, allowing air to pass. Small amounts of head tilt can be used if there is concern regarding cervical spine injury; jaw thrust is an alternative. Use of an oropharyngeal airway is a simple and effective measure for most CPR scenarios, particularly when supplemented with a pocket mask. It should be remembered that an oropharyngeal airway can provoke vomiting. Two-person bag and mask ventilation is easier, and more likely to be successful, for those not regularly using such techniques. More advanced airway techniques might be considered, such as inserting a supraglottic airway device. Nasopharyngeal airways can be useful in the event of oral

---

Box 11.2 Minimum equipment list for an adult psychiatric resuscitation response kit

- Oropharyngeal airways (sizes 2, 3 and 4)
- Nasopharyngeal airways (sizes 6 and 7)
- Clear face masks (sizes 3, 4 and 5)
- Laryngeal mask/supraglottic airway (depends on training)
- Defibrillator and two sets of adhesive pads (type of defibrillator based on local need)
- Emergency drug dose schedule, algorithms, record forms and stationery
- Pocket mask with oxygen port
- Safety pins
- Self-inflating bag and mask (ideally, single-use)
- Scissors
- Ligature knife
- Stethoscope and blood-pressure monitor
- Oxygen mask with reservoir (non-rebreathing) bag
- Magill forceps
- Serviced oxygen tank and regulator
- Sharps container and waste bag
- Lubricating jelly
- Tourniquet
- Two large dressing pads
- Two giving sets
- Selection of syringes and needles
- Intravenous cannulas (selection of sizes)
- Cannula fixing tape/adhesives
- Alcohol wipes
- Intraosseous access device
- 0.9% sodium chloride 1 L (quantity based on local need)
- Gloves, aprons and eye protection
- Portable suction equipment
- Pulse oximeter
- Torch
- Blood glucose analyser and strips
- Specialist holdall/backpack

Source: Adapted from the standards published by the Resuscitation Council (UK) (2014b)

---

trauma or trismus in seizures. Only those who are trained, competent and experienced should attempt tracheal intubation. In patients who have had tracheal intubation, waveform capnography should be regarded as an essential component of emergency care. The skills involved in tracheal intubation are difficult to maintain for most psychiatric in-patient units, although it is recognised that in some instances psychiatric units coexist with acute health facilities. CPR procedures should meet the highest standards locally available. Paediatric life support requires specific training and equipment (Biarent et al, 2010).

For adults, chest compressions should be to a depth of 5–6 cm at a rate of 100–120 compressions per minute. If the rescuer is unable or unwilling to give rescue breaths, continuous chest compressions should be provided, as this is still better than no resuscitation at all. It is important to minimise interruptions to the compressions, although some interruptions (e.g. for ventilation and defibrillation) are inevitable. Providing compressions can be extremely tiring. To avoid this, ideally staff should be rotated every 2 min with the smallest possible pauses between compressions.

There is a trend in UK psychiatric units toward the use of automated external defibrillation (AED) devices. These have the advantage of being portable, being easily maintained, having long service intervals and

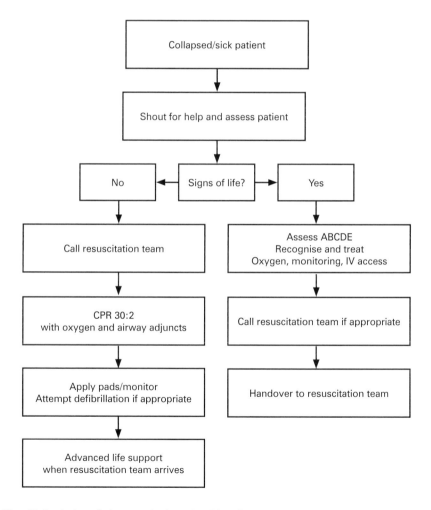

Fig. 11.3 In-hospital resuscitation algorithm (adults). Reproduced with permission from Resuscitation Council (UK) (2010).

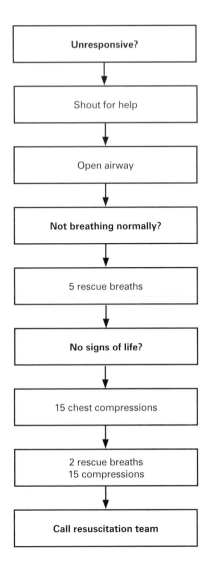

Fig. 11.4 Basic life support algorithm (children). Adapted with permission from Resuscitation Council (UK) (2010).

requiring limited training in their use (Deakin *et al*, 2010). Thus, they might be favoured for infrequent-use scenarios, such as on a psychiatric ward. The National Patient Safety Agency recommends the provision of an AED device to all patient areas in which it is anticipated one arrest might occur every 5 years (National Patient Safety Agency, 2008). Given this, sufficient staff (both clinical and non-clinical) should be trained to allow the first shock to be provided within the goal period of 3 min of cardiac arrest anywhere within a psychiatric unit. The algorithm for resuscitation with an AED device is summarised in Fig. 11.5.

Following the initiation of basic life support or use of an AED device, advanced life support should then follow as quickly as possible. Table 11.1 shows a suggested minimum inventory of drugs for adult in-patient resuscitation on a psychiatric ward.

The decision to terminate or not commence resuscitation is an ethically challenging problem. In some instances, patients might suffer futile attempts

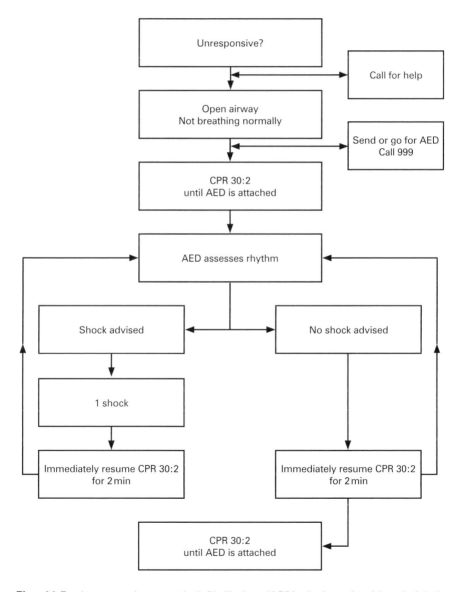

Fig. 11.5 Automated external defibrillation (AED) device algorithm (adults). Reproduced with permission from Resuscitation Council (UK) (2010).

Table 11.1 Suggested minimum drug inventory for adult mental health first line resuscitation.

Drug	Standard emergency dose	Administration	Indication	Minimum stock
Adrenaline	1 mg*	Pre-filled syringe	First-line for cardiac arrest	3
Amiodarone	300 mg	Pre-filled syringe	First-line for cardiac arrest	1
Adrenaline	0.5 mg**	Intramuscular	Anaphylaxis	5
Chlorphenamine	10 mg	Intramuscular or intravenous	Second-line for anaphylaxis	2
Hydrocortisone	100 mg	Intramuscular or intravenous	Second-line for anaphylaxis	2
Salbutamol	5 mg	Nebuliser device	Acute asthma	2
Ipratropium bromide	500 µg	Nebuliser device	Acute asthma	2
Glyceryl trinitrate	400 µg	1–2 sprays, as required	Acute coronary syndrome	1
Aspirin	300 mg	Oral	Acute coronary syndrome	1
Furosemide	50 mg	Intravenous	Congestive heart failure	2
Flumazenil	0.5 mg	Intravenous	Benzodiazepine effect reversal	2
Naloxone	400 µg	Intramuscular or intravenous	Opiate effect reversal	5
Midazolam	10 mg	Buccal	Status epilecticus (unlicensed)	1
Glucagon	1 mg	Intramuscular or intravenous	Hypoglycaemia	2

*10 mL dose contains 1 mg adrenaline as adrenaline 1 in 10 000 dilute
**0.5 mL dose contains 0.5 mg of adrenaline as adrenaline 1 in 1000 dilute
Source: Resuscitation Council (UK) (2014*b*)

to preserve life by CPR, wrongly extending an established dying process where an advance decision could have helped inform care. Information regarding an advance decision not to attempt resuscitation should be readily available for the treating team in an emergency. Where an advance decision exists, it should be clearly documented, with evidence of how this decision was reached, the date of the decision, the reasons and the name and position of the person responsible for the decision. Additionally, the decision should be reviewed regularly or when any changes in the patient's circumstances occur (British Medical Association, 2007). Accurate records should be kept of all resuscitation attempts, together with the electronic data from the AED device, for subsequent audit, training and medico-legal reasons.

Key points

- All potential responders to an emergency should be trained in resuscitation techniques. These should be refreshed at least annually and based on the current evidence-based protocols and national standards.
- Recognition of acutely ill patients is aided by 'track and trigger' tools (e.g. NEWS and PEWS).
- A standardised emergency response should be maintained for suspected cardiac arrest, with standardised equipment available throughout the entire hospital.
- Equipment and drugs should be stored and maintained appropriately.
- All clinical areas for patients should have an AED device ready to deliver a shock, where appropriate, within 3 min of a witnessed collapse.
- Basic life support is a holding process pending further help.
- Advanced life support provision can be variable on a psychiatric ward, but should be sought urgently for cardiopulmonary arrest.
- All resuscitation attempts must be recorded as serious events and appropriate incident forms completed for audit.

Acute upper airway obstruction

Choking

Psychiatric patients and patients with an intellectual disability are more vulnerable to choking (Ruschena *et al*, 2003). The most vulnerable time for patients is while eating, as they can accidentally inhale food. Any mechanism that acts to impede, or alter, the usual swallowing reflex can result in choking. Recognised causes specific to patients in mental health units include slowing of the normal muscular movements of swallowing by neuroleptics (bradykinetic dysphagia), pica and fast eating in intellectual disability patients, and dysphagia in those suffering dementia or other neuropsychiatric syndromes. Intoxication with alcohol or illicit substances might also be a risk factor.

Management

It is important to ask the patient, if conscious, whether they are choking. A verbal response indicates some patent airway and coughing should be encouraged. The importance of asking this question and looking into the face of the patient, even in the face of highly agitated behaviour, cannot be overemphasised. Fig. 11.6 outlines the Resuscitation Council (UK)'s treatment algorithm for adults and Fig. 11.7 the corresponding paediatric algorithm. Choking is highly distressing for the patient and can rapidly progress to respiratory arrest. The patient should not be left alone until either the airway is cleared through coughing or a physical intervention is required. Once the airway is cleared, it is important to assess and support the patient, given the risks of further airway swelling or further injury from a physical intervention.

Laryngospasm

Acute dystonia of the laryngeal muscles is a medical emergency with a similar clinical presentation to choking. There can be a number of possible causes for laryngospasm, but ECT and neuroleptic medication are recognised risk factors for psychiatric patients (Reynolds, 2006). Indeed, any patient who is prescribed neuroleptics and presents with acute breathlessness might be experiencing laryngospasm. Patients using longer-term typical antipsychotics, such as haloperidol and chlorpromazine, are more at risk of this rare, life-threatening side-effect. Other risk factors include young age, male gender, previous acute dystonia, recent cocaine use, hypocalcaemia and dehydration.

Management

An effective short-term treatment is immediate provision of 100% oxygen and the use of intravenous anticholinergic medication (e.g. intravenous procyclidine 5 mg). Subsequently, the patient must be closely monitored in proximity to suitable resuscitation equipment. Further anticholinergic should be provided as necessary and any offending neuroleptic stopped.

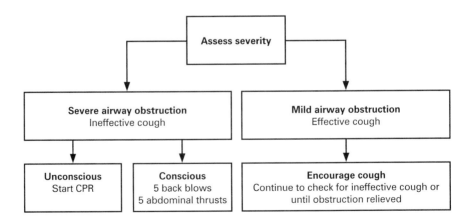

Fig. 11.6 Choking treatment algorithm (adults). Adapted with permission from Resuscitation Council (UK) (2010).

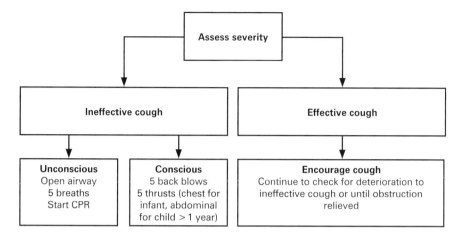

Fig. 11.7 Choking treatment algorithm (children). Adapted with permission from Resuscitation Council (UK) (2010).

Key points

- Psychiatric patients and patients with an intellectual disability should be recognised as being at increased risk of choking and laryngospasm.
- Early rapid recognition and treatment of airway obstruction is crucial.
- All clinical staff should be taught to recognise choking and be familiar with treatment, including when and how to use physical intervention.

Suspected acute coronary syndrome

Acute coronary syndrome (any symptoms that relate to obstruction of the coronary arteries) is a medical emergency. Diagnosis and management involves the recording of a 12-lead ECG and an urgent, detailed, specialist clinical assessment. The effectiveness of many of the treatments is time-dependent. Given this, the emphasis should be on arranging immediate transfer to an acute hospital by emergency ambulance. In addition to the ABCDE approach mentioned previously, there is NICE (2010a) guidance relevant to the immediate management of a suspected acute coronary syndrome.

Management

Pending transfer, where facilities allow, the following key points should be considered in adult patients.

- Provide pain relief – sublingual or buccal glyceryl trinitrate. Consider intravenous opioids such as morphine, particularly if an acute myocardial infarction is suspected.

- Administer aspirin (300 mg) as soon as possible unless there is clear evidence the patient is allergic to it. Record and communicate clearly that this has been given.
- Do not routinely administer oxygen: instead, monitor oxygen saturation using a pulse oximeter as soon as possible. If saturation is falling below 94%, oxygen should be provided to give a saturation of 94–98%. In those specifically with known chronic obstructive airway disease, some caution needs to be exercised, aiming for a target saturation of 88–92% (to avoid hypercapnic respiratory failure) until blood gas analysis is available.
- Take a resting 12-lead ECG if possible and fax the results to the acute hospital before the patient arrives. Recording and sending the ECG must not delay any transfer.
- Remain with and monitor people with acute chest pain, using clinical judgement to decide how often this should be done, until a firm diagnosis is made. Monitoring should include:
  - worsening of pain and/or other symptoms
  - pulse and blood pressure
  - heart rhythm
  - oxygen saturation by pulse oximetry
  - repeated resting 12-lead EGGs
  - checking pain relief is effective.

Cardiovascular shock

Shock occurs when the circulation is inadequate to provide for the metabolic demands of the body. Prompt and sustained resuscitation is required for any shocked patient, together with an assessment and treatment of the cause of shock. The range of signs and symptoms of shock can be varied, related to cause. The causes can be many and include haemorrhage, anaphylaxis, sepsis, toxins and burns. Inadequate circulation usually results in a diminished blood pressure, peripheral cyanosis, reduced conscious level and reduced urinary output. In young adults or children with trauma, lowered blood pressure might be a late sign. Self- harm and suicide attempts can sometimes lead to major haemorrhage through laceration and these patients might present with shock.

Management

Initial management should follow the ABCDE approach, identifying and treating conditions that are immediately life-threatening. Controlling massive haemorrhage by direct pressure and identifying whether anaphylaxis is evident are immediate priorities in shock (Soar *et al*, 2008). A simple measure to restore circulation can be to lay the person flat and raise the legs. However, this must be done with care, as it can worsen any breathing problems. In the case of a pregnant woman (over 20 weeks) a left lateral tilt of at least 15° should be used. Rapid intravenous or intraosseus fluid challenges should be provided if equipment and training in their use exists. Regular assessment of vital signs and monitoring for signs of cardiac failure will be necessary during fluid challenge.

Anaphylaxis

Anaphylaxis is a rare, acute and immediately life-threatening hypersensitivity reaction. Patients with anaphylaxis have life-threatening airway or breathing problems and/or circulation problems, usually associated with skin and mucosal changes. Statistics from the UK's fatal anaphylaxis register (Pumphrey, 2011) indicate that 0.005–0.01% of UK deaths between 1992 and 2005 were due to anaphylaxis. Hypersensitivity reactions to medication, food, immunotherapy or insect stings are the most frequent cause of anaphylaxis. However, in many instances no clear cause can be found. In younger people, food is a common trigger, whereas medication is a more common trigger in older people. The diagnosis is made clinically on the basis of symptoms and history. The cardinal symptoms are acute skin changes, wheezing, inspiratory stridor, hypotension, anxiety, nausea and vomiting.

Management

The diagnosis of anaphylaxis is often not obvious, and initial management should follow the ABCDE approach above for any critically ill patient. The Resuscitation Council (UK) guidelines emphasise that, in all cases of anaphylaxis, treatment should include the provision of immediate life-support techniques and adrenaline (Soar *et al*, 2008). Differential diagnosis for anaphylaxis includes other life-threatening conditions such as septic shock and acute asthma (these can initially be hard to differentiate). The ABCDE approach helps in that, independent of diagnosis, life-threatening problems can be identified and treated in sequence. The key steps in the treatment of anaphylaxis are shown in Fig. 11.8.

A life-threatening asthma attack

A life-threatening acute asthma attack requires urgent treatment in a medical admissions ward or emergency department. Around 1200 asthma deaths occur in the UK each year and as many as 90% of these are thought to be preventable (Royal College of Physicians, 2014). Adverse psychosocial factors, psychiatric illness, intellectual disability, major tranquilliser use and alcohol or drug abuse are all established risk factors for the development of near-fatal or fatal asthma. Most deaths occur before admission to hospital: in two-thirds of cases, the medical standards followed did not match national guidance (British Thoracic Society & Scottish Intercollegiate Guidelines Network, 2014).

It should be remembered that none of the clinical features of asthma, singly or in combination, are specific to make a diagnosis of a severe attack. Any asthma attack should be assumed to be an acute severe attack.

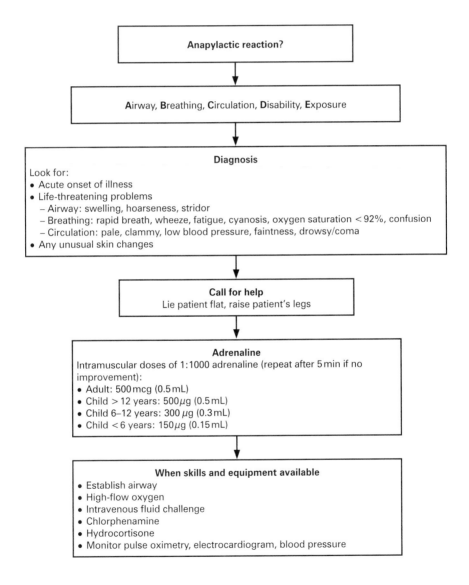

Fig. 11.8 Anaphylaxis treatment algorithm (adults). Adapted with permission from Resuscitation Council (UK) (2008).

The clinical features of acute severe asthma in adults include:

- peak expiratory flow rate > 50% best or predicted
- breathlessness (inability to complete sentences)
- rapid respiratory rate (25 breaths per minute or more in adults)
- fast heart rate (≥ 110 beats per minute in adults).

Life-threatening features in adults and children include:

- peak expiratory flow rate < 33% best or predicted (< 50% in children)
- oxygen saturation < 92%
- poor respiratory effort
- silent chest
- cyanosis
- bradycardia or hypotension
- arrhythmia
- collapse
- agitation or confusion
- coma.

Management

An accurate assessment of severity helps guide initial management. While arranging ambulance transfer, the mainstays of initial treatment are the provision of oxygen to treat hypoxia, an inhaled β2 agonist to treat bronchoconstriction, and steroids (British Thoracic Society & Scottish Intercollegiate Guidelines Network, 2014).

- Oxygen: supplementary high-flow oxygen to maintain an oxygen saturation of 94–99%. Lack of pulse oximetry should not prevent the use of oxygen.
- β2 agonist bronchodilator: this should be should be administered as early as possible (e.g. salbutamol 5 mg or terbutaline 10 mg), ideally through an oxygen-driven nebuliser. The absence of oxygen should not prevent nebulised therapy.
- Steroids: oral prednisolone 40–50 mg or intravenous hydrocortisone 100 mg.
- No sedatives of any kind should be administered.

In the case of life-threatening acute asthma, or if response is poor after 15–30 min, provide inhaled ipratropium bromide 500 μg via oxygen driven nebuliser.

In all cases of acute severe asthma, arrange for immediate hospital transfer. Do not leave the patient, as collapse will require CPR. Call for immediate assistance. Any life-threatening problem should be prioritised according to the ABCDE approach to resuscitation. For children, the same priorities of management exist, with age-appropriate drug-doses.

Delirium (acute confusional state)

Delirium refers to the cluster of neuropsychiatric symptoms seen as a consequence of an acute medical illness. The prevalence of delirium is difficult to estimate in mental health units, but about 1 in 10 of medically hospitalised patients has a period of delirium; this rises to 1 in 3 of elderly hospitalised patients (Brown & Boyle, 2002). It is a medical emergency with urgent need for thorough investigation and treatment. The condition often goes unrecognised and the underlying medical condition remains untreated, potentially leading to coma or death. Particularly for the elderly, early recognition and proactive prevention strategies can reduce the incidence and severity of delirium (Nicholson & Henderson, 2009). Characteristic features are changes in consciousness, perceptual disturbances (particularly visual hallucinations), sudden cognitive change and fluctuating symptoms over time. Three clinical clusters are reported based on psychomotor symptoms (Meagher & Trzepacz, 2000):

1   hyperactive delirium: patients might have heightened arousal, restlessness, agitation and often show hallucinations and delusions;
2   hypoactive delirium: patients might display lethargy, reduced motor activity, incoherent speech and lack of interest;
3   mixed delirium: a combination of hyperactive and hypoactive signs and symptoms.

Hypoactive and mixed states can be more difficult to recognise (Rooij *et al*, 2005).

In mental health units, the identification of delirium can be difficult given the differential diagnosis, which includes dementia, depressive retardation, schizophrenia and the effects of illicit drugs or alcohol. Virtually any medication can cause delirium; medication-induced delirium is more common in the elderly. Scicutella (2006) notes that certain patient groups within a mental health unit might be more vulnerable, given specific risks for developing delirium, including dementia, use of anticholinergic medication, lithium use, polypharmacy and drug withdrawal states. NICE (2010*b*) has published evidence-based guidelines on delirium recommending either the DSM-IV definition (American Psychiatric Association, 2000) or the short Confusion Assessment Method (CAM; Inouye *et al*, 1990) to aid the diagnosis of delirium.

Management

The management of delirium is dependent on identifying and treating the underlying medical condition. Given the multiplicity of possible causes, the first priority is to stabilise the patient's condition and screen for immediate life-threatening problems, using the ABCDE approach, followed by a secondary survey and focused history.

It can take time to identify the cause, and the episode might resolve spontaneously before a cause can be found. The medical management of delirium is complex and relates to initially screening for conditions that, if not treated, can cause irreversible damage and death. Following this, the wider causes can be explored through a careful history, physical examination, detailed review of medication and targeted laboratory investigations. Common contributory causes defined by the British Geriatrics Society & Royal College of Physicians (2006) are:

- infection (e.g. pneumonia, urinary tract infection)
- cardiological illness (e.g. myocardial infarction, heart failure)
- respiratory disorder (e.g. pulmonary embolus, hypoxia)
- electrolyte imbalance (e.g. dehydration, renal failure, hyponatraemia)
- endocrine and metabolic disorder (e.g. cachexia, thiamine deficiency, thyroid dysfunction)
- drugs, particularly those with anticholinergic side-effects (e.g. tricyclic antidepressants, anti-Parkinsonian drugs, opiates, analgesics, steroids)
- drug (especially benzodiazepine) and alcohol withdrawal
- urinary retention
- faecal impaction
- severe pain
- neurological problem (e.g. stroke, subdural haematoma, epilepsy, encephalitis)
- multiple contributing causes.

Practically speaking, confusion can be improved by the provision of familiar nurses, constant reorientation and a quiet and well-lit environment. Low-dose haloperidol or olanzapine may be considered if agitation or aggressive behavioural disturbance requires treatment (NICE, 2010b). However, no consensus exists on the choice or best dose of antipsychotic (Seitz et al, 2007); therefore, ultimately, the choice, route and dose of antipsychotic has to be tailored to the specific clinical circumstances, keeping in mind the drug's pharmacodynamics and potential for side-effects. For cases in which delirium is associated with withdrawal from alcohol or sedatives, benzodiazepines are preferred.

Key points

- Delirium is common, particularly in the hospitalised elderly.
- It can be caused by a variety of medical problems, which might require urgent treatment.
- Delirium can be easily missed, although structured algorithms such as the CAM can improve recognition.
- Management consists of taking all appropriate steps to identify and treat the reversible causes while providing environmental and behavioural support.

The fitting patient

Patients in mental health units are at increased risk of seizures for a number of reasons. Epilepsy is a recognised medical complication in those with intellectual disabilities, with an estimated prevalence of 20–30% (Mellers, 2009). Psychotropic medication is associated with seizures in those with and without epilepsy (Lee *et al*, 2003). Seizures can also complicate withdrawal states in patients with chronic alcohol abuse, particularly in those who also have epilepsy. The fitting patient is at risk of falls, head trauma and other accidental injury. In most instances, seizures self-terminate but in some cases status epilecticus can develop: 30 min or more of unremitting continuous seizures or recurrent seizures with incomplete recovery of consciousness between episodes. About 5% of all adult patients with epilepsy (10–25% for children) will experience at least one episode of status epilecticus (Shorvon, 1994).

Convulsive status epilecticus is a life-threatening neurological condition that can progress to coma and death. The risks of complications and mortality increase the longer the episode goes untreated, and treatment responsiveness reduces as the condition progresses. A prompt and effective response to any convulsive seizure episode can allow more successful treatment of status epilecticus, should it develop. A convulsive seizure is identifiable by a sudden onset of loss of consciousness, cyanosis, jerking movements, possible frothing at the mouth and urinary incontinence. After the seizure, the patient might remain confused and flaccid while regaining consciousness in the post-ictal state. Sleep disorders, syncope, movement disorders and dissociative episodes can sometimes present with seizure-like phenomena (Trimble & Schmitz, 2002).

Management

Management of any fitting patient should start with basic life support and resuscitation measures, as in any other medical emergency. The patient should be protected from accidental injury and the ABCDE approach implemented. No attempt should be made to restrain the patient or put anything in their mouth to prevent them biting their tongue. In most instances, the recovery position is the most effective way to maintain the airway. Oxygen should be provided and physical observations recorded.

Seizures should be timed. Most generalised seizures last for 1–2 min and not more than 5 min (Lowenstein & Alldredge, 1998). Treatment should begin as soon as it seems a seizure is persisting (any tonic–clonic seizure over 5 min in duration). Historically, rectal diazepam has been the drug of choice in pre-hospital care in adults, but concerns about this route of administration for children has led to buccal midazolam being considered for both children and adults where resuscitation facilities are limited. Where any benzodiazepine is given, drowsiness, sleep and even cardiorespiratory collapse can occur, and patients must be monitored, with appropriate resuscitation facilities at hand.

The NICE (2012) recommendation for the first-line treatment of convulsive status epilecticus in adults is summarised in Box 11.3. In most clinical settings, where resuscitation is available and intravenous access is in place, i.v. lorazepam is the preferred antiepileptic, given its long duration of action and good initial effectiveness in controlling seizures (Walker & Shorvon, 2009). However, in mental health units it might only be appropriate to follow the guidance for pre-hospital care for treatment, depending on the available equipment and staff training.

For those presenting for the first time with a seizure, medical transfer should be sought to enable further investigation. Where status epilecticus has developed, urgent medical transfer for intensive support and treatment will be necessary.

Key points

- A seizure of more than 5 min duration is a medical emergency.
- Initial management follows the ABCDE approach, with supportive measures, the administration of oxygen and treatment with a first-line anti-epileptic medication.
- Definitive medical care and investigation will be urgently required in the case of a first-episode seizure or status epilecticus.

Box 11.3 Treating convulsive status epilecticus in adults

Stage 1 (0–10 min)

- Secure airway and resuscitate
- Administer oxygen
- Assess cardiorespiratory function
- Establish intravenous access

Stage 2 (0–30 min)

- Start monitoring (neurological observations, pulse, blood pressure, ECG and temperature)
- Consider the possibility of non-epileptic status
- Start antiepileptic treatment:
  - Pre-hospital care: rectal diazepam (10–20 mg, repeated once after 15 min if necessary) or buccal midazolam (10 mg; unlicensed)
  - In hospital with intravenous access/resuscitation support: intravenous lorazepam (0.1 mg/kg, usually a 4 mg bolus, repeated once after 10–20 min), rate not critical
- Emergency investigations
- Correction of any hypoglycaemia:
  - 50 ml of 50% glucose intravenous injection
  - If there is a history of alcoholism or other nutritional disorders, treat with parenteral administration of vitamins B and C (e.g. Pabrinex)
- Correction of acidosis if severe

Life-threatening self-inflicted injuries, major trauma, poisoning and burns

Fatal or near-fatal self-inflicted injuries, major trauma or accidents are relatively rare events in institutional environments. Nevertheless, such events do occur and effective initial structured response and resuscitation can save lives and lead to better outcomes. Between 2001 and 2010, there were a total of 1,447 in-patient deaths by suicide in the UK, averaging 132 per year (Appleby *et al*, 2013). Methods of suicide and attempted suicide within mental health units tend to reflect the methods available. Ideally, specific policies should be developed for mental health units, outlining special circumstances in which resuscitation might be required (e.g. major blood loss, self-harm, ligature to the neck or hanging), with reference to the current standards of resuscitation in such circumstances (Soar *et al* 2010*b*).

Major trauma, asphyxiation and hanging

Injuries sustained through accidental trauma or self-injury can vary. In the case of major trauma, asphyxiation and hanging, the SAFE ABCDE approach for pre-hospital care should be followed. For all major injuries, the priority is resuscitation and stabilisation, while simultaneously arranging urgent ambulance transfer to the nearest major emergency department. Isolating the patient from further harm and stopping any worsening of an injury are important considerations, together with initial resuscitation. The patient should be handled as little as possible to avoid further spinal injury or haemorrhage (Moss & Porter, 2013). Paramedics, rather than ward-based staff, are often best suited to dealing with these situations, given their rigorous training and experience with pre-hospital care and trauma.

In hanging attempts, particular consideration must be given to cervical spine injury and the potential for airway obstruction from laryngeal oedema or airway swelling. Close airway and ventilation support, cervical spine control and vital sign monitoring must continue, even in the event of recovery, given the potential for airway obstruction to develop or for other, hidden injury to be present.

It is important that pneumothorax and haemothorax are promptly recognised and relieved, bleeding (external or internal) is stopped, shock is recognised and treated promptly with intravenous fluids, spinal-cord, brain and abdominal injuries are recognised and managed, limb-threatening injuries are stabilised, and appropriate pain relief is given.

Poisoning

In the case of self-poisoning, it is difficult to tell with any certainty what has been ingested. Where possible, the exact nature and timing of the poisoning and any witness accounts or evidence (e.g. any packaging, surplus tablets) must be sought. The ABCDE approach should be followed for immediate resuscitation needs and vital signs monitored. Shock, reduced consciousness, impaired respiration, cardiac arrhythmias, an impaired ability to maintain body temperature (hypothermia and hyperthermia), and seizures are all potential initial complications of poisoning.

In an emergency in the UK, advice can be sought from the National Poisons Information Service (0844 892 0111) or, for registered users, TOXBASE (www.toxbase.org). The administration of specific antidotes, supportive treatment and further medical care are all specialist competencies. In the case of any overdose or poisoning, referral for toxicology screening and urgent comprehensive medical care is always recommended.

Burns

Burns can have a variety of causes. The initial rescue and immediate quality of first aid, as well as saving lives, can also limit burn depth, which has profound impact on subsequent mortality and morbidity (British Burns Association, 2001). All patients with major burns should be managed according to resuscitation guidelines, given the potential for life-endangering complications.

Assessment of burn injury takes account of the timing, type, depth, location, extent and depth of burn. Assessment of the extent of skin injury uses the 'rule of nines', where the adult body is divided into anatomical regions representing 9% (or multiples of 9%) of the total body surface:

- head: 9%
- each upper limb: 9%
- each lower limb: 18%
- front of trunk: 18%
- back of trunk: 18%.

In addition, the patient's palm and fingers represent 1% of the total body surface. With knowledge of the burn mechanism and nature, a simple clinical evaluation can help initially categorise an injury. The visual characteristics of various burn depths are shown in Table 11.2.

The type, depth and extent of burn injury are pertinent to both immediate first aid and treatment. Chemical burns may continue to burn and cause more damage. Electrical burns often cause deeper injury, with possible organ damage. If the patient has been exposed to flames, inhalation injury and exposure to carbon monoxide must also be considered. The site of burns is also crucial, with burns involving the face, neck, genitals, hands or feet, or those that are circumferential, being more likely to involve life-endangering complications. A consensus approach for the pre-hospital care of burns is seen in Box 11.4.

Box 11.4 The pre-hospital approach to burns

SAFE approach

- Shout for help: Assess scene: Free from danger: Evaluate
- If electricity involved, isolate the power

Stop the burning process

- Remove the burning source
- If clothing is alight, 'drop and roll'
- Remove burnt/burning clothing (unless adhered to the wound)
- Brush dry chemical powders off the wound; other chemicals might need irrigation and information regarding the type of substance

Assessment and management of immediately or imminently life-threatening problems – ABCDE

- ABCDE (as per resuscitation guidelines)
- Oxygen (not necessary for small burns)

Cool the wound

- Lukewarm water should be applied for up to 20 min; water should be cold but not ice cold
- Be aware of the risk of hypothermia – especially for young or elderly patients

Assessment of burn severity

- Time of burn
- Size of burn (rule of nines)
- Mechanism (flame, flash burn, scald, electrical, chemical)
- Inhalation injury?
- Non-accidental?

Dressings

- Loosely cover the burnt area with clingfilm
- Do not constrict with wrapping
- Take caution with chemical burns, as these might need continuing irrigation
- Powder injuries might worsen with water

Cannulation and intravenous fluids

- Do not attempt if delaying transfer
- 0.9% saline or Hartmann's solution can be started
- Fluid replacement (ideally warmed) must be started for burns > 25% or if time to hospital more than 1 h

Analgesia

- Best achieved by cooling and covering burns initially
- Consider intravenous opiate and an anti-emetic

Transport

- All treatment should be given with the aim of reducing on-scene time and delivering the patient quickly to the nearest appropriate emergency department

Source: Adapted with permission from Allison & Porter (2004)

Table 11.2 Visual characteristics of burn depth classification.

Burn depth	Visual characteristics
Epidermal	Red, no blisters
Superficial dermal	Pink, mottled and small blisters
Deep dermal	Blistering, dry, blotchy and cherry red
Full thickness	Dry, white or black, no blisters
Full thickness +	As above plus fat, muscle and even bone involvement

Key points

- The initial response to a patient with major injury, burns or poisoning should follow the structured approach common to all emergencies (e.g. SAFE, ABCDE).
- A correct initial first-aid response can have a significant effect on recovery.
- Preventing further injury, resuscitation and stabilization is often a holding process while arranging emergency transfer for expert treatment.

References

Aggarwal R, Mytton OT, Derbrew M, *et al* (2010) Training and simulation for patient safety. *Quality and Safety in Health Care*, **19**: i34–i43.

Allison K, Porter K (2004) Consensus on the pre-hospital approach to burns patient management. *Emergency Medicine Journal*, **21**: 112–114.

American Psychiatric Association (2000) *Diagnostic and Statistical Manual of Mental Disorders Fourth Edition (DSM-IV-TR)*. American Psychiatric Association.

Appleby L, Kapur N, Shaw J, *et al* (2013) *The National Confidential Inquiry into Suicide and Homicide by People with Mental Illness Annual Report July 2013*. University of Manchester.

Biarent D, Bingham R, Eich C, *et al* (2010) European Resuscitation Council Guidelines for Resuscitation 2010 Section 6. Paediatric life support. *Resuscitation*, **81**: 1364–1388.

British Burns Association (2001) *National Burn Care Review, Standards and Strategy for Burn Care: A Review of Burn Care in the British Isles*. British Burns Association.

British Geriatrics Society, Royal College of Physicians (2006) *The Prevention, Diagnosis and Management of Delirium in Older People*. Royal College of Physicians.

British Medical Association (2007) *Decisions Relating to Cardiopulmonary Resuscitation*. A joint statement from the British Medical Association, the Resuscitation Council (UK) and the Royal College of Nursing. British Medical Association.

British Thoracic Society & Scottish Intercollegiate Guidelines Network (2014) *British Guideline on the Management of Asthma: A National Clinical Guideline*. Healthcare Improvement Scotland.

Brown TM, Boyle MF (2002) ABC of psychological medicine Delirium. *British Medical Journal*, **21**: 644–647.

Cheung W, Gullick J, Thanakrishnan G, *et al* (2012) Expansion of a medical emergency team system to a mental health facility. *Resuscitation*, **83**: 293–296.

Deakin CD, Nolan JP, Sunde K, *et al* (2010) European Resuscitation Council Guidelines for Resuscitation 2010 Section 3. Electrical therapies: Automated external defibrillators, defibrillation, cardioversion and pacing. *Resuscitation*, **81**: 1293–1304.

Department of Health (2009) *Competencies for Recognising and Responding to Acutely Ill Patients in Hospital*. Department of Health.

Inouye SK, van Dyck CH, Alessi CA (1990) Clarifying confusion: the confusion assessment method. A new method for detection of delirium. *Annals of Internal Medicine*, **113**: 941–948.

Lee KC, Finley PR, Alldredge BK (2003) Risk of seizures associated with psychotropic medications: emphasis on new drugs and new findings. *Expert Opinion on Drug Safety*, **2**: 233–247.

Leonard M (2004) The human factor: the critical importance of effective teamwork and communication in providing safe care. *Quality and Safety in Health Care*, **13**: i85–i90.

Lowenstein DH, Alldredge BK (1998) Status epilecticus. *New England Journal of Medicine*, **338**: 970–976.

Lyketsos CG, Dunn G, Kaminsky MJ, *et al* (2002) Medical comorbidity in psychiatric in-patients: relation to clinical outcomes and hospital length of stay. *Psychosomatics*, **43**: 24–30.

Meagher DJ, Trzepacz PT (2000) Motoric subtypes of delirium. *Seminars in Clinical Neuropsychiatry*, **5**: 75–85.

Mehtonen OP, Aranko K, Malkonen L, *et al* (1991) Survey of sudden death associated with the use of antipsychotic or antidepressant drugs: 49 cases in Finland. *Acta Psychiatrica Scandinavica*, **81**: 372–377.

Mellers JDC (2009) Epilepsy. In *Lishman's Organic Psychiatry: A Textbook of Neuropsychiatry* (4th edn) (eds A David, S Fleminger, MD Kopelman, *et al*). Wiley–Blackwell.

Moss R, Porter KM (2013) *Faculty of Pre-Hospital Care Consensus Statement: Minimal Patient Handling*. Royal College of Surgeons of Edinburgh.

Mukadam N, Sampson EL (2011) A systematic review of the prevalence, associations and outcomes of dementia in older general hospital inpatients. *International Psychogeriatrics*, **23**: 344–355.

National Confidential Inquiry into Patient Outcomes and Death (2012) *Time to Intervene? A Review of Patients who Underwent Cardiopulmonary Resuscitation as a Result of an In-Hospital Cardiorespiratory Arrest*. NCEPOD.

National Institute for Health and Clinical Excellence (2005) *The Short-Term Management of Disturbed/Violent Behaviour (NICE Clinical Guideline 25)*. NICE.

National Institute for Health and Clinical Excellence (2010a) *Chest Pain of Recent Onset: Assessment and Diagnosis of Recent Onset Chest Pain or Discomfort of Suspected Cardiac Origin (NICE Clinical Guideline 95)*. NICE.

National Institute for Health and Clinical Excellence (2010b) *Delirium: Diagnosis, Prevention and Management (NICE Clinical Guideline 103)*. NICE.

National Institute for Health and Clinical Excellence (2012) *The Epilepsies: The Diagnosis and Management of the Epilepsies in Adults and Children in Primary and Secondary Care (NICE Clinical Guideline 137)*. NICE.

National Patient Safety Agency (2004) *Establishing a Standard Crash Call Telephone Number in Hospitals*. National Patient Safety Agency.

National Patient Safety Agency (2008) *Resuscitation in Mental Health and Learning Disability Settings*. National Patient Safety Agency.

National Reporting and Learning Service (2007) *The Third Report from the Patient Safety Observatory: Slips, Trips and Falls in Hospital*. National Patient Safety Agency.

Nicholson TR, Henderson M (2009) Management of delirium. *British Journal of Hospital Medicine*, **70**: 217–221.

Nolan JP (2011) Optimising outcome after cardiac arrest. *Current Opinion in Critical Care*, **17**: 520–526.

Nolan JP, Soar J, Zideman DA, *et al* (2010) European Resuscitation Council Guidelines for Resuscitation 2010 Section 1: Executive summary. *Resuscitation*, **81**: 1219–1276.

O'Driscoll BR, Howard LS, Davison AG (2011) *Emergency Oxygen Use in Adult Patients: Concise Guideline*. Royal College of Physicians.

Pumphrey R (2011) An epidemiological approach to reducing the risk of fatal anaphylaxis. In *Anaphylaxis and Hypersensitivity Reactions* (ed MC Castells). Springer.

Resuscitation Council (UK) (2008) *Emergency Treatment of Anaphylatic Reactions. Guidelines for healthcare providers*. Resuscitation Council (UK).

Resuscitation Council (UK) (2010) *2010 Resuscitation Guidelines*. Resuscitation Council (UK).

Resuscitation Council (UK) (2014a) *Quality Standards for Cardiopulmonary Clinical Practice and Training. Mental Health - Inpatient Care*. Resuscitation Council (UK).

Resuscitation Council (UK) (2014b) *Quality Standards for Cardiopulmonary Clinical Practice and Training. Mental Health – Inpatient Care – Equipment and Drug Lists*. Resuscitation Council (UK).

Reynolds SM (2006) Choking and laryngospasm. In *Handbook of Medicine in Psychiatry* (eds P Manu, RE Suarez, BJ Barnett). American Psychiatric Press.

Rooij SE, Schuurmans MJ, van der Mast RC, *et al* (2005) Clinical subtypes of delirium and their relevance for daily clinical practice: a systematic review. *International Journal of Geriatric Psychiatry*, **20**: 609–615.

Royal College of Physicians (2012) *National Early Warning Score (NEWS): Standardising the Assessment of Acute-Illness Severity in the NHS. Report of a Working Party*. Royal College of Physicians.

Royal College of Physicians (2014) *The National Review of Asthma Deaths*. Royal College of Physicians.

Ruschena D, Mullen PE, Palmer P, et al (2003) Choking deaths: the role of antipsychotic medication. *British Journal of Psychiatry*, **183**: 446–450.

Scicutella A (2006) Delirium. In *Handbook of Medicine in Psychiatry* (eds P Manu, RE Suarez, BJ Barnett). American Psychiatric Press.

Seitz D, Gill S, van Zyl LT (2007) Antipsychotics in the treatment of delirium: a systematic review. *Journal of Clinical Psychiatry*, **68**: 11–21.

Sharp CW, Freeman CP (1993) The medical complications of anorexia nervosa. *British Journal of Psychiatry*, **162**: 452–462.

Shorvon S (1994) *Status Epilecticus: Its Clinical Features and Treatment in Children and Adults*. Cambridge University Press.

Simpson GM, Davis JM, Jefferson JW, *et al* (1987) *Sudden Deaths in Psychiatric Patients: The Role of Neuroleptic Drugs. American Psychiatric Association Task Force Report 27*. American Psychiatric Association.

Soar J, Pumphrey R, Cant A, *et al* (2008) Emergency treatment of anaphylactic reactions – guidelines for healthcare providers. *Resuscitation*, **77**: 157–169.

Soar J, Mancini ME, Bhanji F, *et al* (2010a) 2010 International Consensus on Cardiopulmonary Resuscitation and Emergency Cardiovascular Care Science with Treatment Recommendations. Part 12: Education, implementation, and teams. *Resuscitation*, **81** (Suppl 1): e288–e332.

Soar J, Perkins JD, Abbas G, *et al* (2010b) European Resuscitation Council Guidelines for Resuscitation 2010: Section 8. Cardiac arrest in special circumstances: Electrolyte abnormalities, poisoning, drowning, accidental hypothermia, hyperthermia, asthma, anaphylaxis, cardiac surgery, trauma, pregnancy, electrocution. *Resuscitation*, **81**: 1400–1433.

Trimble M, Schmitz B (2002) *The Neuropsychiatry of Epilepsy*. Cambridge University Press.

Walker M, Shorvon S (2009) Emergency treatment of seizures and status epilecticus. In *The Treatment of Epilepsy* (3rd edn) (eds S Shorvon, E Perucca, J Engel). Wiley–Blackwell.

Weekes R (1999) Scene approach, assessment and safety. In *Pre-Hospital Medicine: The Principles and Practice of Immediate Care* (eds I Greaves, K Porter). Arnold.

Wilkins R (2008) *Resuscitation in Mental Health and Learing Disability Settings Rapid Response Report*. National Patient Safety Agency.

Wilson DN, Haire A (1990) Health care screening for people with mental handicap living in the community. *British Medical Journal*, **301**: 1379–1381.

Windfuhr K, Turnbull P, While D, *et al* (2011) The incidence and associated risk factors for sudden unexplained death in psychiatric in-patients in England and Wales. *Journal of Psychopharmacology*, **25**: 1533–1542.

Woo BKP (2011) Unrecognized medical disorders among older patients in psychiatric emergency service. *International Journal of Geriatric Psychiatry*, **26**: 877–878.

Resources

SABR templates

http://www.institute.nhs.uk/safer_care/safer_care/Situation_Background_Assessment_Recommendation.html

MEWS templates

http://www.rcplondon.ac.uk/resources/national-early-warning-score-news

PEWS templates

http://www.institute.nhs.uk/safer_care/paediatric_safer_care/pews_charts.html

Resuscitation guidelines 2010

http://www.resus.org.uk/pages/guide.htm

Toxbase

http://www.toxbase.org/

CHAPTER 12

Emergencies in intellectual disability psychiatry

David Clarke

In this chapter, the term 'intellectual disability' is used to refer to people with global cognitive problems and associated problems with daily living skills, whose difficulties were apparent before 18 years of age. In the UK, in the past, this group of people were referred to as having a mental handicap. In the USA and many other countries, the term 'mental retardation' is used. The term 'learning disability' is also commonly used in the UK to refer to this group, but in the USA, it refers to people with specific deficits in scholastic skills (e.g. dyslexia, dyscalculia). ICD-10 uses the term mental retardation, but the definition and the sub-classifications set out (mild, moderate, severe and profound) are the same as for intellectual disability in the UK (World Health Organization, 1988; Department of Health, 2001).

Intellectual disability

People with an intellectual disability can experience difficulties leading to an emergency presentation to mental health services for the same reasons as people who do not have an intellectual disability (for example, mood disorders, psychoses). However, their typical presentation might be modified by the presence of intellectual disability (Marston *et al*, 1997; Clarke & Gomez, 1999). They might experience emergencies related to problem behaviours (notably aggressive, self-injurious or sexually inappropriate behaviour) or a seizure disorder. Medical emergencies in people with an intellectual disability can result in a presentation that can be difficult to distinguish from manifestations of psychiatric or behaviour disorder. The special needs or attributes of people with intellectual disability that need to be taken into account when dealing with emergencies comprise the 'four Cs': communication difficulties, capacity to consent, comorbid conditions and complicating effects on symptoms.

Communication difficulties and reliance on other sources of information

A person with intellectual disability might not be able to give an account of recent problems or experiences as easily as a non-disabled person. People with more severe intellectual disabilities might have no, or very limited, ability to use spoken communication. Reliance might have to be placed on non-verbal methods of communication (e.g. appearance, behaviour, body-language, use of signs or pictures to communicate) and on history obtained from carers and other people in close contact with the patient.

Capacity to consent to treatment

The Mental Capacity Act 2005 sets out provisions for dealing with people who lack the capacity to consent to treatment or to make other decisions. The provisions are summarised in the Mental Capacity Act 2005 Code of Practice (Department of Constitutional Affairs, 2007). Some people with intellectual disabilities are able to consent to treatment or other interventions. Guidance about the assessment of capacity to consent is given by Church & Watts (2007), who provide a helpful flow-chart. The stages include assessment of whether there is a disturbance in the functioning of the brain (as is likely in someone with an intellectual disability), clarity about the decision to be made and whether the person can be supported to make the decision, gathering and documenting evidence for a decision-specific test, and testing capacity based on the principles of understanding and believing, retaining and weighing the relevant information.

The code of practice sets out five principles that should always be adhered to when deciding on matters of capacity, which can be remembered using the acronym PLUMB (Department of Constitutional Affairs, 2007).

Presumption of capacity

Every adult with the capacity to do so has the right to make their own decisions. Family carers and medical or social care staff must assume that a person has the capacity to make decisions, unless it can be established otherwise.

Least restrictive alternative

Any act done for, or any decision made on behalf of, someone who lacks capacity should be the option that is the least restrictive of their basic rights and freedoms (if it is still in their best interests).

Unwise decisions should be respected

All adults have the right to make a decision that others might think unwise. A person who makes such a decision should not automatically be thought to lack capacity.

Maximise potential for decision making

People should receive support to help them make decisions. Before concluding that individuals lack capacity, all possible steps should be taken to help them reach their own decision.

Best interests of the person

Any decision made on behalf of, or any act performed for, someone who lacks capacity must always be in their best interests.

Comorbid conditions

People with autistic disorders are prone to anxiety (especially in response to change), mood instability and depression (Stewart *et al*, 2006). Psychotic disorders have also been reported (Clarke *et al*, 1999). It can be difficult to distinguish between behaviour that could justifiably be labelled as a problem (e.g. aggression) and behaviour that communicates distress or pain or results from an altered level of consciousness (e.g. behaviour associated with an acute confusional state or a seizure disorder, or resulting from dental pain). Careful history taking and attempting to gain as much information as possible about the person's psychiatric and medical history is important. Knowledge of specific associations that might explain a change in behaviour (e.g. a liability to infections as well as psychiatric disorder in velo-cardio-facial syndrome) will aid correct assessment.

Complicating (pathoplastic) effects of intellectual disability on the manifestations of psychiatric disorder

It is rarely possible to diagnose schizophrenia in people with severe intellectual disability because of the difficulty in eliciting psychopathology, such as primary delusions, passivity experiences or specific types of auditory hallucinations (Reid, 1972). It might be apparent that a patient is distressed and apparently responding to something they are hearing, and it might be possible for them to describe hearing voices or noises. A diagnosis of psychosis might be possible if other potential causes can be excluded. Depression might have a slightly different symptom profile in people with intellectual disability compared with the general population: lower rates of suicidal ideation and attempted suicide and the emergence or worsening of behaviours such as irritability, psychomotor agitation, screaming and self-injury (Meins, 1995; Marston *et al*, 1997).

Types of emergency

In intellectual disability psychiatry, emergencies can usually be categorised as to do with psychiatric disorders, behaviour disorders, seizure disorders (epilepsy), or some combination of these problems. Any kind of psychiatric disorder might give rise to a need for emergency assessment but, as in the general population, the most common reasons for such an assessment are mood disorders and psychotic disorders, or the suspicion of their presence.

The behaviour that most commonly results in emergency assessment is aggressive behaviour. Occasionally other behaviours, such as severe self-injury, might present as an emergency. The most common seizure disorder resulting in emergency presentation is a prolonged tonic–clonic seizure. The characteristic history and description will usually be available from a witness, but in rare instances the presentation can be in the form of a post-ictal confusional state. A history of epilepsy, especially if there have been similar episodes in the past, might help to clarify the nature of the problem. The management of prolonged seizures or status epilepticus is covered by National Institute for Health and Care Excellence (NICE) guidance (2012), as follows.

- Give immediate emergency care and treatment to children, young people and adults who have prolonged (5 min or longer) or repeated (3+ in an hour) convulsive seizures in the community.

- Only prescribe buccal midazolam or rectal diazepam for use in the community for children, young people and adults who have had a previous episode of prolonged or serial convulsive seizures.

- Administer buccal midazolam as a first-line treatment in the community for children, young people and adults with prolonged or repeated seizures. Administer rectal diazepam if preferred, or if buccal midazolam is not available. If intravenous access is already established and resuscitation facilities are available, administer intravenous lorazepam.

- Treatment should be administered by trained clinical personnel or, if specified by an individually agreed protocol drawn up with the specialist, by family members or carers with appropriate training.

- Care must be taken to secure the child, young person or adult's airway and assess their respiratory and cardiac function.

- Depending on response to treatment, the person's situation and any personalised care plan, call an ambulance, particularly if:
  - the seizure continues 5 min after the emergency medication has been administered
  - the patient has a history of frequent episodes of serial seizures or has convulsive status epilepticus, or this is the first episode requiring emergency treatment
  - there are difficulties monitoring the person's airway, breathing, circulation or other vital signs.

The principles of assessment for the other types of problem are similar.

Assessment

The following information incorporates guidance from the Centre for Addiction and Mental Health (2002) and additional material based on the author's clinical experience.

Optimise the clinical encounter

Adapt your approach to the patient's level of functioning and understanding. Take account of comorbid conditions you know, or suspect, are present (notably, autistic disorders). Language might need to be simplified and very concrete. Effective communication might involve speaking slowly, using simple language, pausing to avoid information overload, and using gestures, pictures or other methods to supplement verbal communication.

Find out about circumstances or factors that might be particularly upsetting for the individual, such as too many questions, using particular types of questions or a certain style of questioning, a noisy environment, use of touch, unusual or strong smells in the environment. A warm and accepting, but not over-familiar, approach usually works best, but this might need to be modified as the interview progresses or in the light of information from informants. Waiting might prove particularly problematic. Try to ensure someone who knows the patient well (and whom they like) is present. Be sensitive to non-verbal communication.

Try to avoid direct questions: these might be perceived as intimidating and be answered to please or to limit the encounter rather than to give the information you are seeking. Respect the patient's personal space, and forewarn them about any procedure that involves personal contact, such as blood pressure measurement. Reassurance by carers might allow procedures to take place if they are absolutely necessary. In some circumstances, anxiolytic medication such as oral lorazepam 1 mg might be necessary for a procedure to go ahead, provided this is medically appropriate and subject to the provisions of the Mental Capacity Act.

Assess symptoms and behaviours relevant to the presentation

A good general guide is to determine whether there has been a change in behaviour (outside the range of normal variation for that individual) lasting at least a week and a definite diminution in level of functioning in self-care, interest in usual activities, need for supervision or a change in social involvement (social withdrawal or abnormal sociability). Psychotic symptoms (especially positive symptoms, such as delusions and hallucinations) might be present for a short period of time and still give rise to an emergency presentation, although a careful history will usually reveal antecedent changes. A sudden onset of apparently psychotic symptoms with a decline in functioning and consciousness level should raise suspicions of an acute confusional state and lead to appropriate examination and investigation. The most common causes are infections (especially urinary or chest infections), post-ictal confusion and toxicity from medication (prescribed or otherwise).

Arrive at a provisional diagnosis

Provisional diagnosis should include consideration of comorbid conditions.

Decide on the most appropriate emergency treatment or management

The first priority is to ensure the safety of the patient, carers and assessing staff. Emergency sedation or restraint might be required, bearing in mind the provisions of the Mental Capacity Act. Restraint should only be used as a last resort – it often escalates, rather than defuses aggressive behaviour and is associated with medical risks. Oral lorazepam 1 mg or oral (or, if justified, intramuscular) diazepam 5–10mg may be used if justified. Other medications sometimes used to manage abnormally aggressive behaviour include typical antipsychotics (Table 12.1).

Off-label use of medication

Risperidone and some other atypical antipsychotics are widely used to treat anxiety and impulsive or aggressive behaviour associated with intellectual disability (especially autistic disorders). Some studies have

Table 12.1 Some antipsychotic drugs licensed for the short-term management of severe behaviour disorders

Drug	Dose	Indication
Chlorpromazine	25–300 mg	Severe anxiety, psychomotor agitation, excitement, violent or dangerously impulsive behaviour
Haloperidol	0.5–15 mg	Psychomotor agitation, excitement, violent or dangerously impulsive behaviour
Pericyazine	5–30 mg	Severe anxiety, psychomotor agitation, violent or dangerously impulsive behaviour
Perphenazine	12–24 mg	Anxiety, severe psychomotor agitation, excitement, violent or dangerously impulsive behaviour
Promazine	400–800 mg	Psychomotor agitation
	25–50 mg	Agitation and restlessness (elderly only)
Trifluoperazine	2–40 mg	Psychomotor agitation, excitement, violent or dangerously impulsive behaviour
Risperidone	0.25–1.5 mg	Persistent aggression in conduct disorder

Sources: www.drugs.com; British Medical Association & Royal Pharmaceutical Society of Great Britain (2011)

shown efficacy (Bokszanska *et al*, 2003), and others have not (Tyrer *et al*, 2008). Risperidone is commonly associated with weight gain and might be associated with hyperprolactinaemia. Other adverse effects seem to be rare, at least during short- to medium-term use. One review of the safety of antipsychotics for people with intellectual disability concluded that 'antipsychotics at the low doses routinely prescribed for people with intellectual disability are generally safe in relation to metabolic adverse effects, even if efficacy remains poorly defined' (Frighi *et al*, 2011).

General advice

In general, emergency management should be confined to the minimum needed to ensure safety and alleviate immediate distress. Guidance has been issued about the use of antipsychotics and other medications to treat behaviour disorders associated with intellectual disability, with recommendations for assessment, prescribing and reviewing, and auditing (Deb *et al*, 2006). It is important to try to find the causes of behavioural problems and to consider other strategies that might be effective, before introducing or changing medication. Underlying medical and dental disorders could be the reason for aggressive behaviour. Consider whether the provision of, or re-assessment by, psychology, communication therapy or community nursing services might be needed instead of (or in addition to) medication. Appropriate recommendations can be incorporated into the follow-up plan discussed above.

It is usually best to avoid changing any medications the patient is already receiving, unless it is clear that they are contributing to the change in functioning that led to assessment. It is best to deal with the emergency and leave regular review of medications to the patient's usual prescriber. Recommendations to consider alternatives can be included in the written communication outlined above. However, increasing the dose of an antipsychotic already prescribed might be a relatively safe and effective emergency response to an increase in aggressive behaviour, provided physical causes for the change in behaviour have been excluded and the dose remains within the recommended range.

When treating abnormally aggressive behaviour associated with intellectual disability, the medication with the most evidence regarding efficacy and safety is risperidone in doses of 0.25–1.5 mg daily. Risperidone should be started in the lowest dose likely to be effective (usually 0.25 mg or 0.5 mg). NICE has issued guidance about rapid tranquillisation, which should only be undertaken in a hospital setting with resuscitation equipment to hand and suitably trained staff (NICE, 2005).

Arrange follow-up

This will usually include written documentation of the assessment, any interventions provided and suggestions for future diagnostic re-evaluation, investigation or management. A letter to a general practitioner or receiving

223

psychiatric team should include as many of the following elements as are relevant to the emergency presentation:

- date of assessment
- basic patient data (date of birth, address)
- NHS number
- diagnosis (provisional or differential diagnosis if appropriate)
- concise summary of signs and symptoms
- statement about relevant risks
- crisis plan if appropriate
- management or medication changes made
- other requests to the general practitioner (e.g. blood tests).

It might also be appropriate to include the local NHS out-of-hours emergency phone number.

Triage

Triage refers to the assessment and categorisation of the urgency of illness. The main function of triage in the context of managing behavioural and psychiatric disorders is to decide where further assessment and treatment can and should take place. The options are in the current living environment, in an alternative living environment, and during in-patient admission. A return to the current living environment is the preferred option, provided risks can be managed and appropriate treatment provided. For people with autistic disorders, change can be a source of anxiety, and options other than a return home (or to another familiar environment) should only be considered as a last resort.

The provision of an alternative living environment might entail access to respite care (sometimes called 'short breaks' within intellectual disability services) or a temporary move to a suitably registered residential home. This is usually organised through the local intellectual disability community team and can take some time to arrange (funding might have to be agreed). Most teams have arrangements to deal with emergencies resulting in someone with an intellectual disability being unable to return to their home environment, and this might be incorporated in their care plan.

In-patient admission should be considered when the risks are such that alternatives are impractical, or when treatment has to be provided that could not be safely or effectively given in another setting. Some people with an intellectual disability will be able to consent to informal admission. For people who lack capacity to consent to admission and meet the criteria for detention under the Mental Health Act 2007, the provisions of the act should be used (see next section). For people who require admission to a psychiatric hospital, but lack capacity to consent and do not meet the criteria for detention under the Mental Health Act, the current advice is to consider using the Deprivation of Liberty Safeguards (a DoLS authorisation). Decisions on capacity are the responsibility of the admitting hospital, but the referrer should make clear their view on the matter.

The Mental Health Act 2007

The Mental Health Act 2007 amends the provisions of the Mental Health Act 1983, but does not replace it. The provisions most commonly used in emergency settings are Section 2 (admission for assessment for up to 28 days, allowing treatment to be provided) and Section 3 (admission for treatment, initially for up to 6 months). The grounds for detention are essentially that the person has a 'disorder or disability of the mind', that treatment in hospital is necessary (because alternatives such as community treatment would not be safe or effective and the patient ought to be detained for their own health or safety or for the protection of others), and that appropriate medical treatment can be provided in the hospital or unit to which the person is being admitted. The concept of medical treatment is wide, and includes aspects such as nursing care and rehabilitation.

A person with an intellectual disability can be admitted on the grounds of the presence of a psychiatric disorder (such as severe depression with food refusal, weight loss and risk of dehydration), without reference to the presence of intellectual disability. Psychiatric disorders include autistic disorders, but other grounds for admission also have to be met: there must be risks justifying admission, other forms of treatment must have been considered and discounted, and appropriate treatment is available in the receiving hospital or home.

Section 2 technically allows someone with intellectual disability to be detained in the absence of abnormally aggressive or seriously irresponsible conduct, but it is difficult to see how the other provisions within the criteria for detention could be met in these circumstances. Such provisions include consideration for the person's health or safety, the need to protect others, and the requirment that treatment could not be provided other than on an in-patient basis.

Section 3 and other sections that deal with longer-term detention allow the detention of a person with an intellectual disability only where the disability is associated with abnormally aggressive or seriously irresponsible conduct. This does not mean that the intellectual disability has to have caused the aggressive or irresponsible conduct. As with Section 2, the presence of a well-evidenced psychiatric disorder would allow the detention of someone who also happened to have an intellectual disability, although the doctor making the medical recommendation would have to be satisfied that appropriate treatment was available (this might entail expertise in intellectual disability as well as management of psychiatric disorder, depending on the needs of the individual patient).

The other provision of the Mental Health Act 2007 that might need to be used in an emergency is Section 5(2): the doctors holding power. This allows for the temporary detention of a hospital in-patient in order to allow time for assessment regarding further detention using the Act. The hospital does not have to be a psychiatric hospital. The patient must be an in-patient (not an out-patient or attending an emergency department) who has not been detained and who wishes to leave. Temporary detention must be in the interests of the patient's health or safety or necessary for the protection of others and it must be impracticable or unsafe to make an application for Section 2 or Section 3. Detention using Section 5(2) can be effected by a registered medical practitioner, an approved clinician or their nominated deputy. Detention is authorised for a maximum of 72 h and treatment can only be given in an emergency within the provisions of the Mental Capacity Act 2005. For detailed advice about the Mental Health Act 2007 see the Code of Practice (Department of Health, 2008).

Conclusions

With the exception of seizure disorders (which should be treated in accordance with NICE guidance), emergencies in intellectual disability psychiatry usually concern the presence of a psychiatric disorder or severe behavioural problems. The most common behaviour resulting in an emergency presentation is aggression. Assessment needs to take into account the preferred style of communication of the person assessed and factors related to the presence of comorbid conditions, such as autistic disorders. Corroborative history and other information from an informant who knows the person well is extremely helpful. Interventions should be confined to those immediately necessary to manage risks and deal with the emergency. Other recommendations about management should be communicated to the general practitioner or psychiatric team providing follow-up. Care should be taken to exclude physical problems as causes or contributory factors in behavioural change. Attention should be given to psychological, communicatory or other methods of reducing problem behaviours or influencing psychiatric disorders.

If medication is required, the impact of potential adverse effects on existing physical or other comorbid conditions should be considered. Changing the dose of medications already prescribed should be considered before introducing new agents. A decision should be made regarding the safety and benefits of returning the patient to their existing residential environment. If necessary, a move to another residential environment can be arranged (often a respite-care facility). Where risks are substantial and cannot be reduced in other ways, hospital admission should be considered. The requirements of the Mental Health Act 2007 and Mental Capacity Act 2005 must be adhered to when making these decisions. The assessing doctor should be aware of their responsibility to act in the best interests of their patient, rather than of services or agencies, at all times.

References

Bokszanska A, Martin G, Vanstraelen M, *et al* (2003) Risperidone and olanzapine in adults with intellectual disability: a clinical naturalistic study. *International Clinical Psychopharmacology*, **18**: 285–291.

British Medical Association & Royal Pharmaceutical Society of Great Britain (2011) *British National Formulary* (62nd edn). BMJ Books & Pharmaceutical Press.

Centre for Addiction and Mental Health (2002) *Guidelines for Managing the Client with Intellectual Disability in the Emergency Room*. Centre for Addiction and Mental Health.

Church M, Watts S (2007) Assessment of mental capacity: a flow-chart guide. *The Psychiatrist*, **31**: 304–307.

Clarke D, Baxter M, Perry D, *et al* (1999) The diagnosis of affective and psychotic disorders in adults with autism: seven case reports. *Autism*, **3**: 149–164.

Clarke DJ, Gomez GA (1999) Utility of modified DCR-10 criteria in the diagnosis of depression associated with intellectual disability. *Journal of Intellectual Disability Research*, **43**: 413–420.

Deb S, Clarke D, Unwin G (2006) *Using Medication to Manage Behaviour Problems Among Adults with a Learning Disability: Quick Reference Guide*. University of Birmingham, Royal College of Psychiatrists & Mencap.

Department of Constitutional Affairs (2007) *Mental Capacity Act 2005 Code of Practice*. The Stationery Office (http://www.justice.gov.uk/downloads/guidance/protecting-the-vulnerable/mca/mca-code-practice-0509.pdf).

Department of Health (2001) *Valuing People: A New Strategy for Learning Disability for the 21st Century*. The Stationery Office (https://www.gov.uk/government/publications/valuing-people-a-new-strategy-for-learning-disability-for-the-21st-century).

Department of Health (2008) *Code of Practice: The Mental Health Act 1983*. The Stationery Office (http://www.dh.gov.uk/en/Publicationsandstatistics/Publications/PublicationsPolicyAndGuidance/DH_084597).

Frighi V, Stephenson MT, Morovat A, et al (2011) Safety of antipsychotics in people with intellectual disability. *British Journal of Psychiatry*, **199**: 289–295.

Marston GM, Perry DW, Roy A (1997) Manifestations of depression in people with intellectual disability. *Journal of Intellectual Disability Research*, **41**: 476–480.

Meins W (1995) Symptoms of major depression in mentally retarded adults. *Journal of Intellectual Disability Research*, **39**: 41–45.

National Institute for Health and Clinical Excellence (2005) *Violence: The Short-Term Management of Disturbed/Violent Behaviour in Psychiatric Inpatient Settings and Emergency Departments (NICE Clinical Guideline 25)*. NICE.

National Institute for Health and Clinical Excellence (2012) *The Epilepsies: The Diagnosis and Management of the Epilepsies in Adults and Children in Primary and Secondary Care (NICE Clinical Guideline 137)*. NICE.

Reid AH (1972) Psychosis in adult mental defectives: II. Schizophrenic and paranoid psychosis. *British Journal of Psychiatry*, **120**: 205–218.

Stewart ME, Barnard L, Pearson J et al (2006) Presentation of depression in autism and Asperger syndrome: a review. *Autism*, **10**: 103–116.

Tyrer P, Oliver-Africano PC, Ahmed Z, *et al* (2008) Risperidone, haloperidol and placebo in the treatment of aggressive challenging behaviour in patients with intellectual disability: a randomised controlled trial. *Lancet*, **371**: 57–63.

World Health Organization (1988) *ICD-10 Classification of Mental and Behavioural Disorders*. WHO.

CHAPTER 13

Emergencies in older persons' psychiatry

Ejaz Nazir

In the UK, the proportion of elderly people in the population has increased dramatically. At the beginning of the 20th century, approximately 4% of people were aged 65 years or over. Today the proportion is approximately 16%. It is predicted that by 2050 the proportion of the UK population aged 65 years and over will increase from the latest figure of 11.1 million to 19 million (AgeDiscrimination.info, n.d.; Cracknell, 2010).

Psychiatric emergencies are common in the elderly. The diagnosis and treatment of psychiatric emergencies in geriatric patients can be challenging, owing to the increased incidence of medical and neurological comorbidities, psychosocial problems and medication-induced adverse events. The most common psychiatric emergencies in the elderly are depression with suicidality, delirium, dementia with behavioural disturbance, substance abuse, elder abuse, conditions resulting from iatrogenic causes, and stupor. Failure to recognise the conditions presenting as psychiatric emergencies in the elderly could lead to the development of complex clinical presentations and increased health expenditure (Borja *et al*, 2007). This chapter discusses the key issues in the diagnosis, assessment and treatment of these prevalent psychiatric emergencies in the elderly.

Depression and suicide

Late-onset depression is a common and potentially life-threatening illness. It remains poorly recognised and undertreated (Borja *et al*, 2007). Symptoms such as loss of appetite, decreased energy, lack of sleep, and multiple psychosomatic complaints tend to overlap in psychiatric and medical illnesses. Moreover, physicians might consider depression in the elderly to be a normal reaction to life events such as the death of a spouse, the development of multiple medical conditions, retirement, becoming increasingly dependent and the loss of purpose in life (Borja *et al*, 2007). Delaying treatment for late-onset depression is associated with increased mortality, functional impairment and use of healthcare resources. Luber and colleagues (2000) found that those with depression had nearly twice as many primary care visits, twice as many referrals to specialists and more than twice as many radiological tests, compared with non-depressed controls.

The prevalence of major depressive disorder in older persons varies, from 1–5% in the community, 5–10% in medical out-patients, 10–15% in medical in-patients and up to 42% in long-term care facilities (Piechniczek-Buczek, 2010). Depression occurs in 85% of elderly suicides and is, therefore, the predominant risk factor for suicide in this population. The rate of completed suicides in the elderly is estimated at 14.3 per 100,000. However, attempted suicide is known to be much less frequent in later life than in younger age groups. This is attributed to various factors, including social isolation, decreased physical resilience and increased use of more violent methods (Piechniczek-Buczek, 2010).

Assessment and diagnosis

Diagnostic assessment consists of a detailed review of medical and neurological problems, current medications, cognition, psychiatric history and social situation. The presence of depressive symptoms should prompt physicians to ask questions about death wishes, suicidal thoughts and intent to self-harm. The suicide ideation scale in the Chronological Assessment of Suicide Events approach can be used to improve detection of suicide ideation (Shea, 1998). Standard screening tools, such as the self-rated Geriatric Depression Scale (30, 15 and 5 items), are widely used to assess mood symptoms and monitor treatment response (Hoyl *et al*, 1999).

Treatment

Pharmacotherapy is the cornerstone of treatment for depression in the elderly. Antidepressants, such as selective serotonin reuptake inhibitors (SSRIs), are generally well tolerated as they have fewer sedative and anticholinergic adverse effects, as well as a lower risk of lethal overdose, than tricyclic antidepressants. Psychotherapeutic interventions that improve adherence to treatment, self-esteem, education and social support and diminish hopelessness are clinically recommended. A large number of studies support the effectiveness of electroconvulsive therapy for treatment of depression in the elderly, but adverse effects such as cardiac complications, cognitive decline and delirium limit its use in some patients.

Aggressive clinical intervention should be undertaken once an older adult is recognised as being suicidal. The intervention should consist of prompt, comprehensive evaluation of the nature and extent of suicidal thoughts and plans, access to means, and any past history of suicidal behaviour. Hospitalisation should be considered if an older person has intent to end their life and refuses to give up the weapon (Borja *et al*, 2007).

Delirium

Delirium is an acute, organic brain syndrome characterised by disturbed consciousness, impaired concentration, hallucinations (usually visual) and associated problems with cognition, attention and psychometric disturbances. Acute confusional state is a term used to describe the same syndrome. Delirium is a common psychiatric emergency, affecting approximately 30–50% of hospitalised elderly patients. It remains undetected in up to 70% of cases and therefore poses a significant diagnostic challenge (Piechniczek-Buczek, 2010). Early detection of delirium and early intervention to address the underlying medical factors reduce its severity and duration and results in improved outcomes for the patient (Saxena & Lawley, 2009).

Clinical presentation varies and can be categorised into three subtypes, on the basis of psychomotor behaviour: hyperactive, hypoactive and mixed. Patients with hyperactive delirium seem restless, agitated and hypervigilant and frequently experience hallucinations and delusions. Patients with hypoactive delirium seem lethargic, somnolent, and subdued, with psychomotor retardation. The hypoactive form often occurs in the elderly and gets frequently overlooked by clinicians. Mixed delirium consists of both hyperactive and hypoactive symptoms (Lipowski, 1983; Fong et al, 2009). The onset of delirium is sudden – this is the hallmark of the presentation – but the course fluctuates.

There are various hypotheses regarding the pathogenesis of delirium. There is a good evidence in support of neurotransmitter disturbances, especially acetylcholine deficiency and dopamine excess (Piechniczek-Buczek, 2010). Further evidence suggests that trauma (such as surgery and infection) can cause increased formation of pro-inflammatory cytokines, resulting in delirium in susceptible individuals (Piechniczek-Buczek, 2010).

Factors that predispose to delirium include older age, pre-existing cognitive impairment and sensory deficits. The aetiology of delirium is organic and frequently reversible, although sometimes delirium is superimposed on chronic organic mental disorder. Common causes include infections, metabolic causes such as hypomanic, electrolyte disturbance or endocrine disorders (e.g. diabetes), vitamin deficiencies (e.g. thiamine deficiency), neurological disorders (e.g. raised intracranial pressure), epilepsy, cerebrovascular disease, head injury, delirium tremens, pain, iatrogenic causes (e.g. from treatment with benzodiazepines, barbiturates, tricyclic antidepressants, anti-Parkinsonian drugs, antipsychotics, cardiac drugs, corticosteroids, or opiates), and illicit drugs.

Assessment and diagnosis

The diagnosis is made on the basis of clinical history, cognitive assessment and behavioural observation. Obtaining a history requires a full review of medical conditions, medication use, and consideration of the risk of withdrawal from drugs or alcohol and change in environment. The Confusion Assessment Method, a standardised, brief, validated algorithm, can help in identifying delirium (Inouye *et al*, 1999). In addition, the Memorial Delirium Assessment Scale is useful in quantifying delirium severity (Farrell & Ganzini, 1995; Lyons *et al*, 2008).

Treatment

Delirium is a medical emergency. It is very important to promptly identify and treat the underlying causes. Pharmacological treatment with a sedative medication can aggravate an acute confusional state and worsen the underlying medical condition, such as hypoxia by sedation. Antipsychotic medication such as haloperidol can be useful if used cautiously. Pay attention to environmental factors, such as keeping the surroundings well lit, reducing noise, and giving reassurance about procedures.

Approximately 30–40% of cases of delirium are preventable. There is increasing evidence to suggest that many non-pharmacological interventions can help prevent delirium (Tabet & Howard, 2009). Modifiable risk factors, such as dehydration, impaired mobility, impaired hearing and eyesight, and insomnia, can be targeted to reduce the risk of delirium.

Dementia

The ICD-10 defines dementia as a progressive condition caused by disease of the brain, characterised by a decline in memory and thinking that is significant enough to impair personal activities of daily living (World Health Organization, 2010). Impairment of memory typically affects the registration, storage and retrieval of new information. There is also impairment of thinking, reasoning, capacity and processing of incoming information.

In 2006, there were an estimated 683,597 people with dementia in the UK (1.1% of the population) and approximately 60% of these had Alzheimer's disease (Knapp *et al*, 2007). The number of people with dementia in the UK is forecast to reach 1,735,087 by 2051 (Knapp *et al*, 2007).

About 97% of patients with dementia develop at least one behavioural or psychological symptom of dementia (BPSD) over a 5-year period (Steinberg *et al*, 2008). These symptoms are challenging to deal with and are associated with clinical depression in carers (Ballard *et al*, 1996). Behavioural symptoms might contribute to transfer of patients into residential care (Alldred *et al*, 2007). BPSD can be divided into three main clusters, although they often co-exist: agitation, psychosis and mood disorder. They can occur at all stages of Alzheimer's disease (Ballard *et al*, 2009).

Assessment and diagnosis

Symptoms and impairment should have been present for at least 6 months in a state of clear consciousness. Several tools have been developed to assess behaviour in dementia. Validated scales for assessing behavioural changes in dementia include the Behavioural Pathology in Alzheimer's Disease rating scale, the Cohen–Mansfield Agitation Inventory and the Neuropsychiatric Inventory (Stoppe *et al*, 1999).

Treatment

The Alzheimer's Society has made recommendations for the best treatment and care of patients with BPSD and published a best-practice guide for health and social care professionals. Person-centred care is a key factor of the guide (Alzheimer's Society, 2011). The particular combination of symptoms that a patient presents with is a key consideration when selecting the most appropriate treatment.

There are serious concerns about the safety of antipsychotics in people with dementia. Side-effects include extra pyramidal symptoms, drowsiness and peripheral oedema (Ballard & Howard, 2006). Risperidone is the only antipsychotic licensed for use in dementia: short-term treatment for up to 6 weeks for persistent aggression in moderate to severe Alzheimer's disease that has not responded to non-pharmacological approaches and where there is a risk of harm to the patient or others.

Meta-analysis has shown a two-fold increase in the risk of cerebrovascular adverse events with antipsychotics (e.g. risperidone, olanzapine, aripiprazole, quetiapine) versus placebo, as well as an accelerated rate of cognitive decline with atypical antipsychotics versus placebo (Schneider *et al*, 2006). Inappropriate antipsychotic prescribing for dementia is associated with an additional 1800 deaths and 1620 cerebrovascular adverse events per year (Banerjee, 2009).

Commissioning community support services can help patients with dementia to stay in their own home. Engaging crisis resolution and home treatment services might prevent unnecessary hospital admission. Commissioners should ensure sufficient capacity in these groups for a 24/7 service. Dementia referral protocols should be jointly developed by mental healthcare providers, acute trusts, adult social services, out-of-hours services, general practices and local implementation (Department of Health, 2009).

Substance abuse

Tobacco, prescribed sedative–hypnotic drugs, and alcohol are the substances most often misused in the elderly. However, alcohol misuse significantly exceeds drug misuse (Atkinson, 1991).

The estimated prevalence of alcoholism among the elderly can vary, because studies assess use differently (self-report versus strict diagnostic criteria) and have included different populations (community versus medical settings). Approximately 2–4% of community dwelling elders, 18% of elderly in-patients in medical wards, 14% of elderly patients in emergency department and more than 20% of elderly in-patients in psychiatric wards meet criteria for alcohol abuse or dependence (O'Connell *et al*, 2003).

Assessment and diagnosis

Standard screening measures such as the four-question CAGE approach might be useful in some settings. Two or more positive answers suggest alcoholism or problem drinking (Ewing, 1984). The Michigan Alcoholism Screening Test – Geriatric Version, developed by Blow and colleagues (1992), is a commonly used assessment tool.

Treatment

Alcohol withdrawal can be treated on an out-patient basis; however, it might be easier to help a patient with detoxification as an in-patient, following the general principle of sedation achieved by regular oral medication, which should be started when there are clear signs of withdrawal. Alcohol withdrawal treatment is discussed more fully in Chapter 4.

Symptoms of withdrawal from alcohol might be present after about 8 h following abrupt cessation of chronic heavy drinking or a week of binge drinking. In some cases, there might be hallucinations, withdrawal seizures and delirium tremens. Delirium tremens usually manifests 3–5 days after withdrawal from alcohol, so it is not prudent to discharge a patient before 5 days of admission. Delirium tremens is associated with high mortality (10%) and therefore must always be treated in hospital (McGrath & Bowker, 1987).

Wernicke's encephalopathy is an acute syndrome resulting from thiamine deficiency consisting of a triad of symptoms such as ataxia, ophthalmoplegia and global confusional state with confusion and memory loss. The condition can be easily missed as the classical signs are not invariably present and there might be a gradual start of symptoms over days. Wernicke's encephalopathy is potentially reversible, if treated with intravenous thiamine and other measures as necessary for treatment of delirium.

Elder abuse and neglect

The term elder abuse usually applies when the victim is of retirement age. Neglect describes the behaviour of an abuser in failing in some way to meet a victim's needs (Jacoby & Oppenheimer, 1991). The American Medical Association defines elder abuse and neglect as an act or omission that results in harm to or threatened harm to the health or welfare of an elderly person (Piechniczek-Buczek, 2006).

Abuse should be suspected if patients present with multiple injuries that are unexplained or in various stages of development. Neglect should be suspected if an elderly person presents with significant negligence in hygiene, medical care and nutrition despite having an assigned carer. Risk factors for abuse and neglect include severe cognitive and functional decline and shared living arrangements with the carer.

There is increasing evidence that abuse, including violence, threats, negligence and restraint, is probably under-reported. There is a risk of professionals overlooking and carers concealing abuse. Elderly people are often ignorant of their legal rights and might be too apathetic, debilitated and cognitively impaired to be able to report the abuse. Physical abuse includes beating, scalding, burning, and poor diet and hygiene (McGrath & Bowker, 1987).

Assessment and diagnosis

Assessment should include taking a detailed history from the patients without the suspected abuser being present. It is important to record the specific circumstances of an injury. Physical examination might show up bite marks, lacerations, abrasions, bruises and burns. Look for signs of confinement by a chain or to a bed, marks due to prolonged sitting on the lavatory, infected wounds, and dirty or urine-soaked clothing. The patient might become frightened and vigilant of those around him. Caretakers might seem withdrawn, aggressive and threatening with the patient.

Treatment

Treatment should consist of emergency assessment recognition of the abuse and engagement with the family. Referral to the specialist services such as the Adult Protection Service for the elderly and the support of carers is imperative.

In the UK, the Mental Health Act can be used to detain victims of abuse with mental illness in a hospital. Abusers who have mental illness may also be treated under the Act. Power of guardianship under the Act would allow a local authority to take responsibility for the care of a mentally ill or disabled elderly person and to direct an elderly person to live in a residential home. Under Section 47 of the National Assistance Act 1948, an elderly person who is neglected to a degree that their habitation is a danger to public health may be placed into permanent care. Under the Mental Capacity Act 2009, abuse and neglect of the elderly is a criminal offence (Fiske *et al*, 2009).

Iatrogenically induced conditions presenting as psychiatric emergencies

Antipsychotics

Life-threatening complications of antipsychotic treatments are found in 1% of treated individuals. Neuroleptic malignant syndrome (NMS), although uncommon, is associated with high-potency neuroleptics such as haloperidol and fluphenazine (Kennedy & Onuogu, 1999). It can also be caused by atypical antipsychotics such as olanzapine (Borja *et al*, 2007). It is characterised by muscular rigidity, autonomic instability, hyperthermia, elevation in creatine phosphokinase and leucocytosis (Neilsen & Bruhn, 2005). Symptoms such as hyperthermia and rigidity might be absent in subclinical presentations, but clinicians should still consider the possibility of NMS because of its potential gravity. Death of the patient can be due to renal failure as a result of rhabdomyolisis, arrhythmia or cardiovascular collapse. The mortality rate of NMS is between 10 and 30% (Tiryaki *et al*, 2006).

Treatment of NMS is mainly supportive, consisting of immediate withdrawal of causative agents, adequate hydration and the application of ice packs and cooling blankets. Benzodiazepine can be prescribed to manage agitation. Bromocriptine and dantrolene can also be used in a specialist medical setting if the supportive measures mentioned are not effective (Sachdev, 2005).

Acute dystonic reaction is another acute adverse effect of antipsychotic use, characterised by spasm of skeletal muscle. Typically involving contraction of the oro-bucco-lingual, extra-occular or neck muscles, it is often extremely alarming and painful. Immediate treatment with anticholinergic agents is indicated and urgent parenteral administration might be necessary (Merson & Baldwin, 1995).

Selective serotonin reuptake inhibitors and serotonin syndrome

Serotonin syndrome is a condition that is mainly caused by selective serotonin reuptake inhibitors (SSRIs) via various mechanisms: blockade of serotonin reuptake, increased production of serotonin, increased serotonin release on direct stimulation of serotonin receptors (Borja *et al*, 2007). It might be difficult to distinguish from NMS as it is also characterised by autonomic instability, confusion, tremor and myoclonus. Concomitant use of antidepressants and antipsychotics mainly atypical antipsychotics such as risperidone and olanzapine might further confound distinguishing between the two conditions. It is important to recognise this condition as severe cases can result in rhabdomyolisis, renal failure, hyperkalaemia, seizures and even death. The treatment includes SSRI withdrawal and use of benzodiazepines for seizure and myoclonus. Tricyclic antidepressants, like SSRIs, can give rise to serotonin syndrome especially in combination with other serotonergic drugs as well as monoamine oxidase inhibitors (Borja *et al*, 2007).

Benzodiazepines

Benzodiazepines are used for treating anxiety and agitation, but they have often caused delirium and worsening of an underlying cognitive impairment; chronic use might result in excessive daytime sleepiness, lethargy, and unsteady gait. This class of psychotropic medication is most often associated with falls and hip fractures. It is best to limit their use to low dose and short-term therapy and encourage the use of agents that are short-acting and have low lipid solubility (Borja *et al*, 2007).

Medication implicated in falls

It is well established that there is a relationship between polypharmacy and falls, but the relationship between specific classes of drugs and falls is not clear. Drug classes that have most commonly been implicated in the aetiology of falls include psychotropic medication, such as hypnotics, anxiolytics, antidepressants and antipsychotics.

Many epidemiological studies that have examined the association between psychoactive medications and falls indicate that there is a two- to three-fold higher risk of falling when using these medications and a two-fold higher risk of experiencing a hip fracture. The use of multiple psychoactive medications has an adverse synergistic effect on the risk of falling (Matters *et al*, 2001).

Stupor

Stupor is defined as the syndrome of akinetic mutism, in which patients are silent and immobile but fully conscious. There are various psychiatric causes of stupor, such as dementia, schizophrenia and depression, as well as neurological causes, such as epilepsy, encephalitis and Parkinson's disease. The clinical features of patients presenting with stupor caused by neurological illness include sudden onset, evidence of abnormality on neurological examination and disturbance of the level of consciousness. By comparison, there is often a recent history of stressful life events and previous similar presentations in patients presenting with stupor caused by psychiatric illness. Patients in a state of stupor should always be regarded as medical emergencies, as it is extremely difficult to distinguish organic from psychiatric causes of stupor. Immediate treatment should include identification of underlying causes, seeking information from other sources such as informants and medical records, and admission to hospital, which might require implementation of the Mental Health Act.

Conclusions

The clinical presentation of elderly people as psychiatric emergencies is complicated by adverse medication-induced events and substance abuse (Chan *et al*, 2009). Behavioural disturbance in the elderly might be secondary to underlying organic conditions (Borja *et al*, 2007). Comorbid medical conditions often result in psychiatric hospitalisation (Lyketsos *et al*, 2002): urinary tract infection, subdural haematoma and thyrotoxicosis are only a few of the illnesses that can cause delusion and agitation that might be mistaken for functional impairment. It is important to note that, in older patients, comorbidity has been the norm rather than exception, resulting in a complicated clinical picture that requires thorough assessment (Borja *et al*, 2007). As older patients are more likely to be medically, as well as psychiatrically, ill, particular attention should be paid to the possibility of adverse drugs reactions and unrecognised medical disorders in elderly patients with behavioural disturbances (Woo *et al*, 2003).

References

AgeDiscrimination.info (n.d.) *Age Discrimination Statistics* (http://www.agediscrimination. info/statistics/Pages/Statistics).

Alldred DP, Petty DR, Bowie P, *et al* (2007) Antipsychotic prescribing patterns in care homes and relationship with dementia. *Psychiatric Bulletin*, **31**: 329–332.

Alzheimer's Society (2011) *Optimising Treatment and Care for People with Behavioural and Psychological Symptoms of Dementia*. Alzheimer's Society.

Atkinson RM (1991) Alcohol and drug abuse in the elderly. In *Psychiatry in the Elderly* (eds R Jacoby, C Oppenheimer). Oxford University Press.

Ballard C, Howard R (2006) Neuroleptic drugs in dementia: benefits and harm. *Nature Reviews Neuroscience*, **7**: 492–500.

Ballard CG, Eastwood C, Gahir M, *et al* (1996) A follow up study of depression in the carers of dementia sufferers. *BMJ*, **312**: 947.

Ballard CG, Gauthier S, Cummings JL, *et al* (2009) Management of agitation and aggression associated with Alzheimer disease. *Nature Reviews Neurology*, **5**: 245–265.

Banerjee S (2009) *The Use of Antipsychotic Medication for People with Dementia: Time for Action*. Department of Health.

Blow FC, Brower KJ, Schulenberg JE, *et al* (1992) The Michigan Alcoholism Screening Test – Geriatric Version (MAST-G): a new elderly-specific screening instrument [abstract]. *Alcoholism: Clinical and Experimental Research*, **16**: 372.

Borja B, Borja CS, Gade S (2007) Psychiatric emergencies in the geriatric population. *Clinics in Geriatric Medicine*, **23**: 391–400, vii.

Chan VT, Woo BK, Sewell DD, *et al* (2009) Reduction of suboptimal prescribing and clinical outcome for dementia patients in a senior behavioural health inpatient unit. *International Psychogeriatrics*, **21**: 195–199.

Cracknell R (2010) The ageing population. In *Value for Money in Public Services*. House of Commons Library Research.

Department of Health (2009) *Living Well with Dementia: A National Dementia Strategy*. Department of Health.

Ewing JA (1984) Detecting alcoholism. The CAGE questionnaire. *JAMA*, **252**: 1905–1907.

Farrell KR, Ganzini I (1995) Misdiagnosing delirium as depression in medically ill elderly patients. *Annals of Internal Medicine*, **155**: 2459–2464.

Fiske A, Wetherell JL, Gatz M (2009) Depression in older adults. *Annual Review of Clinical Psychology*, **5**: 363–389.

Fong TG, Tulebaev SR, Inouye SK (2009) Delirium in elderly adults: diagnosis, prevention and treatment. *Nature Reviews Neurology*, **5**: 210–220.

Hoyl MT, Alessi CA, Harker Jo, *et al* (1999) Development and testing of a five-item version of the Geriatric Depression Scale. *Journal of the American Geriatric Society*, **47**: 873–878.

Inouye SK, Bogardus ST Jr, Charpentier PA, *et al* (1999) A multicomponent intervention to prevent delirium in hospitalised older adults. *New England Journal of Medicine*, **340**: 669–676.

Jacoby R, Oppenheimer C (1991) *Psychiatry in the Elderly*. Oxford University Press.

Kennedy GJ, Onuogu E (1999) Psychiatric emergencies: rapid response and life-saving therapies. *Geriatrics*, **54**: 38–44.

Knapp M, Prince M, Albanese E, *et al* (2007) *Dementia UK. A Report into the Prevalence and Cost of Dementia Prepared by the Personal Social Services Research Unit (PSSRU) at the London School of Economics and the Institute of Psychiatry at King's College London, for the Alzheimer's Society. Summary of Key Findings.* Alzheimer's Society.

Lipowski ZJ (1983) Transient cognitive disorders (delirium, acute confusional states) in the elderly. *American Journal of Psychiatry*, **140**: 1426–1436.

Luber MP, Holtenberg JP, Williams-Russo P, *et al* (2000) Diagnosis, treatment, comorbidity, and resource utilisation of depressed patients in a general medical practice. *International Journal of Psychiatry in Medicine*, **30**: 1–13.

Lyketsos CG, Dunn G, Kaminsky MJ, *et al* (2002) Medical comorbity in psychiatric inpatients: relation to clinical outcomes and hospital length of stay. *Psychosomatics*, **43**: 24–30.

Lyons DL, Grimley SM, Sydnor L (2008) Double trouble: when delirium complicates dementia. *Nursing*, **38**: 48–55.

Matters B, Merry HB, Sherrington C, *et al* (2001) Medications are risk factors for falls. In *Falls in Older People* (eds SR Lord, C Sherrington, HB Merry). Cambridge University Press.

McGrath G, Bowker M (1987) *Common Psychiatric Emergencies*. Butterworth–Heinemann.

Merson S, Baldwin D (1995) *Psychiatric Emergencies*. Oxford University Press.

Neilsen J, Bruhn AM (2005) Atypical neuroleptic malignant syndrome caused by olanzapine. *Acta Psychiatrica Scandinavica*, **112**: 238–240.

O'Connell H, Chin AV, Cunningham C, *et al* (2003) Alcohol use disorders in elderly people: redefining an age old problem in old age. *BMJ*, **327**: 664–667.

Piechniczek-Buczek J (2006) Psychiatric emergencies in the elderly population. *Emergency Medicine Clinics of North America*, **24**: 467–490.

Piechniczek-Buczek J (2010) Psychiatric emergencies in the elderly. *Psychiatric Times*, **27** (7).

Sachdev P (2005) Neuroleptic-induced movement disorders: an overview. *Psychiatric Clinics of North America*, **28**: 255–274.

Saxena S, Lawley D (2009) Delirium in the elderly: a clinical review. *Postgraduate Medical Journal*, **85**: 405–413.

Schneider LS, Dagerman K, Insel PS (2006) Efficacy and adverse effects of atypical antipsychotics for dementia: meta-analysis of randomized, placebo-controlled trials. *American Journal Geriatric Psychiatry*, **14**: 191–210.

Shea SC (1998) The chronological assessment of suicide events; a practical interviewing strategy for the elicitation of suicidal ideation. *Journal of Clinical Psychiatry*, **59** (Suppl 20): 58–72.

Steinberg M, Shao H, Zandi P, *et al* (2008) Point and 5-year period prevalence of neuropsychiatric symptoms in dementia: the Cache County Study. *International Journal of Geriatric Psychiatry*, **23**: 170–177.

Stoppe G, Brandt CA, Staedt JH (1999) Behavioural problems associated with dementia: the role of new antipsychotics. *Drugs and Aging*, **14**: 41–54.

Tabet N, Howard R (2009) Non-pharmacological interventions in the prevention of delirium. *Age and Ageing*, **38**: 374–379.

Tiryaki A, Kandemir G, Ismail AK (2006) The life-threatening adverse effects of psychotropic drugs: a case report [in Turkish]. *Turk Psikiyatri Dergisi*, **17**: 147–151.

Woo BK, Daly JW, Allen EC, *et al* (2003) Unrecognised medical disorders in older psychiatric inpatients in a senior behavioural health unit in a university hospital. *Journal of Geriatric Psychiatry and Neurology*, **16**: 121–125.

World Health Organization (2010) *International Classification of Diseases (10th edn)*. WHO.

CHAPTER 14

Perinatal psychiatric emergencies

Carol Henshaw

The conception rate in most women suffering from a mental disorder is the same as in the general population. Only those suffering from moderate to severe intellectual disability, anorexia nervosa or psychosis have lower rates. However, despite the lower conception rate in women with psychosis, estimates of the number of such women who are mothers range from 56 to 63% (McGrath *et al*, 1999; Howard *et al*, 2002). Women with affective disorders are more likely to be multiparous (Jablensky *et al*, 2005). Therefore, mental health professionals working with women of childbearing potential are likely to have to deal with a psychiatric emergency involving a pregnant or postpartum woman at some point, and many of the women they treat have the potential to become pregnant. This chapter will address the treatment of such patients.

Pregnancy

More than a third of pregnant women suffer from a mental disorder (Kelly *et al*, 2001). Some will be experiencing pre-existing disorders, whereas others will experience a new onset. Pregnancy is a mulitfactorial stressor and might contribute to women with a past history of mental disorder experiencing a recurrence, particularly if medication has been discontinued.

It has previously been thought that pregnancy is protective against relapse; for example, that women with bipolar disorder are less likely to experience an episode of illness during pregnancy (Sharma & Persad 1995; Grof *et al*, 2000). However, a third to half of all bipolar women experience worsened symptoms during pregnancy (Blehar *et al*, 1998; Freeman *et al*, 2002). In the latter study, those who had symptoms in pregnancy were more likely to have a postpartum episode and their episodes were almost exclusively depressive. Akdeniz *et al* (2003) observed that 32% of bipolar women had episodes during pregnancy or postpartum. Viguera & Cohen (1998) identified that episodes during pregnancy are more likely to be depressive or dysphoric mixed states than in manic states. Half of these occurred in the first trimester.

Pregnancy should be considered as a possibility in any woman who presents as a psychiatric emergency, as 50% of pregnancies in the UK are unplanned. A woman who is very unwell might not tell you or even be aware that she is pregnant. The youngest mother in the UK was 11 years old when she delivered and the oldest was in her 60s, so this is not just an issue for psychiatrists treating women of working age.

The Centre for Maternal and Child Enquires (CMACE, 2011) requires that any woman who has a pre-existing, underlying, serious mental health condition or who develops one during pregnancy should be referred to specialist services, and that the referral should be considered as urgent. A woman who requires hospital admission in late pregnancy should be transferred to a mother and baby unit and specialist advice regarding the management of pregnant women should be obtained from the nearest perinatal psychiatry service. Unfortunately, such services are not universal, so it might be necessary to go out of area to access them. By 28 weeks, women with serious mental illness should have a care plan covering the remainder of pregnancy, delivery and the postpartum period; this plan should be held in all versions of their records (paper, hand-held and electronic) and communicated to all professionals involved in their care in primary and secondary care, including maternity services.

When proposing treatment for a woman of reproductive potential, there are several important factors to consider:

- Try to ascertain the date of the last menstrual period and, if she has capacity, ask permission to undertake a pregnancy test before administering medication.
- If the woman lacks capacity, then it is in her best interests for a pregnancy test to be performed.
- Ensure that you know where the nearest sexual health clinic or family planning clinic is, if you are not working in a general hospital setting with easy access to gynaecology.
- Ensure there is access to emergency contraception if a woman has had unprotected intercourse. Levonorgestrel, known as the morning-after pill, is 98.5% effective if used within 72 h and an intrauterine device is almost 100% effective within 5 days.
- Consider the possibility of a sexually transmitted infection and know where to refer to if you need to.

Deliberate self-harm during pregnancy

The rate of attempted suicide (most often assessed by hospital attendance rates) is lower in pregnant women than in the general population. Two studies in the USA estimated it to be about half the rate for non-pregnant women (Greenblatt *et al*, 1997; Weiss, 1999). However, many more cases of deliberate self-harm will not come to medical attention or will have presented at emergency departments and not been admitted.

One small study has found previous loss of a child to be associated with attempted suicide (Lester & Beck, 1988). In Pakistan, domestic abuse, depression and anxiety are the most common risk factors for suicidal thoughts or attempts (Asad *et al*, 2010). In a study of pregnant teenagers in the USA, Bayatpour *et al* (1992) found that the teens with a history of physical and sexual abuse were at high risk for self-destructive behaviours. Farber *et al* (1996) observed that those with a history of physical or sexual abuse are more likely to have suicidal ideation during pregnancy and also more likely to have made a suicide attempt in the past. Marishane & Moodley (2005), reporting on three cases of parasuicide in South Africa, noted they were young (21 years of age or younger), were socioeconomically deprived and had dysfunctional family relationships.

A teratologic evaluation of infants born to mothers who took drug overdoses during pregnancy reported that the rate of congenital anomalies was not significantly higher than in controls (Czeizel & Mosonyi, 1997). Flint *et al* (2002) found that a drug overdose shortly before or during pregnancy was associated with a substantially increased risk of miscarriage, but no increase in fetal pathology among the fetuses surviving until birth. Gandhi *et al* (2006) examined maternal and neonatal outcomes after attempted suicide during pregnancy. It was associated with significantly higher rates of maternal and perinatal morbidity (and in some cases perinatal mortality), including premature labour, Caesarean section, blood transfusion, low birth weight, respiratory distress and neonatal and infant death.

Any woman who self-harms when she is aware she is pregnant should be risk-assessed regarding the safety of the unborn child and referred to safeguarding services where the risk assessment suggests this is needed. However, as such referrals can lead to women disengaging from care, this needs to be managed sensitively and is best done by specialist perinatal mental health teams.

Domestic abuse

Domestic abuse can increase in incidence and severity during pregnancy, and as women who are victims often self-harm and/or have depressed mood, this needs to be considered in assessment. Frequent presentation to emergency departments with minor injuries and complaints, mental health problems or injuries of different ages should raise the possibility of domestic abuse. This should also be suspected if the partner is constantly present at examinations, is domineering, answers all questions for her, is unwilling to leave the room or if the woman seems evasive or reluctant to speak or disagree in front of her partner. Professionals should know what to do if they suspect domestic abuse, including how to help a woman disclose abuse confidentially (using interpreters where necessary) and how to refer to the local multidisciplinary support network if this is required. For more information see Task Force on the Health Aspects of Violence Against Women and Children (2010).

Admitting a pregnant woman

Any pregnant woman admitted to a mental health hospital or home treatment should have an urgent midwifery assessment, as women with serious mental illness are less likely to attend for antenatal care and, when they do, often receive poorer-quality care than women in the general population (Howard, 2005). This is despite the fact that they have an increased risk of complications such as placental abruption, toxic effects of alcohol and illicit drugs, stillbirth, preterm delivery, small-for-gestational-age and low-birth-weight babies, and a higher incidence of congenital anomalies (Nilsson *et al*, 2002; Jablensky *et al*, 2005). Women with particularly chaotic lifestyles might not be registered with a general practitioner or might have failed to attend appointments, fearing that their children could be removed from their care. They can present as emergencies in a late stage of pregnancy. In this case, obstetric advice must be sought.

Any pregnant woman who is still smoking when assessed should be referred for smoking cessation support, and those using illicit drugs or alcohol should be provided with integrated specialist care. They should not be managed solely by their general practitioner or midwife and mental health professionals should not assume, when seeing a woman in an emergency situation, that referral to a specialist service has been made. Integrated care should include addictions professionals, child safeguarding, and specialist midwifery and obstetrics (CMACE, 2011).

Rapid tranquillisation of pregnant women

If a pregnant woman requires rapid tranquillisation, she should be managed according to local policies, which are usually based around national guidelines on the short-term management of disturbed and violent behaviour. However, there are some additional factors to consider, listed below.

- Restraint procedures should take pregnancy into account and not use any forms of restraint that might compromise the fetus. The abdomen should be protected and she should not be laid on her back, as this can cause aorto-caval compression. The left lateral position is preferred.
- She should not be placed in seclusion after rapid tranquillisation.
- Antipsychotics or benzodiazepines with short half-lives are the preferred medication and both at the minimum effective dose. If a benzodiazepine is used in late pregnancy, the risks of floppy baby syndrome must be considered.
- Should a woman require rapid tranquillisation close to term, in labour or soon after delivery, it is advisable to request paediatric and anaesthetic opinions.

243

Postpartum

Overall, 2% of all new mothers will be referred to psychiatric services (not all as emergencies) and 0.2% will suffer from puerperal psychosis. The women most at risk of recurrence of mental illness postpartum, and hence most likely to present as a psychiatric emergency, are those with an affective disorder. However, a substantial minority (21.72%) of women with schizophrenia who have had an admission before pregnancy will also relapse postpartum (Harlow *et al*, 2007).

Up to 67% of women with bipolar disorder will experience a recurrence in the immediate postpartum period (Kendell *et al*, 1987; Terp & Mortensen, 1998; Freeman *et al*, 2002; Robertson *et al*, 2005). Those with a family history of puerperal relapse are particularly likely to relapse postpartum (Jones & Craddock, 2001) and the risk of recurrence seems to be the same in women with either bipolar I or bipolar II disorder; however, recurrence is more likely if they have had more than four episodes (Viguera *et al*, 2000). A history of bipolar disorder was the strongest predictor of psychiatric admission 10–19 days postpartum in a recent study (Munk-Olsen *et al*, 2009).

Postpartum relapse is particularly likely if maintenance medication has been discontinued (Viguera *et al*, 2000). Sometimes the woman herself will have done this, advised by family, friends or a well-meaning health professional who has failed to carry out a full risk–benefit analysis of any potential risk to the fetus against the risks of the untreated disorder. The risk of recurrence remains even if the woman has been well during pregnancy, for many years previously, and has good social support. The time to relapse is shortened if there is a rapid (within 2 weeks) rather than a slower discontinuation of medication (over 2–4 weeks). Cohen *et al* (1995) estimated the relative risk of recurrence for women who did not receive maintenance medication as 8.6 times that of women who did. All women who opt to discontinue medication during pregnancy should have a clear plan for the postpartum risk period, including re-introduction of medication.

The onset of symptoms tends to be rapid: within 48–72 h of delivery if there is a manic relapse, days or weeks after delivery if there is a depressive relapse. Half of all women with puerperal psychosis will have presented within 7 days after delivery and 90% within 3 months (Kendell *et al*, 1987). Mixed affective states might be more common at this time (Wisner *et al*, 1993).

The early signs of illness are often non-specific (e.g. insomnia, agitation, perplexity, excess anxiety, odd behaviour). Such symptoms can easily be overlooked or attributed to postpartum blues or anxiety and their significance not recognised. However, as onset of symptoms and deterioration is frequently rapid, the woman might be floridly psychotic within a few hours. As these illnesses are not very common, this situation can be very unfamiliar to non-specialist psychiatrists and other health professionals. When asked to assess a postpartum woman, it is very important to ascertain psychiatric history and family history and take non-specific or apparently minor symptoms seriously, particularly if there is a relevant history.

Medical professionals face significant pressure to minimise the hospitalisation of mental health patients. CMACE (2011) recommends a lower threshold for admission and rapid response for puerperal women and advises that treatment by multiple teams should be avoided. The pressure to treat at home one psychotic woman with a previous puerperal psychosis and suicide attempt who was preoccupied with her suicide attempt did not result in a positive outcome; introducing two other teams to her care and visiting regularly did not prevent her from killing herself a few hours after a visit (CMACE, 2011).

In low-income countries, there is high comorbidity with physical health problems, including anaemia, infection and oedema proteinuria hypertension gestosis (Ndosi & Mtawali, 2002). However, in the UK, some women have died because symptoms of serious physical illness were misattributed to a mental disorder. This can lead to delays in diagnosis and treatment (for example, admitting a woman who is seriously physically ill to a psychiatric hospital) and are particularly likely to happen when there are unexplained physical symptoms, or when the only symptoms are distress and agitation in a patient who does not speak English. Having a history of psychiatric illness can often lead professionals to assume subsequent presentations are due to a mental disorder. Physical conditions that were attributed to mental disorder and resulted in the death of the patient include subarachnoid haemorrhage, aortic aneurism and pulmonary embolus, epilepsy, an autoimmune disorder, encephalopathy and pneumonia (CMACE, 2011).

Assessing a postpartum woman

It is vital when assessing any mentally unwell postpartum woman to consider not only the risk to herself but also her thoughts regarding her baby and/or other children. Morbid ideas of maternal incompetence and danger to the infant are a common feature of maternal mental illness, and some depressed women experience intrusive obsessional thoughts that their baby will come to some harm. Others will have delusions involving their infants, who might then be at risk. Early symptoms that might indicate the infant is at risk include a feeling that she or he is not really hers, or that the infant is looking at her in a strange way. These symptoms can be followed by frankly delusional ideas.

Many women fear that their children will be removed from their care; therefore, referral to safeguarding teams should not be routine when mothers develop a mental illness. It should only take place as the result of a risk assessment and where the infant has suffered, or is likely to suffer, from harm. When referral to the safeguarding team is necessary, extra vigilance and care are required. Otherwise, referral to social services might result in avoidance of care and necessary treatment and might increase the risk of deterioration in the mother's mental health and suicide. Some mothers, particularly those with substance abuse problems, have killed themselves soon after their child has been removed from their care (CMACE, 2011).

One US study reported that women with a psychiatric disorder have a 27.4-fold risk of hospitalisation following a postpartum suicide attempt, those with substance misuse a 6.2-fold risk, and those with dual diagnosis an 11.1-fold risk (Comtois *et al*, 2008). With very few exceptions, the mothers who have died by suicide in the three most recent UK confidential enquiries had been cared for by non-specialist psychiatric services, underlining the importance of the recommendation that such women should be referred to specialist perinatal mental health services, even if this is outside their own district.

The fact that a woman is in good social circumstances, married, older, well-educated and/or a professional and is well during pregnancy does not protect her from becoming seriously mentally ill after delivery and killing herself. Of the deaths from psychiatric causes recorded in the most recent enquiry (CMACE, 2011), 76% were women who were employed, or whose partner was employed; their median age was 30 years, 41% were educated to at least A-level standard, 28% were in professional occupations and 90% were white. Those assessing postpartum women must remember that not all serious mental illness is associated with social adversity and deprivation.

Postpartum women who attempt or complete suicide are more likely to use violent methods than women in the general population and are, therefore, much more likely to succeed. The most common methods, used by around half of those who have died, are hanging or jumping from a height, followed by self-immolation and drowning.

Medication and breast feeding

All psychotropic medications pass into breast milk and only two (clozapine and lithium) are contraindicated. The guidelines below apply to all others.

If you need to medicate a breast-feeding mother:

- use the same drug as was used in pregnancy (if any), wherever possible
- avoid multiple drug use, either concomitantly or in succession
- use short-acting drugs so that timing of feeds can be when drug levels are lowest, or encourage the mother to express and discard milk at the time of the highest dose
- encourage the mother to consider expressing milk and having someone else do night feeds if sleep deprivation is a problem
- be more cautious if the infant is preterm or sick, and in every case monitor weight gain, feeding and conscious level throughout.

Conclusions

Treating a pregnant or postpartum woman as a psychiatric emergency requires the consideration of many issues beyond the situation many psychiatrists are familiar with. Knowledge of the specific risks involved and acting on these can prevent considerable morbidity and mortality.

References

Akdeniz F, Vahip S, Pirildar S, *et al* (2003) Risk factors associated with childbearing-related episodes in women with bipolar disorder. *Psychopathology*, **36**: 234–238.

Asad N, Karmaliani R, Sullaiman N, *et al* (2010) Prevalence of suicidal thoughts and attempts among pregnant Pakistani women. *Acta Obstetricia et Gynecologica Scandinavica*, **89**: 1545–1551.

Bayatpour M, Wells RD, Holford S (1992) Physical and sexual abuse as predictors of substance use and suicide among pregnant teenagers. *Journal of Adolescent Health*, **13**: 128–132.

Blehar MC, DePaulo Jr JR, Gershon ES, *et al* (1998) Women with bipolar disorder: findings from the NIMH Genetics Initiative sample. *Psychopharmacology Bulletin*, **34**: 239–243.

Centre for Maternal and Child Enquiries (2011) Saving Mothers' Lives: Reviewing Maternal Deaths to Make Motherhood Safer: 2006–08. The Eighth Report on Confidential Enquiries into Maternal Deaths in the United Kingdom. *British Journal of Obstetrics and Gynaecology*, **118** (Suppl 1): 1–203.

Cohen L, Sichel D, Robertson L, *et al* (1995) Postpartum prophylaxis for women with bipolar disorder. *American Journal of Psychiatry*, **152**: 1641–1645.

Comtois KA, Schiff MA, Grossman DC (2008) Psychiatric risk factors associated with postpartum suicide attempt in Washington State, 1992–2001. *American Journal of Obstetrics and Gynecology*, **199**: 120.e1–5.

Czeizel AE, Mosonyi A (1997) Monitoring of early human fetal development in women exposed to large doses of chemicals. *Environmental and Molecular Mutagenesis*, **30**: 240–244.

Farber EW, Herbert SE, Reviere SL (1996) Childhood abuse and suicidality in obstetrics patients in a hospital-based urban prenatal clinic. *General Hospital Psychiatry*, **18**: 56–60.

Flint C, Larsen H, Nielsen GL, *et al* (2002) Pregnancy outcome after suicide attempt by drug use: a Danish population-based study. *Acta Obstetricia et Gynecologica Scandinavica*, **81**: 516–522.

Freeman MP, Smith KW, Freeman SA, *et al* (2002) The impact of reproductive events on the course of bipolar disorder in women. *Journal of Clinical Psychiatry*, **63**: 284–287.

Gandhi SG, Gilbert WM, McElvy SS, *et al* (2006) Maternal and neonatal outcomes after attempted suicide. *Obstetrics and Gynecology*, **107**: 984–990.

Greenblatt JF, Dannenberg AL, Johnson CJ (1997) Incidence of hospitalized injuries among pregnant women in Maryland, 1979–1990. *American Journal of Preventive Medicine*, **13**: 374–379.

Grof P, Robbins W, Alda M, *et al* (2000) Protective effect of pregnancy in women with lithium-responsive bipolar disorder. *Journal of Affective Disorders*, **61**: 31–39.

Harlow BL, Vitonis AF, Sparen P, *et al* (2007) Incidence of hospitalization for postpartum psychotic and bipolar episodes in women with and without prior prepregnancy or prenatal psychiatric hospitalizations. *Archives of General Psychiatry*, **64**: 42–48.

Howard LM (2005) Fertility and pregnancy in women with psychotic disorders. *European Journal of Obstetrics & Gynecology and Reproductive Biology*, **119**: 3–10.

Howard LM, Kumar C, Leese M, *et al* (2002) The general fertility rate in women with psychotic disorders. *American Journal of Psychiatry*, **159**: 991–997.

Jablensky AV, Morgan V, Zubrick SR, *et al* (2005) Pregnancy, delivery, and neonatal complications in a population cohort of women with schizophrenia and major affective disorders. *American Journal of Psychiatry*, **162**: 79–91.

Jones I, Craddock N (2001) Familiality of the puerperal trigger in bipolar disorder: results of a family study. *American Journal of Psychiatry*, **158**: 913–917.

Kelly RH, Zatick D, Anders TF, *et al* (2001) The detection and treatment of psychiatric disorders and substance use among pregnant women cared for in obstetrics. *American Journal of Psychiatry*, **158**: 213–219.

Kendell RE, Chalmers JC, Platz C (1987) Epidemiology of puerperal psychoses. *British Journal of Psychiatry*, **150**: 662–673.

Lester D, Beck AT (1988) Attempted suicide and pregnancy. *American Journal of Obstetrics and Gynecology*, **158**: 1084–1085.

Marishane T, Moodley J (2005) Parasuicide in pregnancy. *International Journal of Gynecology and Obstetrics*, **89**: 268–271.

McGrath JJ, Hearle J, Jenner L, *et al* (1999) The fertility and fecundity of patients with psychoses. *Acta Psychiatrica Scandinavica*, **99**: 441–446.

Munk-Olsen T, Laursen TM, Mendelson T, *et al* (2009) Risks and predictors of readmission for a mental disorder during the postpartum period. *Archives of General Psychiatry*, **66**: 189–195.

Ndosi NK, Mtawali LM (2002) The nature of puerperal psychosis at Muhimbili National Hospital: its physical co-morbidity, associated main obstetric and social factors. *African Journal of Reproductive Health*, **6**: 41–49.

Nilsson E, Lichtenstein P, Cnattingius S, *et al* (2002) Women with schizophrenia: pregnancy outcome and infant death among their offspring. *Schizophrenia Research*, **58**: 221–229.

Robertson E, Jones I, Haque S, *et al* (2005) Risk of puerperal and non-puerperal recurrence of illness following bipolar affective puerperal (post-partum) psychosis. *British Journal of Psychiatry*, **186**: 258–259.

Sharma V, Prasad E (1995) Effect of pregnancy on three cases with bipolar disorder. *Annals of Clinical Psychiatry*, **7**: 30–42.

Task Force on the Health Aspects of Violence Against Women and Children (2010) *Responding to Violence Against Women and Children—the Role of the NHS*. Department of Health.

Terp I, Mortensen P (1998) Post-partum psychosis. *British Journal of Psychiatry*, **172**: 521–526.

Viguera AC, Cohen LS (1998) The course and management of bipolar disorder during pregnancy. *Psychopharmacology Bulletin*, **34**: 339–346.

Viguera AC, Nonacs R, Cohen LS, *et al* (2000) Risk of recurrence of bipolar disorder in pregnant and nonpregnant women after discontinuing lithium maintenance. *American Journal of Psychiatry*, **157**: 179–184.

Weiss HB (1999) Pregnancy-associated injury hospitalizations in Pennsylvania, 1995. *Annals of Emergency Medicine*, **34**: 626–636.

Wisner KL, Peindl K, Hanusa BH (1993) Relationship of psychiatric illness to childbearing status: a hospital-based epidemiologic study. *Journal of Affective Disorders*, **28**: 39–50.

CHAPTER 15

Civilian and military psychological trauma

Martin P. Deahl

Traumatic events are inevitably associated with high-profile accidents and disasters, the military and the 'horrors of war'. However, most trauma goes unseen and unreported within abusive families, following sexual assault and following accidents. Indeed, more than 60% of us suffer potentially traumatising events at some point in our lives (Green, 1994). Many get over their experience and emerge unscathed or even emotionally stronger from their experience. For those who go on to suffer long-term mental health problems, however, the aftermath is often undetected, untreated and, in the case of accident victims, can be more disabling than any physical injury. Physical injuries are visible and these can mask and deflect attention from psychological symptoms, increasing the likelihood of long-term psychological disorder. After road traffic accidents, for example, more than 20% of patients attending the emergency department go on to suffer post-traumatic stress disorder (PTSD; Blanchard & Hickling, 2004), which can be a social handicap and persist for years, despite having made a satisfactory physical recovery. Trauma-related mental health problems are also often mistaken for substance misuse issues or an emotionally unstable personality disorder. Members of the emergency services and clinical staff involved in the management of trauma are themselves at risk and it is particularly important that these groups have access to high-quality supervision and work in an environment where they feel they can talk candidly about the emotional effects of their work. This chapter will consider reactions to traumatic events affecting individuals and groups following disasters and during military conflict, as well as appropriate therapeutic interventions.

Traumatic events

There are two forms of traumatic event: type 1 is a single, 'out of the blue' incident (e.g. an assault or road traffic accident); type 2 is a repeated, ongoing or sustained trauma (e.g. childhood sexual abuse, repeated traumatic events in conflict). Unfortunately, much of the evidence base supporting treatments in the management of trauma is based on type 1 samples (where it is easier to define a homogeneous patient sample). Moreover, many treatment studies specifically exclude patients with comorbidity (often the norm) or other confounding factors, such as alcohol misuse or ongoing litigation (sadly, also common in clinical settings). When evaluating trials of treatment, it is important to look for factors such as the nature and selection of the sample and exclusion criteria before deciding how applicable and relevant any particular treatment is in clinical settings. Unfortunately, a positive treatment response in a trial, although statistically significant, might be clinically inconsequential. Whatever interventions are employed in the management of trauma, it is important to maintain a holistic perspective: treatment is often disjointed and fragmented with, for instance, a psychologist delivering a circumscribed, time-limited intervention (e.g. cognitive–behavioural therapy (CBT), eye movement desensitisation and reprocessing), a counsellor offering practical support and a psychiatrist prescribing and monitoring medication. Under these unsatisfactory circumstances, it is hardly surprising that even treatments with the most robust evidence base can seem ineffective.

What constitutes a traumatic event, disaster, or emergency depends on context: our definition is set very much in the context of an affluent Western society. It is important to remember that in much of the world, there is no clear demarcation between disaster or emergency and ordinary times. Millions of people die every year from famine, from the diseases of poverty and as victims of war; however, from their perspective, this is not an emergency but an unremarkable if tragic part of everyday life. Before considering the medical and psychological interventions to mitigate reactions to traumatic events available to those in a Western society, it is worth bearing in mind those less fortunate – the majority of the global population, for whom trauma is a daily occurrence. Is it appropriate or feasible to apply Western values and medicalise these situations? Even if it is, how could we possibly deliver therapeutic intervention to entire populations? It has been argued that, in these circumstances, security, food, clean water, shelter, warmth and practical support are paramount and that any attempt to provide treatment simply diverts resources from more pressing needs. There is no doubt that where disaster strikes, mental health professionals quickly follow, but how useful or effective they are, and what motivates their enthusiasm to intervene, remains unclear.

Immediate emotional reactions to trauma

A wide range of emotional reactions are seen after physical or psychological trauma. Individuals might show little or no immediate emotion. However, an absence of emotional distress does not mean that an individual is immune to subsequent disorder. Emotional reactions can be delayed or precipitated by secondary events such as anniversaries of the event, media coverage, inquests and police investigations. Intense fear, anxiety and distress are generally short-lived and respond well to reassurance, empathic concern and practical support. It is important not to prematurely medicalise a symptomatic individual, as this might interfere with a patient's own coping strategies, stigmatise their reaction and delay recovery. Mindful watchfulness and reassurance might be all that is necessary. However, brief courses of hypnotic and anxiolytic drugs might be needed for more severe reactions. It is important to monitor the patient's mental state and ensure that symptoms are resolving and that an individual is not resorting to dangerous coping strategies, such as the misuse of alcohol or drugs.

Individual reactions and vulnerability to trauma will vary according to context and someone who copes well on one occasion might, at another point in time, experience a disabling acute stress reaction. For example, an experienced ambulance paramedic (who had also recently become a parent) with many years of trauma experience, well used to dealing with death and grotesque injury, developed a severe acute stress reaction and subsequent PTSD after dealing with a seriously injured baby (of a similar age to his own child) at the scene of an accident. He had coped with many similar situations before, but on this occasion he was unable to maintain his shield of professional detachment because of his own recent parenthood.

Interventions following traumatic events designed to alleviate immediate distress as well as reducing the likelihood of subsequent PTSD and other disorders have a long and very controversial history. There is no evidence to support the use of any early stand-alone psychological intervention such as psychological or critical-incident stress debriefing, which although well-intentioned has been shown to actually worsen the long-term outcome (Mayou *et al*, 2000). One recent initiative, developed within the UK armed forces and now being adopted by other high-risk groups (such as the emergency services), is a management tool known as Trauma Risk Management or TRiM. Currently undergoing trials, but intuitively plausible and based on extensive clinical experience, TRiM is a system of post-incident management that allows managers and commanders to support individuals following traumatic events. Using workplace peers, trained but lay practitioners, TRiM is designed to identify and asses psychological risk to individuals exposed to trauma, according to a number of evidence-based risk factors (Box 15.1). Using brief follow-up interviews, the TRiM practitioners monitor mental state to quickly identify the individuals who, following a traumatic event, will go on to develop a psychological disorder, referring these cases for professional assessment and treatment. TRiM is an occupational tool that avoids unnecessarily medicalising an individual but provides a simple but effective means for an organisation to assess the well-being of its workforce and provide timely help for those who need it. TRiM is still under evaluation; however, where it has been deployed it has proved popular with individuals and organisations and is a pragmatic approach to managing traumatic incidents in high-risk groups.

> **Box 15.1** Individual risk factors for developing later psychological disorder
>
> - The person perceives they were out of control during the event
> - The person perceives their life was threatened
> - The person blames others for what happened
> - Individual shame or guilt for behaviour during an incident
> - Acute distress following the event
> - Exposure to substantial subsequent stress
> - Subsequent problems with day-to-day activities
> - Exposure to previous traumatic events
> - Poor social support (from family, friends, peers)
> - Use of alcohol to relieve distress

In contrast to the above, it is worth noting that NHS staff, particularly doctors and nurses, who are exposed to traumatic events more often than many other groups, often lack adequate support, supervision or access to appropriate treatment following traumatic events. What support is available is often patchy, haphazard and, from an individual perspective, difficult to access. NHS trusts often assert the importance of staff well-being and zero tolerance of assault and the abuse of staff; however, the rhetoric is seldom matched by the reality, which shows the subsequent high rates of long-term sickness absence, burnout, and alcohol and substance misuse among groups of health workers working in high-risk clinical areas. It is ironic that the stigma surrounding mental health problems in society is worst of all within the healthcare profession.

Acute stress disorder

Acute stress disorders (ASD) are defined in DSM-IV (American Psychiatric Association, 1994) as occurring within 4 weeks of a life-threatening traumatic event, lasting for at least 2 days and resolving within that 4-week period. Symptoms include intrusive phenomena (e.g. nightmares, flashbacks), avoidance of reminders of the trauma, hyperarousal, and dissociative symptoms such as emotional numbing and depersonalisation. It is important to distinguish ASD from normal, understandable distress. In the armed forces, ASD is commonly referred to as 'battle shock'. However, the terms are not interchangeable and it is important to remember that battle shock is essentially a functional definition of disorder: an inability to perform one's job because of disabling psychological symptoms, which might be, but are not necessarily, due to ASD.

In conflict situations, it is surprising how even the most severe psychological symptoms can respond to rest, reassurance, respite and simple support without recourse to any formal psychological intervention.

The much-vaunted acronym dating back to the Second World War – PIES, standing for *proximity* (intervention near the site of trauma and not evacuating rearwards), *immediacy* (the earlier the intervention, the better the outcome), *expectancy* (of full recovery) and *simplicity* (avoid medicalising) – has stood the test of time. Moreover, military experience also highlights the importance of more chronic background stressors in determining an individual's response to a type 1 traumatic event. Without doubt, fatigue, ill health, arduous living conditions and domestic welfare concerns all increase an individual's vulnerability to potentially traumatising events. The horrors of war are often simply the straw that breaks the camel's back.

Although ASD often resolves spontaneously, those affected are at greater risk of developing long-term disorders, particularly PTSD, and should be followed up. As many as 75% of patients suffering ASD after traumatic events will suffer from clinically PTSD 2 years later (Harvey & Bryant, 1999). Symptomatic treatment, as above, with anxiolytics and hypnotics can reduce distress and there is evidence that timely trauma-focused CBT, helping to put the event in perspective, can reduce the incidence of subsequent PTSD.

Adjustment disorders

Sometimes symptoms persist, increase in severity, and begin to take on the appearances of more common mental disorders. This is especially the case with patients experiencing social stress or significant life change as a result of traumatic events – for example, as a result of illness or persisting disability. Individuals might develop psychiatric symptoms that, although disabling, are insufficient to meet diagnostic criteria for any other specific psychiatric disorder. These adjustment disorders generally develop within a month or so of a significant life change and typically resolve within 6 months, although they can persist in the face of a persisting stressor. Various clinical features are recognised, but most patients typically manifest either predominantly depressive or anxiety symptoms (Box 15.2).

Adjustment disorders might respond to simple reassurance and supportive counselling, but symptom-targeted treatment with psychotropic drugs such as selective serotonin-reuptake inhibitors (SSRIs), serotonin–noradrenaline reuptake inhibitors or CBT might be indicated in more severe cases.

Post-traumatic stress disorder (PTSD)

The description of PTSD in DSM-III (American Psychiatric Association, 1980) was a landmark in the study of psychological trauma. For the first time, operational diagnostic criteria enabled a well-defined, relatively homogeneous group of patients to be identified, facilitating epidemiological and treatment research. Moreover, the recognition of PTSD as a psychiatric diagnosis did much to validate the suffering of the victims of trauma,

---

Box 15.2 Adjustment disorder (including acute stress reaction)

Presenting complaints:

- Patients feel overwhelmed and unable to cope
- Stress-related physical symptoms such as insomnia, headache, chest pain, palpitations
- Acute anxiety or depression
- Increasing use of alcohol or illicit substances

Diagnostic features:

- Acute reaction to a recent stressful or traumatic event
- Extreme distress resulting from a recent event or pre-occupation with the event
- Symptoms might be primarily somatic

Other symptoms might include the following:

- Low or sad mood
- Anxiety
- Worry
- Feeling unable to cope

Acute reaction usually lasts from a few days to several weeks.

(World Health Organization, 1992)

---

particularly veterans of the Vietnam War, many of whom had become marginalized and socially excluded. The introduction of PTSD into DSM-III owed much to their lobbying. However, the introduction of PTSD as a diagnosis has also had adverse consequences: an overemphasis and narrow focus on PTSD that has resulted in the relative neglect of other post-traumatic disorders. Indeed, from the welter of publications on PTSD since 1980, it would be easy to assume that PTSD was the only long-term consequence of psychological trauma.

Whether an individual develops PTSD (Box 15.3) or another psychiatric disorder after a traumatic event depends upon an amalgam of the event itself, its context and the emotional significance attributed to it by the individual. In addition, several predisposing factors have been identified. These include the emergence of an ASD after the trauma, past history of psychiatric disorder, anxiety-prone personality, exposure to previous traumatic experiences (including childhood abuse), and a perceived threat to life and personal safety at the time of the traumatic event. Important gender differences have been noted: for example, women are more likely than men to develop PTSD after interpersonal, especially sexual, violence. The presence of premorbid vulnerability factors also increases the likelihood of persisting, long-term PTSD and the development of comorbid psychopathology, particularly affective disorder and substance misuse.

Box 15.3   Post-traumatic stress disorder

Presenting complaints:

- Anxious and depressive symptoms linked to a particular trauma of more than 1 month's duration.
- Physical symptoms (e.g. various pains, poor sleep or fatigue) of more than 1 month's duration

Diagnostic features:

- History of an exceptionally traumatic event (brief, prolonged, or repeated) that would probably distress almost anyone
- Intrusive memories, flashbacks and nightmares
- The patient avoids thoughts, activities or situations reminding them of the trauma
- Sense of 'numbness', emotional blunting and detachment from other people
- Patient is unresponsive to surroundings, no longer enjoys anything (anhedonia)
- Autonomic arousal, hypervigilance, increased startle, insomnia, irritability, excessive anger, impaired concentration and/or memory

(World Health Organization, 1992)

A pure PTSD syndrome is unusual, and most likely to be seen in combat-related PTSD in a previously healthy individual. The condition is often complicated by concurrent affective disorders, particularly major depression, generalised anxiety and panic disorder, and alcohol and drug misuse. Other, pre-existing psychiatric disorders can also be significantly exacerbated following psychological trauma. Dysfunctional or delinquent behaviour often coexists and might be the only presenting feature of underlying PTSD. Indeed, PTSD might be identified only after the individuals have entered the criminal justice system. Occupational instability, antisocial behaviour and the breakdown of previously stable relationships also occur frequently and should raise the possibility of PTSD in any individual following traumatic events.

The biology of PTSD

Several enduring biological abnormalities have been identified in individuals with PTSD. Abnormalities of the hypothalamic–pituitary–adrenal axis include hypocortisolaemia and enhanced adrenocorticoid sensitivity to the effects of dexamethasone suppression (super-suppression), which is proportional to the clinical severity of PTSD. It has been suggested that central glucocorticoid-receptor hypersensitivity occurs in PTSD. Other neurochemical findings include evidence of increased central transmitter activity, particularly noradrenaline and 5-HT, playing a part in the encoding and retrieval of memory. Structural neuroimaging techniques such as magnetic resonance imaging have also revealed abnormalities, such as reduced hippocampal volume, in PTSD.

The epidemiology of comorbid disorders

One of the most consistent findings in studies of PTSD is that as many as 80% of sufferers also meet diagnostic criteria for at least one other psychiatric disorder in addition to PTSD. Epidemiological studies reveal that people with PTSD are twice as likely to have some other diagnosis as people without PTSD. In one study, only 16% of patients had PTSD as a sole diagnosis; 56% had one additional diagnosis and 20% had two additional diagnoses (Deahl, 2003). Comorbid diagnoses include depression, alcohol problems, other anxiety disorders, anti-social and emotionally unstable personality disorders, somatisation disorder, and organic mental syndromes. In UK cohort studies of returning troops from Iraq and Afghanistan, depression, substance misuse and other anxiety disorders are much more common than PTSD (Deahl, 2003).

Substance misuse and PTSD

Alcohol and drug abuse have been consistently associated with post-traumatic disorders. Between 21 and 77% of combat veterans with PTSD also meet diagnostic criteria for concurrent substance abuse disorders, with lifetime prevalence rates as high as 91% (Fear *et al*, 2010). The nature of this association is unclear and it has been suggested the substance abuse can variously suppress, exacerbate or perpetuate the symptoms of PTSD. Importantly, substance misuse is an important post-traumatic disorder in its own right and can follow trauma even in the absence of PTSD.

The relationship between PTSD and substance abuse is complex. Individuals with PTSD might use alcohol and illicit drugs as a form of self-medication to help them cope with the symptoms of PTSD. However, the disinhibiting and mood-altering effects of drugs can also aggravate many of the symptoms of PTSD, such as irritability, impaired interaction with others and physiological arousal issues. The chronic effects of drug and alcohol misuse, including withdrawal, tolerance and the effects of repeated intoxication, can interfere with treatment as well as the resolution of post-traumatic psychological and social issues.

Enduring personality change after catastrophic experience

There are no other long-term disorders in DSM-IV caused by traumatic events apart from PTSD. ICD-10 (World Health Organization, 1992), however, alludes to the fact that PTSD can lead to an enduring personality change (F43). In another section, 'enduring personality change after catastrophic experience' is acknowledged (F62.0). Clinical features include social isolation, paranoid thinking, feelings of emptiness, boredom and despair, and a sense of estrangement. Marked hyperarousal is frequently seen, resulting in irritability, impulsivity, emotional lability and socially irresponsible and sometimes aggressive behaviour – features not dissimilar from borderline personality disorder (BPD). Indeed, considering the high incidence of childhood abuse in individuals suffering from BPD, it has been suggested that perhaps BPD itself is a trauma-related condition caused by the impact of traumatic events on the developing brain. This clinical syndrome was recognised during DSM-IV field trials and included in the epithet DESNOS (disorders of extreme stress not otherwise specified) that, despite being widely recognised by researchers, was not included in DSM-IV. Considerable controversy exists over the diagnostic criteria for PTSD, as well as over the validity and status of these other trauma-related syndromes and it is likely that future editions of DSM and ICD will see a number of important changes reflecting the continuing debate.

Other psychological responses to trauma

Anxiety disorders

A wide range of anxiety disorders has also been reported following traumatic events. Generalised anxiety disorder has been reported in as many as 46% of individuals following traumatic events (Kessler *et al*, 2005) and might be just as common as PTSD, if not more so. Specific phobias are common and can occur independently of PTSD. Following traffic accidents, driving phobias might be more than twice as common as PTSD, yet frequently go undetected, particularly when a patient has suffered concomitant, and more obvious, physical injuries. Agoraphobia, social phobia, panic disorder and obsessive–compulsive disorder have all been reported following trauma, either comorbid with PTSD or as post-traumatic disorders in their own right.

Somatoform disorders

The hysterical conversion disorders associated with the First World War, also known as shell shock, are well known but seen infrequently today. Although less dramatic than shell shock, a number of studies report an excess of unexplained physical symptoms following trauma. Disorders such as irritable bowel syndrome, unexplained chest pains and other somatic complaints are frequently reported following traumatic events and have been particularly associated with sexual assault in ethnic minority populations.

Psychotic disorders

There is no convincing evidence that trauma alone can cause schizophrenia, although it can certainly be a precipitating factor in those with an underlying vulnerability. A number of studies written before the definition of PTSD suggest that schizophrenia might have been misdiagnosed (Deahl, 2003). It has been suggested that what was once diagnosed as hysterical psychosis might, with hindsight and contemporary diagnostic criteria, be diagnosed as PTSD today.

Mechanisms of comorbidity with PTSD

Four alternative hypotheses have been proposed to explain the high rates of comorbidity seen with PTSD.

- Pre-existing disorders constitute a vulnerability for PTSD.
- Other disorders are subsequent complications of PTSD.
- The disorders co-occur because of shared risk factors.
- Considering that none of the psychopathology seen in PTSD is unique to the disorder, it has been suggested that perhaps PTSD does not really exist as a distinct entity and is merely a *forme fruste* of anxiety or affective disorder pathoplastically modified by culture, context and traumatic events.

If comorbid disorders constitute a predisposition to or vulnerability for PTSD, then elevated levels of other disorders prior to exposure to a traumatic stressor should be expected. If the comorbid disorders are a complication of PTSD, one would expect the associated disorder to emerge after trauma exposure. If comorbid disorders and PTSD share risk factors, one would expect approximately simultaneous onset of both. Studies investigating dates of onset for these various disorders suggest that the onset of comorbid disorders increases following trauma exposure and is closely associated with the development of PTSD (Kessler *et al*, 2005). These findings suggest that comorbid disorders (and especially major depression) are complications of PTSD. Other disorders develop concurrently with PTSD.

This is an important diagnostic issue, considering that PTSD is responsible for increasing numbers of disability claims. If PTSD mimics or presents with the features of other disorders, patients might be mistakenly misdiagnosed with a condition unrelated to trauma. It is therefore important to specifically enquire about the onset of any psychopathology in relation to potentially traumatising events, as well as about the features of PTSD itself, in patients presenting with ostensibly unrelated disorders. Conversely, in patients diagnosed as suffering from PTSD it is important to detect any associated treatable comorbidity, as it is known that these cases are more likely to become chronic and are associated with a particularly poor outcome.

Perhaps the time might soon come when the term PTSD is discarded in favour of the broader concept of post-traumatic disorders. Virtually no treatment studies have looked at the impact of therapeutic interventions on these disparate disorders, and their epidemiology is still poorly understood, as is the extent to which any premorbid vulnerability determines whether an individual goes on to develop which post-traumatic disorder or which combination of post-traumatic disorders. PTSD has served its time (i.e. the post-Vietnam 1980s) and purpose well, but researchers must now look beyond PTSD to further advance our understanding of the human response to trauma.

Management of psychological responses to trauma

Primary prevention

True prevention involves reducing trauma by measures such as improving safety in the workplace, on the roads and in the home, crime prevention and preventing war. Specific measures include preparing emergency service workers, soldiers and others routinely exposed to traumatic events to cope with the anticipated trauma. Thorough recruit selection to screen out vulnerable individuals (i.e. those with a past psychiatric history) is important; there is no evidence that more general screening for particular personality styles has any validity, and where this has been undertaken (e.g. in the US military in the Second World War), it has failed dismally. Realistic training and establishing tightly knit cohesive teams within high-risk groups can mitigate against the effects of trauma. Stress-inoculation programmes are often used in training; these programmes include the exposure of prospective body-handlers to human remains and post-mortem examinations and educational briefings before combat that explain the probable effects of trauma to servicemen and tell them when, where, and how to access support and help.

Secondary prevention

Healthcare professionals are most likely to encounter victims of trauma in the emergency department. Following traumatic events, there are a number of measures that reduce immediate distress and possibly help reduce the incidence of subsequent post-traumatic illness. General measures ('tea and sympathy') might seem intuitively obvious but can be easily overlooked following a major incident, when staff are understandably preoccupied with major trauma rather than minor physical injuries or emotional distress. However, in the immediate post-trauma period, the psychological needs of the patient are often inversely proportional to the extent of any physical injury: those with minor injuries often require proportionately more psychological support.

Although timely psychiatric liaison is important, mental health professionals are generally neither welcome nor required following major incidents. Patients brought to the emergency department following traumatic events should be made as physically comfortable as possible as quickly as possible: for example, by expediting physical and forensic examinations and allowing the patient privacy and the opportunity to remove wet or soiled clothing and wash themselves. Allocating a specific staff member to supervise the patient facilitates a therapeutic relationship and provides an opportunity for the patient to discuss their experience and feelings, should they wish to do so. Simple support is not only a matter of kindness but also allows an opportunity to make a brief mental state assessment. After major incidents, telephones should be made available for patients to contact friends and family and let them know they are safe and make arrangements to be collected. Acutely distressed patients or those with marked emotional numbing or other dissociative symptoms should not be allowed to leave the department unescorted.

The general public are unlikely to have access to organisational tools such as TRiM. The only possibility for supervison is their general practitioner (GP), so perhaps the GP of any patient involved in a traumatic event should be informed, no matter how trivial the physical injury, and requested to review the patient in the coming weeks to monitor well-being and the emergence of any psychological disorder. The GP should be provided with some brief information regarding what to look for, such as changes in personality, a deterioration in relationships, social or occupational functioning, excessive alcohol or substance misuse, and obvious signs of psychological disorder. Any one or more of these signs should alert the GP to the possibility of an underlying post-traumatic illness; this should trigger a more detailed examination and specialist referral if necessary. General practitioners often find access to appropriate local mental health services confusing and they should also be advised where to seek specialist advice and when to refer the patient to mental health services.

Treatment of established PTSD

Many psychological interventions and pharmacological treatments have been shown to relieve at least some PTSD symptoms. The diversity of available treatments is an indication that none in isolation is particularly effective, and an eclectic approach combining psychotherapy, drug treatments and social support is most likely to succeed. PTSD victims can be difficult to engage and are often reluctant to discuss symptoms or seek help. Time should be taken to establish a good therapeutic relationship with the patient before embarking on specific therapies. The therapist should also be prepared to be proactive and include facilities for community outreach. PTSD creates secondary victims among families and it is important to involve significant others wherever possible in any treatment programme. It is important to identify, address and treat at the outset any comorbidity, such as alcohol misuse, that is likely to undermine any attempts to treat a PTSD itself.

Psychological therapies

A variety of psychological treatments have been advocated in the treatment of PTSD. Group-based therapies can be particularly useful when dealing with the victims of a shared trauma, such as soldiers or disaster-rescue workers. Cognitive techniques and exposure-based behavioural interventions are popular and have proven efficacy. Anxiety management programmes used alone are probably less effective. Audiotape desensitisation is an effective and commonly used technique based on the principle of 'imaginal' exposure. The patient writes a detailed script, describing not only events but also the feelings, sights, sounds and smells of the trauma. These are then recorded onto audiotape. Repeated exposure to the recording often reduces symptoms of hyperarousal to tolerable levels within a few weeks. Eye movement desensitisation and reprocessing is a popular but controversial technique that nevertheless has a firm evidence base, in which the patient relives traumatic memories while the therapist induces saccadic eye movements that in some cases can produce rapid symptom relief. Its mechanism of action is uncertain but exposure in a safe, supportive setting almost certainly plays an important role. In some cases, it can produce a rapid and dramatic improvement.

Pharmacological treatment

Medication can alleviate some of the symptoms of PTSD, although it is not generally as effective as psychological treatment and should generally be combined with psychotherapy. Medication tends to be most effective with acute PTSD and is of particular benefit in reducing positive symptoms such as nightmares and intrusive thoughts. Comorbid depression and other psychiatric disorders are also indications for pharmacological treatment.

Medications that act on central serotonergic transmission seem to have the most beneficial effects on the symptoms of PTSD. These include SSRIs such as fluoxetine. Doses considerably in excess of those used to treat depression are commonly required and treatment is maintained for 2 months or more before the full therapeutic effect is observed. Recent studies have shown that MDMA (3,4-methylenedioxy-N-methylamphetamine) might be one of the more effective pharmacological treatments for PTSD (Carhart-Harris *et al*, 2014); however, its illegal status in the UK and many other countries will make further evaluation very difficult. Benzodiazepines are occasionally useful in reducing symptoms of hyperarousal but they should generally be avoided, particularly if there is a concurrent problem with substance misuse.

A variety of other medications have been used to some effect, including more sedative antidepressants acting primarily on 5-HT systems (e.g. nefazadone), tricyclic antidepressants, monoamine-oxidase inhibitors and non-psychotropic drugs (e.g. clonidine) that act by reducing central noradrenergic activity. The 5-HT antagonist cyproheptadine is occasionally useful in preventing nightmares.

Military service and mental health ... not always as it seems

Mental health problems amongst serving and veteran armed forces personnel can present in a variety of ways: domestic and occupational breakdown, social exclusion, criminality, homelessness, self-harm and substance misuse. This group also suffers from an excess of medically unexplained symptoms; this has been reported during and after all recent conflicts but especially by veterans from the 1991 Gulf War. Symptoms include fatigue, dizziness, nausea, and gastrointestinal complaints, for which there is no (as yet) known biomedical aetiology.

The explanation for this complex help-seeking behaviour and frequently veiled presentation of psychopathology include ignorance (on the part of both healthcare professionals and patients), stigma, pride, a lack of insight, and an inability on the part of veterans to communicate their difficulties. Moreover, there are positive benefits of the sick role, which include status, recognition, and (sometimes) financial gain. Finally, chronic psychopathology amongst some veterans might be an integral (and indispensable) element of their core identity, and worn as a badge of honour.

The failure to understand the problems facing serving and veteran armed forces personnel reflects a lamentable educational shortfall, particularly because they are such a large (and expanding) group. Many health professionals are simply unaware that their patients are veterans. Psychiatric textbooks and postgraduate training programmes generally neglect military psychiatry, and the average psychiatric trainee sees little PTSD. Small wonder, then, that civilian mental health professionals experience such difficulty in accurately assessing and addressing the needs of veterans. Moreover, even when a veteran does seek help, a lack of understanding of the military culture, ethos, the specific problems of service life, and transitional adjustment issues frequently result in misdiagnosis, particularly in terms of an over-diagnosis of PTSD.

A preoccupation with PTSD amongst the academic community has led some to imagine that military psychiatry and PTSD are synonymous, and has deflected attention from the less tangible, less quantifiable, and more difficult to define adjustment issues. Equally, even when a correct diagnosis is made, it is often wrongly attributed to military service, or specifically to combat experience, which can be a convenient scapegoat for problems that antedated military service or are not combat related at all. It is understandable that, without an awareness of these broader contextual issues, health professionals might reach a spurious conclusion and make a diagnosis of PTSD for a patient who is more than willing to accept a diagnosis that is arguably one of the least stigmatising of psychiatric disorders. This diagnosis conveniently avoids painful introspection and consideration of the above factors, which are more difficult to articulate, lack an obvious diagnostic label, are more difficult to treat, and might threaten an individual's core identity.

Conclusions

Psychological trauma is common and disabling, yet still poorly understood among mental health professionals. Stigma, shame and the avoidance symptoms associated with PTSD mean that patients all too often suffer in silence or present with dysfunctional social lives and a variety of diverse and seemingly unrelated difficulties. Many cases go undetected and a high index of clinical suspicion is required – particularly in high-risk groups such as emergency service workers, participants in combat, and rape and accident victims – to enable them to have access to treatment and therapeutic facilities. Health professionals are not immune to the psychological effects of trauma. They are also more likely to deal with their difficulties by self-medicating with drugs and alcohol than face the stigma and professional opprobrium associated with seeking help. Conversely, mental health problems in serving armed forces personal or veterans should be carefully evaluated and not swayed by the popular stereotype that they must all have PTSD.

Public attitudes towards psychological trauma are ambivalent and at times downright hostile (e.g. 'after all, they're lucky to be alive', 'they're malingerers only after compensation'). Contrary to popular opinion, when litigation follows trauma, a successful resolution for the plaintiff seldom brings about any significant clinical improvement. In the aftermath of traumatising events, psychological symptoms are easily disregarded.

There can be no room for complacency and symptoms should not be dismissed merely because they are understandable in the context of trauma. Any patient with significant psychological distress more than 6 months after a traumatic event, or whose symptoms are socially handicapping, should be referred for a psychiatric assessment. The earlier the treatment of psychological trauma, the more effective it is likely to be; trauma victims should not have to wait for a crisis before receiving help.

References

American Psychiatric Association (1980) *Diagnostic and Statistical Manual of Mental Disorders Third Edition (DSM-III)*. American Psychiatric Association.

American Psychiatric Association (1994) *Diagnostic and Statistical Manual of Mental Disorders Fourth Edition (DSM-IV)*. American Psychiatric Association.

Blanchard EB, Hickling EJ (2004) *After the Crash (2nd edn)*. American Psychological Association.

Carhart-Harris RL, Murphy K, Leech R (2014) The effects of acutely administered 3,4-methylenedioxymethamphetamine on spontaneous brain function in healthy volunteers measured with arterial spin labelling and blood oxygen level-dependent resting-state functional connectivity. *Biological Psychiatry*, doi: 10.1016/j.biopsych.2013.12.015.

Deahl M (2003) Non-PTSD post-traumatic disorders. *Psychiatry*, **2**: 26–28.

Fear NT, Jones M, Murphy D, *et al* (2010) What are the consequences of deployment to Iraq and Afghanistan on the mental health of the UK armed forces? A cohort study. *The Lancet*, **375**: 1783–1797.

Green BL (1994) Psychosocial reserach in traumatic stress: an update. *Journal of Traumatic Stress*, **7**: 341–362.

Harvey AG, Bryant RA (1999) Acute stress disorder across trauma populations. *Journal of Nervous and Mental Disease*, **187**: 443–446.

Kessler RC, Chiu WT, Dernier O, *et al* (2005) Prevalence, severity and comorbidity of 12 month DSM IV disorders in the National Comorbidity Survey replication. *Archives of General Psychiatrey*, **62**: 617–627.

Mayou R, Ehlers A, Hobbs M (2000) Psychological debriefing for road traffic accident victims: three year follow-up of a randomised controlled trial. *British Journal of Psychiatry*, **176**: 589–593.

World Health Organization (1992) *ICD-10 Classification of Mental and Behavioural Disorders*. WHO.

CHAPTER 16

Emergencies in liaison psychiatry

Christian Hosker

Clinicians working in general hospitals can expect to see the full spectrum of psychiatric and psychological presentations, ranging from time-limited distress through to highly disturbed behaviour caused by serious mental or medical illness. The general hospital is a particularly challenging environment in which to diagnose and treat mental illness, both in terms of the types of disorders that present and the nature of the hospital environment itself.

In this chapter, I will focus on a number of disorders that commonly present in an acute manner to the general hospital, including medically unexplained emergencies and presentations for which the presence of physical disorder is a complicating factor in terms of aetiology or management.

Behavioural disturbance in the general hospital

A request for assessment of an acutely disturbed patient, such as the one shown in case study 1, is among the most common reasons for referral to a liaison psychiatry team (Bronheim *et al*, 1998). A recent survey of general hospital wards in Leeds found that the prevalence of disturbed behaviour, as identified by senior nursing staff, was 4% and that the management of this behaviour consumed a disproportionately high amount of nursing time (Kannabiran *et al*, 2008).

Case study 1

A 40-year-old woman who is undergoing potentially curative chemotherapy for leukaemia is admitted to the acute oncology ward, having developed problems swallowing. The cancer nurse specialist who has met her on several previous occasions notices that the patient has been more irritable and withdrawn than usual during the first 24 h of her admission. This irritability slowly increases over the ensuing days and culminates in the patient becoming hostile and aggressive to staff, attempting to pull out her central line and trying to leave the isolation area in which she is being treated. The patient is likely to die if the chemotherapy is not given.

Psychiatric staff are generally familiar with the challenges that patients with disturbed behaviour present in the psychiatric setting, but managing such challenges in the general hospital environment can be difficult. General hospital staff are far less likely to be familiar with disturbed behaviour and can find such presentations highly anxiety provoking. This is partly because they typically lack the training required to help them deal with it, but other factors, such as the comparatively low patient to nurse ratio on general wards and the presence of other vulnerable and incapacitated patients, are also relevant. Consequently, the level of disturbed behaviour that can normally be tolerated in general hospital settings will differ from that that can be tolerated in psychiatric units.

Presentation

Types of disturbed behaviour can be grouped as follows:

- acts of verbal or physical aggression directed at staff or other patients and carers
- self-injurious behaviour
- inappropriate interference with their own or others' medical treatment (e.g. by removing intravenous infusions)
- wandering
- expressions of high levels of emotion.

As in case study 1, it might be that the patient will display more than just one of these types of behaviours.

Aetiology

There are many different potential causes of disturbed behaviour in general hospital settings. The most likely are listed below:

- delirium
- dementia
- intoxication due to alcohol or other psychoactive substances
- severe mental illness
- disturbed behaviour that is not the result of mental disorder.

Assessment and management

On first receiving a call for assistance, an assessment should be made as to whether the immediate situation has been made safe and security staff should be deployed if necessary. As disturbed behaviour is likely to present with associated risks, these cases should be given the appropriate priority. General hospitals differ from psychiatric units in that ward staff are not trained in restraint techniques and rely on security staff for the immediate containment of disturbed behaviour. When receiving a request for consultation regarding a disturbed patient, such as the one in case study 1, it is therefore essential to ensure that appropriate measures have been implemented to maintain the immediate safety of the patient and others, and that hospital security is either aware of or already involved in the situation.

Precise information should be obtained regarding the nature of the disturbance and the medical condition of the patient. Psychiatric clinicians should be prepared for the fact that such situations can be highly charged. Non-psychiatric staff might jump to conclusions when witnessing a patient suddenly becoming incoherent and aggressive and attribute the behaviour to an underlying mental illness rather than an organic cause. It is important, therefore, that a calm approach is maintained and that the patient's medical condition is clearly established. Attempts should be made to both engage and assess the patient directly with a view to formulating the extent to which medical, psychiatric and interpersonal factors are contributing to the presentation.

The overarching purpose of the assessment is to identify risks and to ensure they are appropriately managed. It is important to think widely when carrying out a risk assessment of the situation, so as to ensure that risks that might be unique to the particular medical condition and setting are considered. For example, are other sick patients at risk from the behaviour? Is the patient's behaviour compromising the management of their own physical health condition? Is the disturbed patient being treated on a ward from which they could fall by opening or smashing a window?

Where violence or significant aggression has occurred in the context of mental illness, the algorithm for the short-term management of disturbed or violent behaviour offered by the National Institute for Health and Care Excellence (NICE, 2005) should be followed (Box 16.1). Assessment and management of each case will depend upon the underlying cause and, as such, different approaches are outlined in this chapter.

The disturbed, delirious patient

Cases of delirium can result in profoundly challenging behaviour erupting quite suddenly in a previously cooperative patient. Understandably, the emergence of such behaviour can prove highly alarming to general hospital staff.

Case study 2

A 60-year-old man with lung cancer is admitted to hospital for pain management. His oral opiate analgesia is switched to a fentanyl patch. When his family visit the following evening, he seems agitated and confides in them that he has heard the nursing staff talking about their intention to 'finish him off'. These concerns are passed on to the medical team. However, when they come to review him he is asleep and the staff report that he has been settled. Later that evening, the patient leaves hospital and attempts to take a bus home dressed only in his hospital gown. The patient is returned to the ward. Investigations reveal that he has a mildly raised white cell count and a new area of consolidation in his diseased lung. The fentanyl patch is removed, he is switched to an alternative lower-potency opiate and he is treated with antibiotics for a chest infection. He agrees to take a low dose of haloperidol. Over the following 12 h, the paranoid ideas and agitation completely resolve and the haloperidol is withdrawn after a further 12 h, with no symptoms returning.

Delirious patients display sudden changes in presentation, such as fluctuating levels of consciousness and psychomotor activity, cognitive impairment and sleep disturbance. It is the combination of these symptoms that can result in severe behavioural disturbance and risks. Discriminating between cases of delirium and cases of dementia should be possible by obtaining a collateral history of the time course of onset and also by looking for features, such as impairment of consciousness level and perceptual abnormalities, that are more suggestive of delirium than dementia. It should be remembered, however, that the former can frequently be superimposed on the latter.

As there is always an underlying cause of delirium, the ultimate aim of management is to identify the cause and reverse it wherever possible. Laboratory tests are crucial in achieving this aim (Table 16.1). It might be, however, that the patient is too disturbed for testing to be practical without measures to reduce agitation being implemented first. De-escalation

---

Box 16.1 Key features from the NICE guidance on short-term management of disturbed/violent behaviour

- Risk assessments should be conducted where appropriate to predict and prevent occurrences of aggression.
- Staff should be aware of warning signs that may herald the escalation to aggression.
- When aggression occurs, de-escalation techniques that calm down an escalating patient should be employed.
- Observation of the patient might be required to manage disturbed or violent behaviour and prevent self-harm.
- Physical intervention and rapid tranquillisation should only be used if de-escalation techniques have failed to calm the situation.
- Physical restraint should be avoided if at all possible, should not be used for prolonged periods and should be ceased at the earliest opportunity.
- If rapid tranquillisation is employed, the potential risks should be considered and extra care taken in the presence of QTc prolongation or if other QTc-prolonging medications have been taken.
- Oral medication should be offered before parenteral routes are considered and intravenous administration should be avoided.
- In the non-psychotic context, oral or intramuscular lorazepam is preferred.
- In the psychotic context, an antipsychotic in combination with lorazepam should be given in the first instance (intramuscular olanzapine or lorazepam should not be given within 1 h of each other).

Source: NICE (2005)

Table 16.1 Investigations for delirious patients

Investigation type		Cause of delirium
Brain imaging	Computed tomography/magnetic resonance imaging	Trauma Intracranial mass Stroke Infection Degenerative change
Blood studies	Full blood count and differential	Anaemia Infection (leukocytosis) Agranulocytosis HIV
	Serum electrolytes Sodium Potassium Calcium Chlorine Phosphate	Electrolyte imbalance
	Urea and creatinine	Renal failure
	Bilirubin Liver enzymes Ammonia	Liver failure
	Thyroid-stimulating hormone Thyroxine Glucose level Cortisol/adrenocorticotrophic hormone	Endocrinopathy
	Vitamin B6 Vitamin B12 Folate	Vitamin deficiency
	Syphilis serology	Neurosyphilis
	HIV testing	HIV delirium
	Urine toxicity	Illicit drug intoxication
	Urine culture	Urine infection
Other studies	Cerebrospinal fluid	Raised intracranial pressure Infection Syphilis Protein Haemorrhage
	Vital signs	Infection
	Heart rate	Arrhythmias Infection Metabolic disturbance
	Respiratory rate and oxygen saturation	Hypoxia

techniques should be used in the first instance. If these are unsuccessful, NICE (2010) recommends that haloperidol or olanzapine should be considered to correct perceptual abnormalities and reduce agitation. The presence of an acute physical illness will affect the pharmacokinetics of these agents and, as such, the lowest therapeutic doses should be used initially, with doses increased subsequently according to the patient's response. Such an approach should reduce the chance of side-effects.

The patient's case should be regularly reviewed so that the dose can be modified and so that the patient does not remain on a potentially harmful antipsychotic for longer than is necessary. Consideration should also be given to the preferred route of administration. Oral administration is the ideal but not always possible, in which case either intramuscular or intravenous routes might have to be used. Haloperidol can also be administered via a subcutaneous driver or injection for agitated but debilitated patients.

Despite delirium being common on general hospital wards, staff can still be alarmed by its presentation. Therefore, following the immediate measures described above, staff should be reminded about their role in the patient's treatment and recovery. The patient should ideally be nursed in a side room, proximal to the nursing station. The number of different members of staff caring for the patient should be minimised to provide consistency. Lighting should be managed to reduce the potential for perceptual abnormalities to occur and aids such as clocks and papers should be on hand to orientate the patient. A step that is often neglected is that of explaining to carers about delirium to ensure that they understand what is happening and that the presentation does not herald the presence of an enduring mental illness.

The disturbed patient with dementia

For a comprehensive overview of emergencies related to dementia, please see Chapter 13 in this book. In this section, the acute management of cases of dementia in the general hospital, such as the one described in case study 3, is considered.

Case study 3

A 92-year-old patient is admitted to hospital from home with pressure sores following the death of her husband. She is clearly confused and the general practitioner confirms that she had been diagnosed with dementia several years previously. There are no signs of infection or biochemical disturbance. The patient is reasonably calm when left alone in bed but becomes highly agitated when any attempts are made to examine her. She attempts to scratch and bite staff when they come within reaching distance of her.

All hospital patients with suspected dementia should be thoroughly assessed for reversible causes and receive treatment for concurrent illnesses and evidence-based interventions for the underlying disorder. Ideally, this will involve referral to a specialist hospital-based older-adults liaison psychiatry team. Occasionally, factors such as the stress of hospitalisation or the presence of physical illness will result in the behaviour of a patient with dementia becoming challenging and precipitate a crisis in a general hospital. As is the case in case study 3, this might make examination impossible. The types and frequencies of behaviours that are likely to be displayed are shown in Table 16.2.

Challenging behaviour in a patient with known dementia can often be anticipated by those who know the patient well. A crisis could be prevented by the use of a pre-formulated treatment plan that caters for the possibility of disturbed behaviour. Sometimes, however, a disturbance will occur in the absence of such a plan. In such instances, a rapid assessment should be carried out to consider possible causes, potential risks and measures that will be needed to manage the behaviour. The ABC assessment framework offers a useful approach to assessment (Stokes, 2000).

A – Antecedents or triggers – What was happening before the behaviour occurred? Who was present? When and where did it occur?

B – Behaviour – What exactly is the specific behaviour that is causing concern? Is this new behaviour? What form did it take? How long did it last?

C – Consequences of the person's behaviour – What risks are associated with the behaviour?

This approach helps to identify the exact nature of the behaviour, whether it really is a problem and whether actions really need to be taken to modify it. In case study 3, the behaviour is occurring when attempts are made to examine the patient. The behaviour is extreme and distressing and the consequence is that treatment of acute problems, such as the bed sores, is not possible.

Table 16.2 The frequency of troublesome behaviours found in a sample of patients with dementia

Behaviour	Frequency (%)
Angry outbursts	51
Dietary change	46
Sleep disturbance	45
Paranoia	32
Phobia	25
Delusions and hallucinations	22
Assault/violent behaviour	21
Bizarre behaviour	21
Incontinence	17

Swearer *et al* (1988)

Once the initial assessment has been carried out, a useful approach to immediate management is offered by Cohen-Mansfield (2000), who put forward an unmet-needs model for agitation, in which behaviours are viewed as an indication of an underlying unmet need. This model proposes that disturbed behaviours arise from three domains: attempting to meet a particular need (e.g. pacing up and down the ward for stimulation); communicating a need (e.g. repeatedly asking the same question); an unmet physical need (e.g. pain, thirst, hunger). In case study 3, the aggression might be resulting from a failure to reassure the patient that attempts to examine her are not intended to hurt her. Family members could be useful to provide familiarity and reassurance, but ultimately tranquillisation might be required.

General hospital staff are often uncertain about how to manage challenging behaviour in dementia patients, and the role of the psychiatrist will be to develop a treatment plan in cooperation with them to ensure that appropriate measures, such as a consistent approach to nursing, reality orientation and a degree of tolerance of behaviours, are incorporated. In general, the options for management will be behavioural interventions, environmental interventions and, if absolutely necessary, the use of medication.

If medication is required for behavioural disturbance, this will normally be either the cautious use of an antipsychotic or a benzodiazepine. A short-acting benzodiazepine, such as lorazepam, might be preferable where Lewy Body dementia cannot be excluded. The Committee on Safety of Medicines (2004) produced an alert highlighting the risk of stroke in patients with dementia treated with atypical antipsychotics. They cited a threefold increase in risk from 1.1 to 3.3%. It seems that this risk also applies to typical antipsychotics. Consequently, their use should be avoided if possible. The Royal College of Psychiatrists (2004) produced guidance on this matter and suggested a 'three Ts' approach (target, titration, time), as follows:

- drug treatments should have a specific target symptom
- the starting dose should be low and then be titrated upwards if necessary
- drug treatments should be time-limited.

The disturbed, psychotic patient

Treating the acutely disturbed, psychotic patient on a general hospital ward produces some additional factors for consideration. Referrals in such cases, as is the case in case study 1, usually arise because of a need for behaviours to be controlled and the associated distress and risks quelled so that the patient can receive the treatment for which they are in the general hospital in the first place. If the patient is suffering from a medical condition, this might have implications in terms of the use of antipsychotic or other psychotropic medication and the environment in which treatment will have to be administered.

The same step-wise approach to general management should be used as that already described above. A careful assessment should be conducted and any signs of delirium noted, as delirium will be the most likely alternative diagnosis to psychosis, and will require different treatment.

Once the diagnosis has been established, the psychiatrist should seek a good understanding from the treating team of the patient's medical condition and the organs that are affected, as this will influence how psychotropics can be used. The nature of the physical illness might dictate the choice of antipsychotic with, for example, sulpiride, which is almost exclusively renally excreted, being preferred where there is significant liver failure but avoided when renal failure is an issue. Similarly, a low platelet count could contraindicate the use of intramuscular preparations, as they could result in compartment syndrome. In general, in the presence of acute illness, initial psychotropic doses should be low and subsequently titrated according to response. While a response is awaited, safety should be maintained by ensuring that security staff are present, if necessary. Depending on the level of physical need, it might be possible to transfer the patient to a psychiatric setting; however, this is often not possible. If it is not, the aim should be to ensure that the patient's psychiatric needs are met while they remain in the general hospital by providing both medical and nursing psychiatric input as required.

The patient whose disturbed behaviour might be due to drug or alcohol intoxication

Acute alcohol intoxication is a common presentation in emergency departments, but rarely requires psychiatric assessment. A psychiatric opinion might be requested, however, when a patient is expressing suicidal ideation or actively self-harming, for instance. In such cases, it is important the patient is allowed to return to a sober condition in a safe environment before a psychiatric assessment is attempted, as mental state examinations of intoxicated individuals will not be valid. Patients who are clearly intoxicated are unlikely to be capacitous and, as such, can be detained in hospital against their wishes if there is a probable risk to themselves or others. While the patient remains in the hospital, the potential for harm through falls, respiratory depression, inhalation of vomit and hypothermia should be managed.

The psychoactive effects of recreational drugs can also result in aggressive and disturbed behaviour. The use of amphetamines, cocaine and crack (chemically pure) cocaine can all result in a form of psychosis in which paranoia and subsequent aggression are prominent. The psychosis will usually resolve once ingestion stops; however, rapid tranquillisation techniques might have to be employed if behaviour cannot be contained in the interim by a calm approach and de-escalation techniques. Benzodiazepines, rather than antipsychotics, should be the rapid tranquillisation medication of choice, as the psychosis should be self-limiting and most patients are likely to be neuroleptic-naive. Additionally, there is the possibility of arrhythmias being induced by the combination of stimulant drugs and antipsychotics.

The hallucinogenic properties of lysergic acid diethylamide (LSD) and phencyclidine can also result in patients presenting with disturbed behaviour. Again, the usual de-escalation techniques should be employed, with benzodiazepines and antipsychotics reserved for cases where behavioural disturbance is unresponsive to these techniques, prolonged or particularly disturbed.

Substance withdrawal is also a common cause of disturbed behaviour in general hospitals. Alcohol withdrawal is the most common type and the opportunity to treat pre-emptively might be missed by a failure to ask patients about their drinking habits or inadequate dosing of chlordiazepoxide once dependency has been revealed.

The patient whose disturbed behaviour is not due to mental disorder

Illness and hospitalisation can place considerable stress on patients and family members. Occasionally, this can result in displays of hostility or aggression towards staff or fellow patients. NHS institutions have a zero-tolerance approach to aggression; however, this black-and-white view doesn't always allow for complex situations, where distress and aggression lie on a spectrum.

Hospital wards tend to be highly structured environments in which various norms are expected and rules, both explicit and implicit, exist. The usual expectation is that patients will remain in or near to their bed, adhere to treatments as prescribed and request help in a way that takes into consideration the needs of fellow patients and of busy clinical staff. If patients fail to stick to these rules, conflict can ensue.

Case study 4

A 40-year-old man is admitted to hospital with an exacerbation of chronic obstructive pulmonary disorder. He is extremely overweight and has become immobile because of muscle loss secondary to inactivity. He wished to be placed in a nursing home, but attempts to find a suitable placement that can cater for his unique needs have resulted in a prolonged hospital stay. The patient requires a high level of nursing input, which is made difficult as he is frequently rude and abusive to staff. He will often call for assistance when staff are trying to help other patients and will threaten to 'shout the place down' if staff do not respond to his requests immediately. The staff feel that he could do more for himself and some of them have become so worn down by his abuse that they have taken time off work.

The role of the psychiatrist is to assess situations where aggression and hostility have occurred, to determine whether there is any evidence of mental illness and additionally, even when mental illness is excluded, to attempt to make some sense of the behaviour by taking into consideration the factors that are at play. Non-tolerance might be the answer in some cases, but in other instances empathy and engagement might be more appropriate – or perhaps the only available option, if discharge is not possible. As with other causes of disturbed behaviour, establishing the exact behaviour that is the source of concern is a crucial step. Frequently, reports of disturbed behaviour will be second-hand, having occurred during the previous nursing shift and, therefore, care should be taken to establish the true facts and circumstances.

The next step is to meet with the patient to hear their perspective. This assessment should encompass the situation that has arisen and also a background history. It might become apparent that the patient is prone to impulsivity, dependence or other traits that might explain why conflict has arisen. It is often useful to take the position of a diplomat, with the aim of mediating between patient and staff and improving understanding between the two sides. It might be possible to negotiate with staff to implement boundaries around the behaviour of concern, or to encourage staff members who have found it easier to deal with the patient to become the main point of contact for the patient while they remain in the hospital. The concept of splitting is also highly relevant on hospital wards, where different groups of staff might find that they have contrasting feelings about a patient. This should be addressed by organising debriefing sessions for staff working with particularly difficult patients. Family members can also be a useful resource, as they are likely to be experienced in dealing with a relative's behaviour and can pass on useful strategies.

The difficulties described above might be particularly challenging for patients with mild or borderline intellectual disabilities. They might find the environment especially threatening because they find it even harder to understand. Asking about the individual's routine at home and, in particular, how they cope with stressful situations will be helpful in seeing how ward rules and routines might be provoking or maintaining certain behaviour. Negotiations will again be important to see if the patient can be awarded flexibility regarding visiting times or time allowed off the ward.

The patient refusing treatment

English law is eminently clear on the right of patients to accept or refuse treatment as long as they are capacitous, acting voluntarily and appropriately informed. In some cases, the refusal of treatment is fully understandable and the legal tests described above are easily satisfied without the involvement of a psychiatrist. In other instances, however, the context of the immediate situation or the patient's previous history might lead the medical team to request a psychiatric opinion.

A psychiatric opinion might be requested, for example, in the following situations:

- a patient with known or suspected mental illness refuses treatment for a medical condition

- a patient makes an unexpected decision to disengage from treatment
- a patient who has intentionally self-harmed refuses treatment for those injuries.

The last of the three scenarios is a particularly frequent occurrence and can cause considerable anxieties for staff, who must deal with both the acute situation and the potential long-term consequences. Case study 5 illustrates such a case.

Case study 5

A 30-year-old woman is rushed to the emergency department by an ambulance after her husband became aware that she had taken an overdose of 20 paracetamol tablets. She had written a suicide note and another letter, which stated that she intended to die and did not want to have any treatment that would resuscitate her or reverse the effects of the overdose. The letter was signed and dated. The date was the same day as the presentation and overdose. On arrival in the department, the patient shouts that she does not want any treatment. The patient has previously attended the department following overdoses and has required in-patient psychiatric treatment on at least one occasion in the past.

The general approach to this and other acute situations is considered below. This is intended as a guide only, and where doubt exists about how to proceed for a particular case, senior clinicians should become involved. These clinicians, in turn, might need to seek advice from their hospital trust's legal department.

When a psychiatric opinion is requested, the first task will be to determine the urgency of the request so that cases such as that in Case study 5, which require an immediate response, receive one. It is also crucial to discuss with the most informed member of the medical team the intended benefits of the proposed treatment, the potential side-effects, the time-frame for which the treatment can be delayed and the consequences of ultimately refusing it. If at all possible, it is desirable that this same member of the medical team participates in the part of the assessment where the patient's decision-making process is tested.

The exact nature of the assessment in different countries will be dictated by the legislation that relates to refusal of medical treatment in that particular jurisdiction. In England and Wales, this is the Mental Capacity Act 2005 and its associated Code of Practice (Department of Constitutional Affairs, 2007). Readers from other regions should refer to their own legal statutes.

Patients who refuse treatment fall into a number of groups: those who have made a rational, capacitous decision; those for whom decision-making is impaired by the presence of a mental illness or a condition affecting the brain; and those for which the decision to refuse treatment is based on poor judgement or strong emotion, to the extent that capacity is questionable (but not necessarily lacking).

Assessment should, therefore, aim to do more than simply establish the presence or absence of mental illness and capacity. It should also aim to understand the patient's rationale for refusing treatment and the psychosocial context of the decision and to empathise with the patient as far as is possible. In some cases it might become apparent that the patient's refusal of treatment is due to exasperation with the burden of ongoing interventions and investigations, or is a manifestation of interpersonal difficulties, and an empathetic approach might re-engage the patient and lead to the resumption of treatment. An awareness of the therapeutic window of opportunity for the proposed treatment is important as, if there is the potential for the patient to delay a decision, this might offer the opportunity to remove some of the anxiety from a stressful situation and allow the patient the welcome chance to exert some control over what is happening to them.

When faced with a difficult choice, individuals can feel pulled in opposite directions. This is a particularly uncomfortable situation when there is pressure to make a choice – the end result can be that people attempt to cope by becoming over-definite in one direction. This is illustrated by a familiar scenario in which a patient seeks help by presenting at an emergency department having self-harmed, only to then refuse any medical intervention. This decision can arise from a desire to minimise the difficult emotions associated with either option (that is, dying or continuing to live). It is important to explore the process that has led someone to make a particular decision by, for example, asking them who they have discussed the decision with. It may be that the patient has not discussed the decision at all, which is understandable, given that discussion is likely to add to the uncertainty. If this is the case, they should be encouraged to discuss it further.

In some cases, the patient will remain steadfast in their refusal of treatment or the immediacy of the situation is such that a precipitant decision is needed. In these situations, an assessment of the patient's decision-making capacity is required. In this process, the task for the psychiatrist will be to establish whether the patient is suffering from an impairment or disturbance of mental functioning and whether this affects their ability to understand, retain, use and weigh up information and to communicate their intent.

Determining the presence of an impairment or disturbance of mental functioning will require a mental state examination and collateral information. If an impairment or disturbance is identified, the next question will be whether it renders them incapable of making the decision to refuse treatment. The assessor should, therefore, have a discussion with the patient to ascertain whether they are able to understand, retain and weigh up the relevant information. It should be noted that the patient's level of understanding only needs to be that of an informed layperson, rather than a medical expert, and as such it should be ensured that the patient has been informed at an appropriate level to their needs. It is desirable that the medical professional who is offering the treatment is available to take part

---

Box 16.2 The applicability and validity of advance decisions in England and Wales

An advance decision is not valid if the patient has:

- withdrawn the decision at a time when they had capacity to do so
- conferred authority on the donee, under a lasting power of attorney created after the advance decision was made, to give or refuse consent to the treatment to which the advance decision relates
- done anything else clearly inconsistent with the advance decision.

An advance decision is not applicable to the treatment in question if:

- at the material time, the patient has capacity to give or refuse consent to it
- the treatment is not the treatment specified in the advance decision
- any circumstance specified in the advance decision is absent
- there are reasonable grounds for believing that circumstances exist that the patient did not anticipate at the time of the advance decision and that would have affected their decision had they anticipated them.

For an advance decision to refuse life-sustaining treatment to be valid:

- it must include a statement by the patient stating that it is to apply even if life is at risk
- it must be in writing
- it must be signed by the patient or by another person in the patient's presence and by the patient's direction
- the signature must be witnessed.

---

in this process, as they are best placed to check the patient understands aspects of treatment that a psychiatrist is unlikely to be familiar with.

Where capacity is deemed to be lacking and advance decisions either have not been made or are not valid in the given context (Box 16.2), any necessary urgent treatment should be provided as per the patient's best interests. The General Medical Council has stated that, in an emergency, where there is doubt or disagreement about the validity or applicability of an advance refusal of treatment but no time to investigate further, the presumption should be in favour of providing treatment (General Medical Council, 2010).

The means of determining the patient's best interests might differ depending on the urgency of the situation. The ideal is for a meeting to be convened, during which the patient's wishes (present and past) are heard, in addition to the views of carers and health professionals, but this might not always be possible. If time allows, the preferred course of action might be to delay treatment until the patient regains capacity. If the lack of capacity is due to the presence of a mental illness, this illness should be treated appropriately.

Even if the patient is deemed to have passed the legal test for capacity, the psychiatrist's involvement should not necessarily end at that point. If the refusal of treatment has potentially distressing consequences, the patient might still require emotional support, as might carers and members of staff. In the case of a patient who has self-harmed and is refusing treatment, consideration should also be given to the use of the Mental Health Act 1983.

Medically unexplained symptoms

The umbrella term 'medically unexplained symptoms' describes the presentation of physical symptoms in the absence of tissue pathology. Patients presenting with medically unexplained symptoms are a common phenomenon, accounting for approximately a quarter of consultations in general practices (Bridges & Goldberg, 1985) and half of those in secondary care (Nimnuan *et al*, 2001). As might be expected, presentations that are purely medically unexplained are less common in patients admitted to hospital wards, although the relatively small numbers of these patients who are admitted tend to use a disproportionately high amount of healthcare resources (Fink, 1992).

Medically unexplained symptoms potentially incorporate a wide spectrum of patients, ranging from primary care attendees who are easily reassured about their time-limited physical symptoms through to individuals who are severely disabled by more persistent symptoms. The focus in this section will be upon presentations at the latter end of the spectrum that occur in emergency departments or medical admission units.

Classification and terminology

The term 'medically unexplained symptom' is not used in the classification systems of ICD-10 (World Health Organization, 1992) and DSM-V (American Psychiatric Association, 2013). It is beyond the scope of this chapter to discuss the merits of the term or the classification approaches taken, other than to say that both systems have increasingly different approaches to the classifying presentations of physical symptoms in the absence of tissue pathology. Table 16.3 provides an overview of the approaches used in ICD-10 and DSM-V.

Medically unexplained symptoms in the psychiatric and emergency context

Specialist mental health interventions will not be required for the vast majority of patients with unexplained symptoms, as most presentations will be isolated, time-limited and minor. However, some patients will need a more specialist level of input, and this might sometimes be requested on an urgent basis because of high levels of distress, loss of function associated

Table 16.3 The classification of persistent medically unexplained symptoms in ICD-10 and DSM-V

ICD-10		DSM-V
F44	**Dissociation [conversion] disorders**	**Dissociative disorders**
F44.0	Dissociative amnesia	Dissociative amnesia +/- fugue
F44.1	Dissociative fugue	Dissociative identity disorder
F44.2	Dissociative stupor	Depersonalization/derealization disorder
F44.3	Trance and possession states	Other specified dissociative disorder
F44.4	Dissociative motor disorders	Unspecified dissociative disorder
F44.5	Dissociative convulsions	
F44.6	Dissociative anaesthesia and sensory loss	
F44.7	Mixed	
F44.8	Other Ganser's syndrome Multiple personality disorder Transient dissociative disorders occurring in childhood and adolescence Other specified	
F44.9	Dissociative disorder unspecified	
F45	**Somatoform disorders**	**Somatic symptom and related disorders**
F45.0	Somatization disorder	
F45.1	Undifferentiated somatoform disorder	
F45.2	Hypochondriacal disorder	Illness anxiety disorder
F45.3	Somatoform autonomic dysfunction	
F45.4	Persistent somatoform pain disorder	
F45.8	Other somatoform disorders	
F45.9	Somatoform disorder unspecified	
		Conversion disorder
		Psychological factors affecting other medical conditions
		Factitious disorder
F68	**Other disorders of adult personality and behaviour**	
F68.1	Intentional production or feigning of symptoms or disabilities, either physical or psychological [factitious disorder]	

Sources: World Health Organisation (1992), American Psychiatric Association (2103)

with the presentation or a need to reduce the potential for harm from unnecessary investigations (or a combination of these factors).

Examples might include:

- acute medically unexplained symptoms (e.g. pain, breathlessness)
- medically unexplained loss of consciousness, stupor or seizure
- profound loss of function (e.g. paralysis, blindness)
- medically unexplained cognitive difficulties (e.g. fugue states).

Assessment and management of medically unexplained symptoms

Patients with complex and enduring symptoms will require long-term engagement and therapy; however, there are certain practical preventive and reactive steps that can easily be deployed in the emergency setting.

The role of general hospital staff

Successful management calls for close collaboration between the patient, general hospital staff, general practitioners and, if needed, mental health specialists. Usually, even in urgent cases, by the time a psychiatrist becomes involved, the patient has received some form of assessment from general hospital staff and might have presented in a similar manner on previous occasions. It is important, therefore, to consider the wider context of assessment and management and to ensure that general hospital staff receive adequate training on how to deal with such presentations. A typical scenario might be a patient who presents repeatedly with chest pain and is highly anxious because of their belief that they are about to have a heart attack and die.

The clinician's aim should be to understand the symptoms from the patient's perspective. Illness representation is a useful concept that can guide this approach (Petrie *et al*, 2007). It suggests that patients will often attach a meaning to the symptoms they are experiencing, on the basis of the perception they have of its identity, symptoms, cause, consequence, time course and controllability. General hospital staff should therefore be encouraged to determine not only what the symptoms are but also the patient's understanding of and preconceived ideas about them.

The patient's general practitioner should be contacted at an early stage to ensure that information is shared. This aids the provision of consistent messages across different health settings and can prevent the repetition of unnecessary investigations. Modern medical informatics should also make it possible to flag up frequent attendees so that the reasons for the frequent attendance can be explored at an early stage, with a view to attending to any psychosocial factors and consequently preventing iatrogenic harm through unnecessary investigations and interventions.

Ambulance crews are often the first point of contact for medically unexplained presentations. Liaison psychiatry services should therefore communicate with ambulance staff to ensure that patients who frequently attend emergency departments via the ambulance service receive a psychiatric assessment when appropriate. These patients can be provided with tailored crisis plans that detail alternative courses of action to follow, such as employing relaxation techniques, when they are considering calling an ambulance.

The role of the mental health specialist

Broadly, referrals that require specialist mental health assessment will consist of cases where there is a high level of distress associated with the medically unexplained symptoms (for which anxiety might be the underlying issue), or cases where there is a sudden and dramatic loss of function to the point where the patient is unresponsive, paralysed or has lost the ability to speak or see. In either scenario, the mental health specialist should not assume that the processes of listening and understanding described above have already been adequately carried out.

The mental health specialist should manage both time and the environment to ensure that they can offer the patient an open, confidential and un-rushed opportunity to discuss their presentation and what they understand about it. The aim of this discussion is to arrive at a shared understanding of the situation. This might be the first time that the patient has been afforded such an opportunity within a hospital system, where doctors can routinely arrive en mass, with little other than bed curtains to shroud hurried, didactic conversations.

One aim of the assessment is to screen the patient for the presence of a psychiatric illness, given their known association with medically unexplained symptoms (Van Hemert *et al*, 1993). This should not, however, be the only aim of the assessment, as in many cases a psychiatric diagnosis will not be present. A thorough assessment must therefore go beyond simply screening for psychiatric pathology and explore all the longitudinal psychosocial factors and potentially abnormal illness beliefs that could have led to and be maintaining the presentation.

The ultimate aim of the assessment is to achieve a collaborative formulation of the patient's situation. It can offer both the patient and involved carers a way of understanding the situation and be a vehicle for change. This collaborative approach is crucial, as patients will otherwise find themselves in a frustrating battle to obtain answers and explanations from health professionals who do not have them.

Management of somatoform and dissociative disorders

Somatoform disorders

The general measures described above are highly applicable for patients in this group. Patients with somatization disorder are usually chronically impaired and rapid change following an urgent referral should not be expected. The aims of urgent intervention are to prevent iatrogenic damage once pathology has been adequately excluded and to lay the groundwork for engagement with a therapeutic process (for those willing to engage). Longer-term, specific therapies might include cognitive–behavioural therapy (Sharpe, 1995), interpersonal therapy (Guthrie, 1995) and group therapy (Kashner *et al*, 1995), but these will not be accessible or possible in the acute setting.

Acute dissociative/conversion disorders

Acute dissociative/conversion disorders can be divided into those producing motor symptoms (e.g. aphonia, paralysis, seizure), those producing sensory symptoms (e.g. blindness, deafness, sensory loss) and those producing individual symptoms (e.g. amnesia, stupor, fugue). In each instance, the sudden and dramatic nature of the presentation can prove challenging for general hospital teams and might provoke a referral to psychiatry.

As with other forms of medically unexplained presentations, symptoms are often minor, short-lived and time-limited and patients and treating teams should both be provided with empathetic reassurance to this effect. Treatment approaches should follow the general schema described above, with care taken to assess for comorbid psychiatric disorders and psychosocial stressors that might have led to or be maintaining the presentation.

One important aspect of care is the prevention of secondary complications, such as atrophy of muscle groups and contractures, that can result from disuse. Physiotherapy, therefore, should be an important part of a goal-driven treatment plan. Other allied health professionals, such as speech therapists, might be useful, depending upon the nature of the loss of function.

Abreaction, which involves patients being interviewed while under the influence of drugs, has been commonly used in the past as a treatment for conversion disorders. Such a therapy consists of components such as catharsis, suggestion, exploration and rehabilitation. The technique is uncommon in most practices. A recent meta-analysis showed that there is a lack of research in this area and the authors called for more work to be done on exploring the benefits of this possibly efficacious treatment (Poole *et al*, 2010).

In large urban areas, it is not unusual for cases of fugue states to present via transport hubs. For example, an individual might be found wandering in a train station, saying that they do not know who they are. Such patients should receive all the assessments, investigations and interventions described above. Additionally, they should be made aware that if the police are not already involved, they will have to be contacted and informed.

Factitious disorder

This disorder describes the conscious, deliberate production of symptoms or signs of illness for unconscious reasons. In order to make the diagnosis, there must be convincing evidence that the signs or symptoms have been deliberately engineered. When patients with the disorder are confronted with evidence of their behaviour, they will frequently discharge themselves, only to re-present in a similar manner elsewhere.

The evidence that the patient has deliberately feigned illness should be reviewed, as if conclusions have been wrongly drawn, the therapeutic relationship with the patient could be irrevocably damaged. Equally, the patient should be screened for other mental illnesses that could be driving the behaviour. If the patient has induced a medical condition, then this will require appropriate treatment. Otherwise, further investigation and treatment should be avoided.

Although research on this disorder is sparse, there is some evidence that confronting patients in a non-punitive and supportive way does not result in immediate self-discharge, additional psychological harm or suicide (Sutherland & Rodin, 1990) and might, in a small number of cases, lay the way for further engagement. Attempts should be made, therefore, to engage the patient in follow-up therapy with the aim of addressing the maladaptive behaviour. Unfortunately, however, many patients decline such opportunities and the aim might then have to be damage limitation, using hospital alert systems in an attempt to prevent repeat admissions.

References

American Psychiatric Association (2013) *Diagnostic and Statistical Manual of Mental Disorders Fifth Edition (DSM-V)*. American Psychiatric Association.

Bridges KW, Goldberg DP (1985) Somatic presentation of DSM-III psychiatric disorders in primary care. *Journal of Psychosomatic Research*, **29**: 563–569.

Bronheim HE, Fulop G, Kunkel E, *et al* (1998) The Academy of Psychosomatic Medicine Practice guidelines for psychiatric consultation in the general medical setting. *Psychosomatics*, **39**: S8–30.

Cohen-Mansfield J (2000) Use of patient characteristics to determine non-pharmacologic interventions for behavioural and psychological symptoms of dementia. *International Psychogeriatrics*, **12** (Suppl 1): 373–380.

Committee on Safety of Medicines (2004) *Atypical Antipsychotic Drugs and Stroke*. Committee on Safety of Medicines.

Department of Constitutional Affairs (2007) *Mental Capacity Act 2005 Code of Practice*. The Stationery Office (http://www.justice.gov.uk/downloads/guidance/protecting-the-vulnerable/mca/mca-code-practice-0509.pdf).

Fink P (1992) Surgery and medical treatment in persistent somatising patients. *Journal of Psychosomatic Research*, **36**: 439–447.

General Medical Council (2010) *Treatment and Care Towards the End of Life: Good Practice in Decision Making*. GMC.

Guthrie E (1995) Treatment of functional somatic symptoms: psychodynamic treatment. In *Treatment of Functional Somatic Symptoms* (eds R Mayou, C Bass, M Sharpe). Oxford University Press.

Kannabiran M, Deshpande S, Walling A, *et al* (2008) Cross-sectional survey of disturbed behaviour in patients in general hospital in Leeds. *Porstgraduate Medical Journal*, **84**: 428–431.

Kashner T, Rost K, Cohen B, *et al* (1995) Enhancing the health of somatization disorder patients. *Effectiveness of short-term group therapy. Psychosomatics*, **36**: 462–470.

National Institute for Health and Clinical Excellence (2005) *Violence. The Short-Term Management of Disturbed/Violent Behaviour in In-Patient Psychiatric Settings and Emergency Department (NICE Clinical Guideline 25)*. NICE.

National Institute for Health and Clinical Excellence (2010) *Delirium. Diagnosis, Prevention and Management (NICE Clinical Guideline 103)*. NICE.

Nimnuan C, Hotopf M, Wessely S (2001) Medically unexplained symptoms: an epidemiological study in seven specialities. *Journal of Psychosomatic Research*, **51**, 361–367.

Petrie KD, Jago LA, Devcich DA (2007) The role of illness perceptions in patients with medical conditions. *Current Opinion in Psychiatry*, **20**: 163–167.

Poole N, Wuerz A, Agrawal N (2010) Abreaction for conversion disorder. A systematic review with meta analysis. *British Journal of Psychiatry*, **197**: 91–95.

Royal College of Psychiatrists (2004) *Atypical antipsychotics and behavioural and psychiatric symptoms of dementia. Prescribing update for old age psychiatrists*. Royal College of Psychiatrists.

Sharpe M (1995) Cognitive behavioural therapies in the treatment of functional somatic symptoms. In *Treatment of Functional Somatic Symptoms* (eds R Mayou, C Bass, M Sharpe). Oxford University Press.

Stokes G (2000) *Challenging Behaviour in Dementia: A Person-Centred Approach*. Winslow Press.

Sutherland AJ, Rodin GM (1990) Factitious disorders in a general hospital setting: clinical features and review of the literature. *Psychosomatics*, **31**: 392–399.

Swearer JM, Drachmann DA, O'Donnell BF, *et al* (1988) Troublesome and disruptive behaviours in dementia – relationships to diagnosis and disease severity. *Journal of the American Geriatrics Society*, **76**: 784–790.

Van Hemert AM, Hengeveld MW, Bolk JH, *et al* (1993) Psychiatric disorders in relation to medical illness among patients of a general medical out-patient clinic. *Psychological Medicine*, **23**: 167–173.

World Health Organization (1992) *ICD-10 Classification of Mental and Behavioural Disorders*. WHO.

CHAPTER 17

Psychiatric emergencies in deaf people

Manjit Gahir, Simon Gibbon and Brendan Monteiro

Deafness is a blanket term that covers many different conditions. Some people are born deaf and others become deaf at some stage in their lives. Age at onset, degree of deafness and level of functional impairment can all influence a deaf person's self-image, communication preferences and cultural identity (Baines, 2007). There are different implications of deafness for those deaf from birth or an early age (pre-lingually deaf) and for those who have acquired deafness at a later stage, when verbal language might be present (Table 17.1). It is difficult to precisely define deafness, as hearing itself encompasses complex characteristics such as intensity, loudness, pitch and frequency, and is very much a subjective experience. However, there is a general consensus on differentiating hearing loss on the basis of intensity or loudness on a continuum: mild (25–40 dB), moderate (41–70 dB), severe (71–95 dB) and profound (>96 dB).

Partial deafness is said to affect those with mild, moderate or severe hearing loss who might benefit from hearing aids or cochlear implants to hear speech. Some might internalise verbal language (use of words) and, therefore, gain some benefit from lip-reading. It is important to realise that these people might have specialised communication needs and experience difficulties when in groups or when there is background noise. Profound deafness affects people who have little or no hearing for speech, who might obtain some benefit from hearing aids for environmental sounds. It occurs in approximately 8 in 1000 (0.8%) of the population, with this having its onset in early childhood in 1 in 1000. Of the children who are born deaf (congenital deafness) approximately 50% will have a genetic cause for this, that is some chromosomal disorder which included deafness as one of its symptoms, and the other 50% with have a different cause such as maternal infection with rubella or influenza, or some sort of birth injury.

Around 20% of the general population have a hearing loss of >20 dB, and this proportion rises to 75% of those over 75 years of age. However, these are people who are described as 'deafened' or 'hard of hearing', and their hearing loss is part of the normal ageing process. They might have some residual hearing and essentially they belong to the wider hearing community.

Table 17.1 Differences between pre-lingual and post-lingual deafness

Pre-lingual	Post-lingual
Onset at birth/early age; difficult to acquire speech and verbal language	Onset after speech and verbal acquisition of language
Communication based on sign language/ gesture	Communication based on speech and written word
Early development influenced by communication difficulties between hearing parents and deaf child	Early development not affected as parents and child share same language
Deafness affects emotional, social, psychological, linguistic and educational development	Deafness does not affect social, psychological, linguistic or educational development
Person identifies with deaf community and deaf culture	Person often does not identify with deaf culture

It is estimated that approximately 700 000 people in the UK are either severely or profoundly deaf, of whom approximately 50 000 are British Sign Language (BSL) users (Royal National Institute for Deaf People, 2011). The vast majority (approximately 90%) of deaf children are born to hearing parents and only 10% are born to deaf parents. There is evidence that deaf children of deaf parents are much better adjusted, have much better communication skills and might have a lower incidence of mental illness than deaf children of hearing parents. In this chapter, the word 'Deaf' (as opposed to 'deaf') is used to describe a subsection of the population who use a signed language; in Britain, this is usually BSL.

Doctors and mental health professionals who have little or no understanding of deafness might feel deskilled when they encounter deaf people in mental health or criminal justice settings. Schlesinger & Meadow-Orlans (1972) have described a 'shock–withdrawal–paralysis syndrome' to describe a sense of inadequacy and paralysis experienced by professionals when assessing a deaf client. These professionals can find themselves unable to use well-established diagnostic and therapeutic skills to assess and treat deaf people.

Communication preferences

Not everyone who has a degree of hearing loss will use a signed language to communicate. There are a variety of communication methods that can be employed, and some deaf people, especially those with post-verbal or acquired deafness, might have learnt English as their first language. However, children who are pre-lingually deaf cannot acquire speech or verbal language normally. At around the end of the first year of life, the hearing child begins to imitate speech, but without understanding. They soon begin to associate names and words with people and objects, and so begin the internalisation of verbal language. By 4 years of age, the child will have grasped most of the complexities of spoken language and will become literate and express complex ideas and concepts using speech and words.

The deaf child is seriously disadvantaged in this regard and the majority of deaf children do not develop intelligible speech, as they cannot imitate speech or monitor their own voices. As verbal language cannot develop through auditory mechanisms, there is no basis on which to develop literacy skills (Denmark, 1978). The deaf child has to develop language through vision, either by lip-reading or by written word. Lip-reading is very difficult because of its inexactitude: for example, some speech sounds are not associated with lip movements and some lip patterns are the same for different words. It also presupposes some knowledge of verbal language that, in the case of the pre-lingually deaf child, is poorly developed or absent. Equally, developing verbal language through the written word might be impossible, as reading and writing skills have a basis in auditory language, such that even a hearing child with well-developed auditory language is not capable of literacy in their early years.

Most deaf children are born to hearing parents and are not exposed to a signed language in their early years, thus limiting their ability to access an appropriate communicatio method at a crucial developmental time. This has been compounded by historical educational policies (some still present in certain areas of the UK) that have insisted on deaf children being taught verbal speech and being discouraged or punished for using sign language. Deaf children receive special education, either as part of mainstream schooling, in small units attached to schools or in specialist deaf schools, where education is provided via the oral/aural method or BSL. Despite specialist education, however, deaf children are more likely to achieve poor levels or English literacy, and the average reading age of deaf school leavers was found to be 8–9 years of age (Conrad, 1977).

Deaf people often use sign language to communicate with each other, and some acquire this language without the help of formal education. BSL has now achieved formal recognition as the fourth official language in the UK and is a rule-governed, fully developed language using the hands, facial expression, lip pattern and movements to convey information. It is not a universal language, since regional variations exist within the UK and other countries have developed their own form of sign language. Significant differences exist between the different sign languages, for example French and American Sign Languages communicate using the fingers of one hand, whereas in BSL, both hands are used. Consequently, although a hearing person visiting the USA will have little difficulty in understanding others and being understood, a deaf visitor will be faced with a completely different language.

Not all deaf people have the same ability to use sign language. Their ability depends on a number of factors, including the cause of deafness, intellectual ability, exposure to sign language at a critical phase of language development, education methodology and involvement in the deaf community. A small but significant group of deaf people have little or no sign language (known as minimal language skills), and require careful assessment and specialist interpreting skills/communication support. There are a number of reasons why a deaf person might have minimal language skills – for example, a technical problem related to sensory impairment, neurological problems affecting receptive or expressive communication (Hyvarinen *et al*, 1990), intellectual disability, or another disorder that might affect language acquisition, such as autistic spectrum disorder, aphasia, attention–deficit hyperactivity disorder or blindness.

Deafness and disability

Culturally, deaf people do not see themselves as disabled, but there are a variety of disabilities that can co-exist with deafness (Fortnum *et al*, 1996):

- visual problems
- neuro-motor problems
- cerebral dysfunction
- cognitive deficits
- cranio-facial abnormalities
- systemic disorders
- named syndromes.

The first four of these have implications for communication and language development. There are a variety of inherited syndromes that involve deafness and blindness, of which Usher syndrome is the most common. This syndrome is characterised by congenital deafness and retinitis pigmentosa – a degenerative condition of the retina that leads to night blindness and tunnel vision. Intrauterine infections, such as rubella embryopathy or cytomegalovirus, are associated with visual problems, behavioural difficulties and intellectual impairment, and might also be related to mental illness in later life (Brown *et al*, 2000).

Deafness and mental health

There is increasing recognition of the difficulties faced by deaf people regarding mental health and access to treatment (Fellinger *et al*, 2012; The Lancet, 2012). Deaf people require special psychiatric services, because there is a serious risk of misdiagnosis when they are assessed by mental health professionals who have no understanding of the psychological, cultural and sociological aspects of different types of deafness and who cannot communicate using sign language.

Communication is of vital importance in all medical practice, but in psychiatry it assumes central importance. The clinical interview is the main tool of assessment and treatment in psychiatry (Rutter & Cox,

1981). Communication is also crucially important if the mental health professional is to put the patient at their ease and enlist their cooperation. If the patient is profoundly deaf from birth or an early age, has poor speech, poor verbal language, and relies on sign language for communication, most mental health professionals find it difficult to examine the patient properly and make an accurate diagnosis. See Fig. 17.1 for a guide to assessing the possibility of effective communication with a deaf patient and when to request an interpreter.

There are three main areas of possible misdiagnosis:
1   deafness can be mistaken for intellectual impairment;
2   mental illness can be missed;
3   mental illness can be diagnosed where none exists.

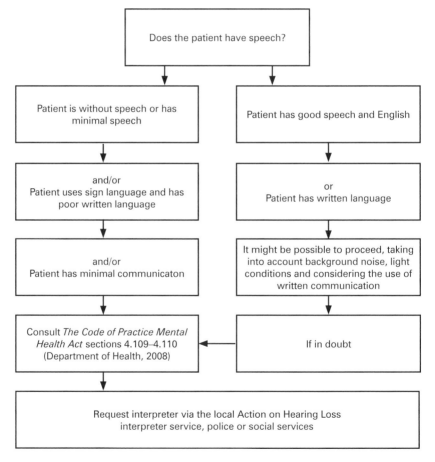

Fig. 17.1 Assessing whether an interpreter is needed to communicate effectively with a deaf patient.

The study of the incidence and prevalence of mental disorder in deaf adults is fraught with difficulty, and most studies have been based on referrals to specialist services. A study of mental disorder in Deaf people (Denmark, 1985) found that, of 250 referrals to the department of psychiatry for the deaf at Whittingham Hospital, only 104 had a diagnosable mental illness, 48 had a developmental disorder of communication and 58 had problems directly related to deafness (including behavioural problems, depression due to acquired deafness and alcoholism).

The relationship between Deafness and schizophrenia remains unclear and an early study (Houston & Royse, 1954) suggested that the rate of schizophrenia is higher in Deaf people than in hearing people. However, other studies (Cooper, 1976; Cooper et al, 1976) do not support this, although an increased incidence of paranoia has been noted. The mode of action proposed by these authors is that changes in psychological functioning and social adaptation take place over a prolonged period of time and result in interference with attention, perception and communication processes. More recently, it has been suggested that Deaf people have the same incidence of schizophrenia as the general population (du Feu & Fergusson, 2003) and that they can experience hallucinations in all modalities, including auditory hallucinations, although the way in which the symptoms are expressed might be unusual (Thacker, 1994; du Feu & McKenna, 1999).

Deaf people are thought to suffer major affective disorders with the same frequency as hearing people, although a comparative study of Deaf and hearing in-patients in the USA found that Deaf patients were almost twice as likely to suffer from a serious mood disorder and four times as likely to suffer from an anxiety disorder, especially post-traumatic stress disorder (Black & Glickman, 2006). Equally, a study of Deaf people in the community in Norway also found an increased incidence of depression and anxiety (Kvam et al, 2006). However, the concept of depression can be difficult to discuss with Deaf patients, who might have limited communication. They might describe sadness (i.e. everyday mood changes due to situational factors), and it might be difficult to assess the degree of depression. It is important to be aware that what might be thought of as depressive symptoms, such as sadness, agitation, withdrawal and being uncommunicative, might be due to frustration and not actually indicative of a depressive illness. Features related to organicity, including distractibility, disinhibition and hyperactivity, might be misdiagnosed as mania. A careful history about the onset of these features and their causation should be taken, and recent changes should be carefully noted and evaluated over a period of time. Biological symptoms, diurnal variation of mood, self-neglect, threats of self-harm and persistent somatic complaints can be helpful in arriving at a diagnosis.

It is important to assess the risk patients pose to themselves. The risk of suicide and deliberate self-harm is not known in the Deaf population

(Turner *et al*, 2007) and the evaluation of risk is fraught with difficulties. For example, information given by relatives and friends, who are not always able to communicate appropriately with the Deaf person, might be inaccurate. However, the increased incidence of depression, other medical problems and difficulty in accessing help might increase the risk of suicide and self-harm.

Psychiatric emergencies in Deaf people

Psychiatric emergencies in Deaf people can occur in a variety of different settings, such as the community, hospitals (both general and psychiatric) and prisons, to name but a few. In some ways, the emergencies will be similar to those occurring in the hearing population (e.g. in terms of the acuteness of the presentation), but matters will be compounded by a higher prevalence of mental disorder in the Deaf, different expression of symptoms, inability to explain what is being experienced and the linguistic and cultural barriers to being understood.

It is well established that Deaf people are less likely than the general population to visit their general practitioner, while, conversely, they are more likely to suffer from poor physical and mental health (Sign Health, 2008). Once they are seen, there might be difficulties in establishing what exactly is wrong and in dealing with them appropriately, especially if communication support is not available.

In 1998, a homicide was committed in London by an 18-year-old, mentally ill, profoundly deaf man. The homicide was the subject of an independent inquiry chaired by a leading barrister (Mishcon *et al*, 2000). It was found that, despite having extensive input from psychiatric services for the Deaf, there were significant failings in communication between different clinical teams involved in his care. A number of recommendations were made by the inquiry team, including the need for a coordinated national strategy for deaf people with mental health problems, robust emergency assessment and admission arrangements to specialised deaf services and the need for all mental health professionals to participate in multi-agency training on information sharing.

Another homicide was committed by a profoundly deaf man in 2000 and was again the subject of an independent inquiry (Downham *et al*, 2004). Although in this case the perpetrator did not have a formal diagnosis of mental illness, he did have contact with the community psychiatric nurse for the deaf in Nottingham and was receiving support for his marital difficulties. He was seen 6 days before and the day after the killing, at which times there was no evidence of any disorder and he did not disclose his intention to commit the offence. Although the inquiry team found that nothing in this homicide was predictable, they did comment on the difficulties in conducting an out-of-hours psychiatric assessment in an emergency department. Unfortunately, although there was already a contract in existence with the local Deaf Society for accessing BSL interpreters, this was not well publicised and staff were unaware that this could be done. This resulted in the unacceptable situation where his wife was asked to interpret for him, even though some of the questions were about his thoughts of self-harm and alleged threats to stab her.

Again, a number of recommendations were made, including the need for a local policy to address the needs of Deaf patients, 24-hour access to BSL interpreters and the suggestion that health and social care services for the Deaf should be integrated. A further comment was made around the need for Care Programme Approach documentation and risk assessments to be completed and circulated at the point of discharge rather than later on.

In 2002, a consultation document was launched to address the mental health needs of Deaf people, including a BSL version designed to be accessible to Deaf people (Department of Health, 2002). Following a lengthy consolation period, a final best-practice guidance document was published (Department of Health, 2005). It included 27 recommendations regarding the assessment needs of Deaf children and adults, accessibility to appropriate services, use of technology (including video conferencing), minicoms and BSL/English translation software, staff training in BSL and increased access to specialist assessment for Deaf prisoners.

Working with interpreters

The ideal situation is for assessment to be conducted by a mental health professional with the necessary communication skills and an understanding of deafness. Unfortunately, there are currently very few mental health professionals with these skills in the UK, so almost invariably non-signing mental health professionals will conduct the assessment. When dealing with deaf people with poor or minimal sign-language skills, it is often necessary to use an additional deaf professional person to help in simplifying the standard BSL to a more understandable format. These professionals are known variously as deaf communication support workers or deaf relay interpreters and have a vital role in aiding communication.

With the changes to the Mental Health Act in 2007 and the introduction of the Mental Capacity Act 2005, there is an increasing role for independent advocates, and a legal responsibility on the part of mental health trusts to ensure that advocates are available. Ideally, this should include Deaf advocates (e.g. those provided by the Sign Health charity), although their services might be expensive and are often not immediately available. When working with interpreters, it is important to bear in mind that many will not have any knowledge or training in mental health matters, and might not have the knowledge or linguistic skills to undertake the interpretation of a detailed psychiatric evaluation. Although it might not be possible in an emergency situation (e.g. when conducting a Mental

Health Act assessment out of hours), as far as possible, a mental health trained interpreter should be used.

Deaf prisoners

There is currently limited research into the number and specific needs of deaf prisoners. Various estimates have been made of how many prisoners in the UK are deaf or hard of hearing, and these figures vary between 66 and 139. Unfortunately, research into this area is limited by the lack of formal data kept by the Ministry of Justice. Although the reception screening questionnaire (administered to all prisoners on the day of remand into custody) now asks a specific question about the presence of all disabilities, including deafness, there is little evidence of data collection or of this information being used to influence prison policy.

A survey of all prisons and young-offender institutions in England and Wales (Gahir *et al*, 2011) identified 139 Deaf or hard-of-hearing inmates. Prison staff reported that the main difficulties in dealing with deaf inmates related to lack of access to sign-language interpreters and a lack of specialist assessments. It was noted that the clinicians conducting this research were aware of a number of instances where deaf prisoners were not appropriately diagnosed or treated, as they had not been formally assessed in BSL by deaf-aware professionals.

There are a number of specialised secure units for deaf people but as yet there is no community forensic deaf provision. Equally, there are only two prisons in England that regularly receive psychiatric input from professionals with specialist deaf knowledge, Her Majesty's Prison (HMP) Manchester and HMP Moorlands near Doncaster, although a sex-offender treatment programme in BSL has recently been developed at HMP Whatton in Nottinghamshire.

The lack of a single prison that deals with deaf prisoners can arguably lead to them being disadvantaged, as they might be isolated, geographically distant from their family and unable to communicate with prison staff, and might not have access to sign-language interpreters or (very importantly) not be able to access appropriate offence-focused courses in BSL. The in-reach to Manchester and Moorlands prisons was begun with the intention of providing specific therapies to deaf people, including sex-offender treatment and anger-management programmes. Unfortunately, although the regional sex-offender prison in Nottinghamshire houses a number of deaf prisoners, they do not have access to regular sex-offender work in BSL at this time.

There are a number of potential difficulties in providing this specialist input to prisons, not least of which is the cost and the fact that deaf people are distributed widely throughout the prison system. The need for specialist input might not be recognised, as not all Deaf prisoners are identified as such, or interviews might not be adequately conducted in BSL such that mental disorder is not appropriately recognised or treated.

Conclusions

Psychiatrists and other professionals need to be aware of the particular needs of deaf people with mental disorder, both in terms of the possible different presentation of disorders but also in terms of the cultural and linguistic context.

Although psychiatric emergencies seem unlikely to occur more frequently in deaf people, the true emergency occurs when adequate assessment is not undertaken. It is essential that Deaf people are interviewed with an appropriately trained sign-language interpreter and that referral to a specialist mental health service for deaf people is made at the earliest practicable point in the assessment and treatment process.

References

Baines D (2007) *Unravelling the anomaly of deafness*. In *Deafness and Challenging Behaviour* (eds S Austen and D Jeffrey). Wiley.

Black P, Glickman N (2006) Demographics, psychiatric diagnoses and other characteristics of North-American deaf and hard-of-hearing inpatients. *Journal of Deaf Studies and Deaf Education*, **11**: 303–321.

Brown AS, Cohen P, Greenwald S, *et al* (2000) Nonaffective psychosis after pre-natal exposure to rubella. *American Journal of Psychiatry*, **157**: 438–443.

Conrad R (1977) The reading ability of deaf school leavers. *British Journal of Educational Psychology*, **47**: 138–148.

Cooper AF (1976) Deafness and psychiatric illness. *British Journal of Psychiatry*, **129**: 216–226.

Cooper AF, Garside RF, Kay DW (1976) A comparison of deaf and non-deaf patients with paranoid and affective psychoses. *British Journal of Psychiatry*, **129**: 532–538.

Denmark JC (1978) Early profound deafness and mental retardation. *British Journal of Mental Subnormality*, **24**: 81–89.

Denmark JC (1985) A study of 250 patients referred to a Department of Psychiatry for the Deaf. *British Journal of Psychiatry*, **146**: 282–286.

Department of Health (2002) *A Sign of the Times. Modernising Mental Health Services for People who are Deaf*. Department of Health Publications.

Department of Health (2005) *Mental Health and Deafness. Towards Equity and Access*. Department of Health Publications.

Department of Health (2008) *Code of Practice Mental Health Act 1983*. Department of Health Publications.

Downham G, McKenna J, Jamil M, *et al* (2004) *Report of the Independent Inquiry into the Care and Treatment of Sarawat Al-Assaf*. Gedling Primary Care Trust.

du Feu M, Fergusson K (2003) Sensory impairment and mental health. *Advances in Psychiatric Treatment*, **9**: 95–103.

du Feu M, McKenna P (1999) Prelingually profoundly deaf schizophrenic patients who hear voices: a phenomenological analysis. *Acta Psychiatrica Scandinavica*, **97**: 1–9.

Fellinger J, Holzinger D, Pollard R (2012) Mental health of deaf people. *Lancet*, **379**: 1037–1044.

Fortnum H, Davis A, Butler A, *et al* (1996) *Health Service Implications of Changes in Aetiology and Referral Patterns of Hearing Impaired Children in Trent Region, 1985–1993*. MRC Institute of Hearing Research and Trent Health.

Gahir MS, O'Rourke S, Monteiro BT, *et al* (2011) The unmet needs of deaf prisoners: a survey of prisons in England and Wales. *International Journal of Mental Health and Deafness*, **1**: 58–63.

Houston F, Royse AB (1954) Relationship between deafness and psychotic illness. *British Journal of Psychiatry*, **100**: 990–993.

Hyvarinen L, Gimble L, Sorri M (1990) *Assessment of Vision and Hearing of Deaf–Blind Persons*. Royal Victorian Institute for the Blind.

Kvam MH, Loeb M, Tambs K (2006) Mental health in deaf adults: symptoms of anxiety and depression among hearing and deaf individuals. *Journal of Deaf Studies and Deaf Education*, **12**: 1–7.

Mishcon J, Sensky T, Lindsey M, *et al* (2000) *Report of the Independent Inquiry Team into the Care and Treatment of Daniel Joseph*. Merton, Sutton and Wandsworth Health Authority, Lambeth, Southwark and Lewisham Health Authority.

Royal National Institute for Deaf People (2011) *Facts and Figures on Deafness and Tinnitus*. RNID (http://www.actiononhearingloss.org.uk/supporting-you/factsheets-and-leaflets/deaf-awareness.aspx).

Rutter M, Cox A (1981) Psychiatric interviewing techniques: I. Methods and measures. *British Journal of Psychiatry*, **138**: 273–282.

Schlesinger HS, Meadow-Orlans KP (1972) *Sound and Sign: Childhood Deafness and Mental Health*. University of Berkley Press.

Sign Health (2008) *Why Do You Keep Missing Me? A Report into Deaf People's Access to Primary Health Care*. Beaconsfield.

Thacker AJ (1994) Formal communication disorder. Sign language in deaf people with schizophrenia. *British Journal of Psychiatry*, **165**: 818–823.

The Lancet (2012) The health of deaf people: communication breakdown. *The Lancet*, **379**: 977.

Turner O, Windfuhr K, Kapur N (2007) Suicide in deaf populations: a literature review. *Annals of General Psychiatry*, **6**: 26.

CHAPTER 18

Mental health law

Dawn Crowther

Legislation pertaining to the care and treatment of individuals presenting with mental disorders is constantly evolving. Legal provision can be traced back to the Madhouses Act of 1774 but, until 1845, the law was mainly concerned with the licensing and inspection of madhouses and asylums. In 1845, the Lunacy Commission was established, with jurisdiction over the detention and treatment of persons of unsound mind throughout England and Wales. This year also saw the requirement to establish county asylums throughout the two countries, via the Lunatics Asylums Act 1845. The Idiots Act 1886 further permitted local authorities to build special asylums for 'idiots' or 'mental defectives'. The Lunacy (Consolidation) Act 1890 allowed for four methods of admission to an asylum, all of which required certification; this Act was somewhat updated by the Mental Deficiency Act 1913, which defined four grades of mental deficiency (idiots, imbeciles, feeble-minded persons and moral defectives) and the Mental Treatment Act 1930, which for the first time made provision for the voluntary admission of individuals who were able to make a written application and be received as a patient without a reception order. The Lunacy (Consolidation) Act 1890 was not repealed until 1959.

The Mental Health Act 1959 (the 1959 Act) brought major changes to the rules surrounding the assessment, detention, care and treatment of those deemed to be suffering from mental disorders and mental deficiency, repealing all previous legislation in this regard. Building on advances in psychiatric treatment, the 1959 Act introduced the concept that mental health patients should be treated no differently to other patients. Patients could be cared for in the community if hospital treatment was not required, and if it was, this did not need to be under compulsion unless treatment was deemed urgently necessary and the person refused to accept informal admission and their clinician's advice with regard to treatment. It was intended that most patients would be admitted informally, and this represented a major shift in focus from 'asylum' for patients to care, treatment and individual rights. The 1959 Act introduced a definition of mental disorder: 'mental illness, arrested or incomplete development of mind, psychopathic disorder, and any other disorder or disability of mind'. Mental Health Review Tribunals were also introduced to review cases of compulsory detention when requested by patients and their relatives.

Mental Health Act 1983 and Mental Capacity Act 2005

Current statutory provision in England and Wales is afforded under the Mental Health Act 1983 (the 1983 Act). The Department of Health (2008a) has produced a reference guide with information on use of the legislation, and separate codes of practice for England and Wales (Department of Health, 2015; Welsh Assembly Government, 2008). The Mental Capacity Act 2005 (the 2005 Act), introduced in 2007 together with a code of practice (Department for Constitutional Affairs, 2007), imposes additional safeguards for those who lack capacity to consent to certain care and treatment. The Mental Health Act 2007 (the 2007 Act) made amendments to both of these Acts, in particular updating the 1983 Act to reflect changes in practice in mental health and social care and the impact of human-rights legislation over the 25 years since it was enacted. These amendments also made provision, under Section 4A of the 2005 Act, for additional procedural requirements for individuals not detained under the 1983 Act who lack capacity to consent to care and treatment that amounts to a deprivation of their liberty – safeguards introduced as a remedy for the breaches identified in what is known as the Bournewood case (*HL v United Kingdom* (45508/99) [2005]), where it was found that Mr L had been detained as an informal patient at the Bournewood Hospital in violation of his right to liberty and security under Articles 5(1) and 5(4) of the European Convention on Human Rights. A code of practice accompanies the additions to the 2005 Act (Ministry of Justice, 2008).

Article 5(1) of the Convention ensures a 'right to liberty and no-one shall be deprived of this save in the following cases and in accordance with a procedure prescribed by law... (e) the lawful detention of persons for the prevention of the spreading of infectious diseases, of persons of unsound mind, alcoholics or drug addicts, or vagrants'. Article 5(4) ensures that 'everyone who is deprived of his liberty by arrest or detention shall be entitled to take proceedings by which the lawfulness of his detention shall be decided speedily by a court and his release ordered if the detention is not lawful'. It is these articles that permit and shape detention, care and treatment under the 1983 and 2005 Acts.

Although the 1983 and 2005 Acts have very different aims, the former focusing on risks to the health and safety of individuals and protection of the wider public with the use of compulsion where necessary, and the latter on enabling and supporting individuals to make their own decisions, these two key pieces of legislation together enable professionals to facilitate care of those who might require treatment for a mental disorder. It is not possible to cover all legal provisions in depth in this short chapter, but I hope the reader will find it a simple guide to help inform practice.

When a person presents with a mental disorder that professionals believe requires intervention, the starting point is whether they have capacity to consent to the treatment or care recommended. The 2007 Act applies to those over 16 years of age and has five guiding principles.

1   There is to be a presumption of capacity.
2   Individuals have the right to be supported to make their own decisions.
3   Individuals have the right to make an unwise decision.
4   Any act or decision made on behalf of a person who lacks capacity must be in their best interests.
5   Any act or decision made on behalf of a person who lacks capacity must be the least restrictive of their rights and freedom of action.

The question of capacity is always issue-specific; for example, can the individual consent to a certain proposed medication, or admission and care in hospital? The impairment can be permanent or temporary and the question is decided on the balance of probabilities.

Assessment of capacity should be carried out wherever there is a concern that the individual might lack the ability to consent to treatment. The person carrying out the assessment should be the person proposing to make the decision or act on behalf of the individual in question (the decision-maker). There might be occasions where a psychiatrist or other mental health specialist is brought in to advise on a particular assessment, but the ultimate say-so lies with the decision-maker. In the case of *PC v City of York Council* [2013] EXCA Civ 478 MHLO 61, the Court of Appeal found that the approach to applying the capacity test should differ to that set out in the 2005 Act's code of practice (Department for Constitutional Affairs, 2007), the stages of the assessment reordered.

Section 3 of the 2005 Act should first be applied.

- Is the individual able to understand the information relevant to the decision (provided in a manner appropriate to their circumstances)?
- Can the individual retain the information (for long enough to make the decision)?
- Can the individual use or weigh that information as part of the process of making the decision (including believing the information)?
- Can the individual communicate their decision (whether by talking, using sign language, or any other means)?

They must also be able to reasonably foresee the consequences of deciding one way or another or of failing to make the decision.

If the individual is unable to do any of the above, the assessor must then address Section 2 of the 2005 Act and determine whether any inability to do so is due to an impairment of, or disturbance in the functioning of, the mind or brain. The Court of Appeal found that the presence or absence of the causative nexus is significant – any inability to decide on the matter in question must be because of the impairment or disturbance. Assessments should be recorded in line with local record-keeping protocols and the greater the consequences of the decision, the more robust the recording should be.

A person who is assessed as having capacity to consent to the care and treatment proposed for a mental disorder, including admission to hospital, can only have their refusal overridden by implementation of the 1983 Act. Where it is deemed that the person lacks the capacity to consent to treatment, further questions must be asked before it can be provided.

Does the person have a valid and applicable advance decision or statement?

An advance decision relates to a refusal of treatment and is legally binding on the professionals responsible for providing care. An advance decision does not have to be in writing unless it relates to withholding or withdrawing life-sustaining treatment – in which case, it must be in writing, signed and witnessed. A statement might be, for example, a request for certain care or treatment; professionals have a duty to consider the request, but are not bound by it.

Where one exists, consideration must be given to whether the decision or statement mirrors current circumstances, whether the individual is now acting in a manner incompatible with the decision or statement, whether it has been withdrawn while the individual has capacity, whether, since making the decision, they have given an attorney authority to make such decisions on their behalf and whether there have been developments in the person's personal life or in medical treatment that they might not have foreseen and would be likely to affect their decision. Note that an advance decision to refuse basic care or to go into a care home does not have any legal standing.

Does the person have a lasting power of attorney or a court-appointed deputy who is able to make the decision on their behalf?

A lasting power of attorney (LPA) is a legal document made by an individual over 18 years of age while they have capacity. It grants decision-making powers in respect of property, financial affairs and personal welfare (including healthcare and consent to treatment) to an attorney or another person and must be registered with the Office of the Public Guardian before it can be used. An individual can place restrictions on the attorney's powers; therefore, it is important to be confident that the attorney has the right to make the decision in question. A copy of the LPA should be requested if there is any doubt.

An attorney will only have the right to consent to or refuse life-sustaining treatment if this is specifically stated in the LPA document. The Court of Protection has the power to appoint deputies to make decisions on behalf of an individual who lacks capacity. These can be limited in scope and duration and can apply to financial and/or personal-welfare decisions so, again, it might be necessary to clarify the extent of the deputy's power. If there is a dispute as to whether an attorney or deputy's decision either prevents life-sustaining treatment being given or might cause a serious deterioration of a patient's condition, action can be taken to sustain life or prevent serious deterioration while the dispute is referred to the Court of Protection.

The Court of Protection, part of Her Majesty's Courts Service, has the power to make declarations on whether a person has capacity to make a particular decision and can rule whether an act proposed or performed on behalf of a person who lacks capacity is lawful. It is important, therefore, to be aware of any ruling in relation to the individual. The court's jurisdiction does not extend to authorisation of the use of powers under the 1983 Act.

The 2005 Act imposes an obligation on those making a decision on behalf of an incapacitated individual to do so in their best interests.

- Is it likely that the individual will at some time have capacity in relation to the matter in question?
- If it seems likely that they will, can the decision be postponed until that time?
- The individual should be permitted and encouraged to participate as fully as possible in the decision.
- The individual's past and present wishes, feelings, beliefs and values likely to influence their decision, so far as is reasonably ascertainable, should be considered.
- If practicable and appropriate, the views of anyone named by the person as someone to be consulted or anyone engaged in caring for the person or interested in his welfare should be taken into account.

Patients with no person to speak for them

Where the individual is found to have no person who can speak for them and the decision to be made is in respect of 'serious medical treatment' or long-term placement, an independent mental capacity advocate (IMCA) must be consulted. The aim of the IMCA service is to provide independent safeguards for people who lack capacity to make certain important decisions. An IMCA must be instructed, and then consulted, whenever an NHS body is proposing to provide, withhold or stop serious medical treatment, or whenever an NHS body or local authority is proposing to arrange accommodation (or a change of accommodation) in a hospital or a care home, and the person will stay in hospital longer than 28 days (or in the care home for more than 8 weeks) and the treatment or placement is not authorised by the use of the 1983 Act.

Serious medical treatment is defined as involving giving new treatment, stopping treatment that has already started, or withholding treatment that could be offered in circumstances where (a) if a single treatment is proposed, there is a fine balance between the probable benefits, the burdens to the patient and the risks involved, (b) the decision between a choice of treatments is finely balanced, or (c) what is proposed is likely to have serious consequences for the patient. Serious consequences are those that could have a serious impact on the patient, either from the effects of the treatment itself or from its wider implications. This treatment can include therapies that cause serious and prolonged pain, distress or side-effects. Any information or reports provided by an IMCA must be taken into account when working out whether a proposed decision is in the person's best interests.

Taking into consideration the above requirements, Section 5 of the 2005 Act provides legal protection from liability for carrying out certain actions in connection with the care and treatment of people who lack capacity, provided that an assessment of capacity has been carried out, that it is reasonably believed that the person lacks capacity in relation to the matter in question, and that the action taken is in the best interests of the person – however, there are limitations to this protection.

Deprivation of liberty and restraint

Section 6 of the 2005 Act dictates that restraint can only be used when the person using it reasonably believes that it is necessary to prevent harm and its use is proportionate to the likelihood and seriousness of the harm (i.e. the least intrusive and minimum amount necessary to prevent the harm occurring). Less-restrictive options must always be considered before using restraint. The restraint must be in the person's best interests and the level of restraint should lessen as the risk of harm diminishes. Restraint covers a wide range of actions, including the use of, or threat of, force to do something that the person concerned resists. Acts of restraint might include holding or steadying someone's arm to enable an injection to be given safely, holding a person down while administering a sedative, or using reasonable force to take a person to hospital to receive necessary treatment. Sections 5 and 6 together might provide the authority required to take an incapacitated person to a hospital and treat them.

Thus, the 2005 Act can be used to treat people when they cannot consent to the treatment because they lack capacity and where the treatment is in their best interests. However, there is no protection afforded for actions that result in someone being deprived of their liberty, as defined by Article 5(1) of the European Convention on Human Rights. In *Storck v Germany* [2005] 43 EHRR, it was ruled that deprivation of liberty has three elements:

- the 'objective element of confinement to a certain limited place for a not negligible length of time'

- the 'additional subjective element [that] they have not validly consented to the confinement in question'
- the confinement must be 'imputable to the State' (i.e. a public authority is directly involved).

Historically, court judgments on what constitutes deprivation of liberty have been closely focused on the facts of each particular case. However, in the joined cases of *P (by his litigation friend the Official Solicitor) (Appellant) v Cheshire West and Chester Council and another (Respondents)* and *P & Q (by their litigation friend, the Official Solicitor (Appellants) v Surrey County Council (Respondent)*[2014] UKSC 19, the Supreme Court found two key elements:

- the person is subject to constant supervision and control
- they are not free to leave (it does not matter whether they are compliant and not trying or voicing a desire to leave – the question is, whether they would be free to leave if they wanted to).

The common-law defence of necessity cannot be relied upon to authorise short-term deprivation of liberty to respond to an emergency where the 1983 or 2005 Act applies. The Court of Appeal, in the case of *Commissioner of the Police for the Metropolis v ZH* [2013] EWCA Civ 69, found that restraint at a pool side for 15 min and then in a police van for 25 min amounted to a deprivation of liberty. This case referred to the earlier case, *R (Sessay) v South London and Maudsley NHS Foundation Trust and another* [2011] EWHC 2617 (QB); [2012] QB 760, where the Divisional Court held that the scheme of the 1983 Act was such that the concept of necessity did not apply so as to give a defense to a claim of false imprisonment or unlawful detention where a person was detained pending completion of an application under the provisions of Section 2 of the 1983 Act. This decision means that where there is a legal process that can be followed under either the 1983 or 2005 Act, this should be done.

Least-restrictive options should always be practised. Where there is no alternative way of providing care or treatment other than by depriving the person of their liberty, that deprivation must be authorised to be lawful, either under the Deprivation of Liberty Safeguards (DoLS) contained in the 2005 Act, under the 1983 Act or through an application to the Court of Protection. Decision-makers must focus on the reason the patient should be deprived of their liberty by asking a series of specific questions (see *GJ v The Foundation Trust* [2009] EWHC 2972 (Fam)).

- What care and treatment should be provided for:
  - physical disorders or illnesses that are unconnected to and unlikely to affect the patient's mental disorders
  - mental disorders
  - physical disorders or illnesses that are connected to them and/or that are likely to directly affect their mental disorders?
- If the need for the package of physical treatment did not exist, would the patient be deprived of liberty in a hospital?

The patient would only be eligible to be held under DoLS if the need to be in hospital is not connected to treatment of their mental disorder. Where it is considered that a person might need to be detained for treatment for mental disorder, an assessment under the 1983 Act should take place.

The use of the 1983 Act must be considered in every case of deprivation of liberty in a hospital where the person requires care and treatment for their mental disorder before moving on to DoLS. It must be demonstrated that the regime for in-patients not detained under the 1983 Act is distinct and different to the regime for those who are detained under that Act. Otherwise, a person who lacks capacity to consent, even when they are not objecting, is likely to be deprived of his liberty simply by being an in-patient. An application can only be made under the 1983 Act if the decision-maker thinks the criteria in Section 2 or 3 are met.

The case of *AM v South London & Maudsley NHS Foundation Trust & Secretary of State for Health* [2013] UKUT 0365 (ACC); [2013] COPLR 510 sets out three questions that should be considered when deciding whether an individual should be detained under the provisions of the 1983 or 2005 Act.

1   Do they have capacity to consent to admission as an informal patient?
2   Could they be lawfully assessed/treated under the provisions of the 2005 Act (i.e. they are deemed to lack capacity to consent but are not objecting to care and treatment for their mental disorder)?
3   Which is the least-restrictive method of achieving the proposed assessment/treatment?

Whether the person is or is not deemed to have capacity to consent to assessment or treatment for their mental disorder, any objection or non-compliance should result in an assessment under the 1983 Act. Fig. 18.1 provides further guidance on whether the 1983 or 2005 Act should be considered.

Where the implementation of DoLS procedures are necessary, local guidance should be followed, as processes can vary. Where use of the 1983 Act is thought to be required, a full Mental Health Act assessment should be arranged. Local procedures will differ but in most areas it will be the local approved mental health professional (AMHP) (Department of Health, 2008*b*,*c*), either in a dedicated team or within a community or crisis team who will coordinate the assessment.

Applications for detention under the 1983 Act

Applications for detention under the 1983 Act may be made by an AMHP or the nearest relative of the patient, as defined by Section 26 of the Act. In reality, it is the AMHP who is normally best placed to carry out this role, because of their professional training and knowledge of legislation and resources. An application by a nearest relative is an extremely rare occurrence.

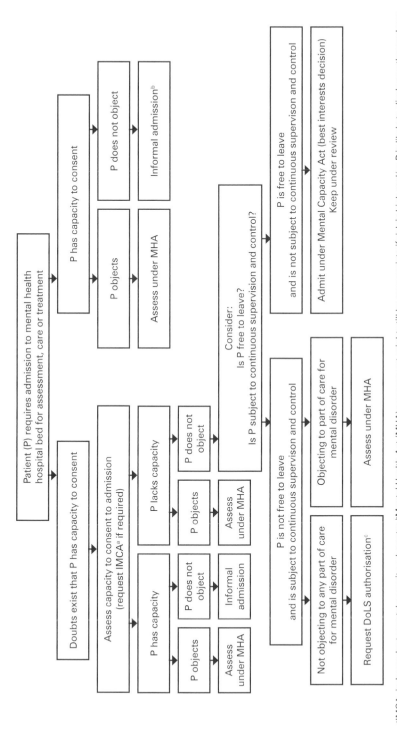

Fig. 18.1 Legal considerations regarding admission to in-patient mental health settings.

[a]IMCA, independent mental capacity advocate; [b]Mental Health Act (MHA) assessment might still be appropriate if risk is high and/or P is likely to discharge themselves; [c]Deprivation of Liberty Safeguards (DoLS) only authorises deprivation of liberty, not treatment. Consider using Mental Capacity Act for specific treatment.

Applications for detention must be based on recommendations from two medical practitioners and, therefore, the recommendations must be dated before or on the same date as the application. This requires the attendance of two fully registered medical practitioners (see the Medical Act 1983), one of whom must be approved under Section 12(2) of the 1983 Act as having special experience in the diagnosis or treatment of mental disorders. In addition, one must preferably have had previous acquaintance with the patient (Department of Health, 2008a). To make a recommendation for detention under Section 2 or 3 of the 1983 Act, the medical practitioners must personally examine the patient, either together or, where this is not possible, with no more than 5 days between the examinations. Where problems arise over access to a patient on private property and there are serious concerns for the patient's mental state, an AMHP might consider applying to a magistrate for a warrant under Section 135 of the 1983 Act, providing authority for police to enter the premises. This allows the patient to be taken to a place of safety for the examination and assessment to be carried out, although local policies differ on the execution of this function.

Section 12A of the 1983 Act prohibits registered medical practitioners making recommendations if they have a conflict of interest in the case; such circumstances are laid out in the regulations for both England and Wales (Department of Health, 2008d,e). Both doctors should not routinely work for the same team, and one doctor may not direct the work of the other proposing to make a recommendation, a requirement that should be observed particularly where a rota is used out of normal working hours (as this is likely to operate under a hierarchy system and, therefore, a consultant would be directing the work of a lesser-grade doctor on the rota). Chapter 14 of the 1983 Act's code of practice contains guidance on applications and undertaking assessments for detention in hospital (Department of Health, 2015). Where a patient is under 18 years of age, or has a learning disability, at least one of the professionals carrying out the assessment should have expertise in that field, and where this is not possible, consultation with such experts should take place.

Although a joint assessment with all parties present is always preferable, both doctors and the AMHP should apply their own professional judgement and reach an independent decision on whether detention is appropriate. Such assessments will also take into consideration what alternatives are available, such as home treatment and crisis intervention. There are no age limits for detention in hospital under the 1983 Act (though in criminal proceedings, age of responsibility must be taken into account), and detention may be considered for a child or young person under 18 years of age where the primary purpose is to provide medical treatment for their mental disorder. Where detention or secure accommodation alone is required for disturbed behaviour, consideration should be given to using Section 25 of the Children Act 1989. There are special considerations when applying the 1983 Act to children and young people under 18 years of age, and specialist, age-appropriate accommodation will normally be required. Where it is necessary to send a minor to an adult mental health bed, this will normally be treated as an untoward incident.

Which Section should be used?

Section 2 of the 1983 Act may be used to admit someone to hospital from the community or to detain someone who might already be in hospital, where those carrying out the assessment believe the individual requires admission for assessment and treatment of their mental disorder. The related code of practice (2015) indicates that:

'Section 2 should only be used if

- the full extent of the nature and degree of a patient's condition is unclear;

- there is a need to carry out an initial in-patient assessment in order to formulate a treatment plan, or to reach a judgement about whether the patient will accept treatment on a voluntary basis following admission; or

- there is a need to carry out a new in-patient assessment in order to re-formulate a treatment plan, or to reach a judgement about whether the patient will accept treatment on a voluntary basis.'

Detention under Section 2 lasts for up to 28 days and is not extendable. When calculating duration, the first day is included and the detention period will always cease at midnight on the 28th day.

Section 3 can be used to admit someone to hospital from the community or to detain someone who might already be in hospital, including those who might already have been detained under Section 2 but require further detention for treatment for a mental disorder. Section 3 should be used where the nature and current degree of the patient's mental disorder, the essential elements of the treatment plan to be followed and the likelihood of the patient accepting treatment as an informal patient are already sufficiently established to make it unnecessary to undertake a new assessment under Section 2 (Department of Health, 2015). Section 3 requires that appropriate treatment is available for the patient's mental disorder. It must be available in actuality, rather than in theory, and must take into account the individual's mental disorder and all other circumstances of their case. The recommendations from both doctors must agree on and name the hospital where the appropriate treatment is available. It is the role of the doctors involved in the assessment to secure a suitable hospital bed where admission is required; many areas arrange this through Crisis Teams and local protocols will dictate how this is carried out (Department of Health, 2015). Where bed availability is an issue, more than one hospital can be named – however, the detention will be invalid if the patient is admitted to a facility that is not named on the recommendations. A Section 3 application can be objected to by the patient's nearest relative and where this occurs the AMHP might have to consider whether steps to remove them from that role via an application to the magistrates should be taken in order for the detention to go ahead. Detention under Section 3 can last for up to 6 months in the first instance and is renewable for a further period of 6 months, and 12 months thereafter.

There is provision in the 1983 Act for an emergency application for admission under Section 4, in exceptional circumstances, where it is of urgent necessity for a patient to be admitted for assessment (observing the criteria laid out in Section 2 of the 1983 Act) and it would cause an undesirable delay in the admission process to await the attendance of a second doctor. In this case, the doctor making the recommendation does not have to be Section 12(2) approved. The detention will last for 72 h from the time of admission to hospital and can be converted to a Section 2 by the completion of a second medical recommendation within this time period (by a Section 12(2) doctor, if the doctor completing the Section 4 medical recommendation was not one).

When completing the necessary recommendations for detention, doctors must use English forms if carrying out the assessment in England and Welsh if in Wales; however, an AMHP must make their application using the relevant form for where the admitting hospital will be (i.e. English if the hospital is situated in England and Welsh if situated in Wales).

Where medical recommendations are completed, an AMHP has 14 days in which to make an application, although in most cases, prompt action will be required. The AMHP holds the authority to convey the patient to the hospital named in the application and arrange appropriate transportation. The power to detain the patient at the named hospital commences only when accepted by a person authorised to do so on behalf of the hospital managers.

The 1983 Act requires that all patients subject to detention under the Act are allocated a responsible clinician with overall responsibility for their mental health care. This responsible clinician must hold approved clinician status (Department of Health, 2008f,g) and it should be clearly established what local cover arrangements are in place for those who might require admission to general healthcare facilities in the first instance. Although this will be a straightforward process for admissions to mental health facilities, it will be relatively rare for medical staff of general hospitals to hold such status. A further point of note when allocating a responsible clinician is the clear requirement for an approved clinician to be approved in England if the responsible hospital is in England and to be approved in Wales if the responsible hospital is in Wales (Department of Health, 2008h).

Part IV of the 1983 Act specifies what treatment for mental disorder may be imposed on patients subject to detention under the Act (chapters 23 to 25 of the code of practice and chapters 16 and 17 of the reference guide give further guidance and requirements; Department of Health, 2008a, 2015). Medical treatment is defined as being for the purpose of alleviating or preventing a worsening of a mental disorder, or one or more of its symptoms or manifestations, and this includes nursing, psychological intervention and specialist mental health habilitation, rehabilitation and care, in addition to medication.

Although use of the 1983 Act might be considered appropriate for the treatment of a person's mental disorder, the 2005 Act will continue to apply for treatment and welfare decisions that fall outside the remit of the 1983 Act: that is, treatment for physical disorders unconnected with the pre-existing mental disorder. The case of *B v Croydon Health Authority* [1995] 1 All E.R.683 (feeding of a patient suffering from borderline personality disorder by nastogastric tube) established that a range of acts ancillary to the core treatment (concurrent with, or as a necessary prerequisite to, core treatment) can fall within the definition of 'medical treatment' under Section 145(1) of the 1983 Act. This might include nasogastric feeding of a patient with anorexia nervosa, blood monitoring for a patient prescribed clozapine, and medical or surgical treatment for self-harm as a result or symptom of a patient's mental disorder.

Patients subject to Sections 2 and 3 can generally be given treatment for their mental disorder for up to 3 months from the date medication was first administered during their period of detention. After this time, their formal consent or authorisation by a second-opinion appointed doctor (SOAD) will be required for any further treatment. There are special provisions in place under Section 58A, however, for administration of electroconvulsive therapy (ECT) at any point in a patient's detention. This will always require the patient's consent or a SOAD certificate. (A SOAD certificate is always necessary for any patient under 18 years of age, irrespective of whether they are capable of consenting.) Advance decisions need to be taken particular note of when considering ECT, as the existence of a valid and applicable advance decision refusing ECT will mean that a course of treatment might not be authorised. It could only be given if the clinician in charge of the treatment believes it is necessary to save the patient's life or prevent a serious deterioration in their condition (and it would only be permissible to give the treatment while those circumstances apply). In general, when a patient is detained, any valid and applicable advance decision refusing treatment must be taken into account when planning care and treatment. However, should no reasonable alternative treatment be deemed appropriate, medication for their mental disorder may be administered, provided the prescription of it complies with the requirements of the 1983 Act and associated guidance.

The 1983 Act provides for emergency measures to be taken in circumstances other than the use of Section 4 above. Under Section 5(2), where a patient is already admitted to a hospital bed, they can be prevented from leaving the hospital before necessary assessments are completed, if the registered medical practitioner (or approved clinician) in charge of their treatment, or their nominated deputy, considers that an application under Section 2 or 3 is required. This effectively 'holds' the person for a period of 72 h in order for an assessment for detention to be carried out.

Where a patient is already in a hospital bed receiving treatment for their mental disorder on an informal or voluntary basis, they can also be held for a period of 6 h by a nurse of the prescribed class (mental health or learning disabilities registration) making a report under Section 5(4) for the purpose of securing the attendance of a doctor or approved clinician in order to complete a Section 5(2) (Department of Health, 2008*i,j*). The nurse must consider that the patient is suffering from a mental disorder to such a degree that it is necessary for the patient's health or safety, or for the protection of others, that they be immediately restrained from leaving the hospital. Section 5(4) is the one section where the power to detain becomes effective as soon as the nurse makes the report.

The police are also provided with powers under Section 136 to detain a person who is in a place to which the public have access, seems to be suffering from mental disorder and is thought to be 'in need of immediate care and control'. They are able to remove the person to a place of safety (normally a designated facility within mental health services, an emergency department or, in exceptional circumstances, a police station), for a period of up to 72 h so that they can be assessed by a registered medical practitioner and (where appropriate) an AMHP, and necessary arrangements made for their treatment or care.

In these three scenarios, as with Section 4, treatment is not authorised under the 1983 Act and any treatment given must be under the provisions of the 2005 Act, if the patient is incapable and the treatment is in their best interests, or under common law, if the patient is mentally capable of consenting to the treatment. Where a patient subject to supervised community treatment under Section 17A of the 1983 Act comes to the attention of services as requiring further treatment in hospital, either in an emergency or in a planned review, and it is deemed inappropriate for this to be provided on an informal basis, then they must be recalled to hospital by their responsible clinician in accordance with the provisions of Section 17E.

As stated throughout, in addition to legal provisions and guidance there will be local protocols and procedures to assist professionals when assessing and planning a patient's care and treatment for a mental disorder. Though it might not be possible to plan for every eventuality, it is recommended that professionals find out who to contact and where to look for guidance in their local area.

This book was sent to press after the 15 January 2015 publication of the revised English Mental Health Act 1983 Code of Practice (due to come into force on 1 April 2015, subject to parliamentary approval). All references to the English code are from the 2015 version. The Reference Guide (Department of Health (2008*a*) is also being revised; however, actual content was not available to include at the time of print. In addition, the Welsh version of the code of practice (Welsh Assembly Government, 2008) is being revised, with anticipated completion in 2015.

References

Department for Constitutional Affairs (2007) *Mental Capacity Act 2005: Code of Practice.* TSO (The Stationery Office).

Department of Health (2008a) *Reference Guide to the Mental Health Act 1983.* TSO (The Stationery Office).

Department of Health (2008b) *Mental Health (Approved Mental Health Professionals) (Approval) (England) Regulations 2008 (SI 2008/1206).* TSO (The Stationery Office).

Department of Health (2008c) *Mental Health (Approval of Persons to be Approved Mental Health Professionals) (Wales) Regulations 2008 (SI 2008/2436 (W.209)).* TSO (The Stationery Office).

Department of Health (2008d) *The Mental Health (Conflicts of Interest) (England) Regulations 2008 (SI 2008/1205).* TSO (The Stationery Office).

Department of Health (2008e) *The Mental Health (Conflicts of Interest) (Wales) Regulations 2008 (SI 2008/2440 (W.213)).* TSO (The Stationery Office).

Department of Health (2008f) *Mental Health Act 1983 Approved Clinician (General) Directions 2008.* TSO (The Stationery Office).

Department of Health (2008g) *Mental Health Act 1983 Approved Clinicians (Wales) Directions 2008.* TSO (The Stationery Office).

Department of Health (2008h) *The Mental Health (Mutual Recognition) Regulations 2008 (SI 2008/1204).* TSO (The Stationery Office).

Department of Health (2008i) *Mental Health (Nurses) (England) Order 2008 (SI 2008/1207).* TSO (The Stationery Office).

Department of Health (2008j) *Mental Health (Nurses) (Wales) Order 2008 (SI 2008/2441 (W.214)).* TSO (The Stationery Office).

Department of Health (2015) *Code of Practice: Mental Health Act 1983.* TSO (The Stationery Office).

Ministry of Justice (2008) *Mental Capacity Act 2005: Deprivation of Liberty Safeguards – Code of Practice to Supplement the Main Mental Capacity Act 2005 Code of Practice.* TSO (The Stationery Office).

Welsh Assembly Government (2008) *Mental Health Act 1983: Code of Practice for Wales.* The Stationery Office.

Cases

AM v South London & Maudsley NHS Foundation Trust & Secretary of State for Health [2013] UKUT 0365 (ACC); [2013] COPLR 510.

B v Croydon Health Authority [1995] 1 All E.R.683.

Commissioner of the Police for the Metropolis v ZH [2013] EWCA Civ 69.

GJ v The Foundation Trust [2009] EWHC 2972 (Fam).

HL v United Kingdom (45508/99); sub nom. *L v United Kingdom* (45508/99) (2005) 40 .H.R.R. 32.

P & Q (by their litigation friend, the Official Solicitor (Appellants) v Surrey County Council (Respondent)[2014] UKSC 19.

P (by his litigation friend the Official Solicitor) (Appellant) v Cheshire West and Chester Council and another (Respondents).

PC v City of York Council [2013] EXCA Civ 478 MHLO 61.

R (Sessay) v South London and Maudsley NHS Foundation Trust and another [2011] EWHC 2617 (QB); [2012] QB 760.

Storck v Germany [2005] 43 EHRR.

CHAPTER 19

Self-poisoning: aspects of assessment and initial care

Kevin Nicholls

Self-poisoning is defined as the intentional self-administration of more than the prescribed dose of any drug, whether or not there is evidence that the act was intended to cause self-harm (Hawton *et al*, 1997). About 80% of self-harm episodes are self-poisoning (Hawton *et al*, 2007). Basic medical management of overdose is lent more space here than is usual in a psychiatry text, for the benefit of those practising in isolated circumstances or low-resource communities. In such situations, time might be of the essence and knowledge of simple therapeutic measures and how to avoid pitfalls is essential. In the UK, acute facilities are usually readily available, but this is not invariably the case. Parts of mid-Wales, for example, are over 1 h away from the nearest district general hospital (not allowing for ambulance attendance time).

The role of an attending psychiatrist is to arrange urgent transfer to an appropriate emergency department before competently assessing the patient in the time available and administering basic life support if necessary. Elementary expediencies should not be overlooked: for example, placing an intoxicated patient in the recovery position.

The prevalence of different substances used for self-poisoning recorded at the John Radcliffe Hospital in Oxfordshire is shown in Fig. 19.1. Paracetamol accounts for almost 50% of overdoses (Hawton *et al*, 2011a). Self-poisoning is more prevalent in women (57%), with two-thirds under 35 years of age. Women aged 15–19 years make up the largest group (Hawton *et al*, 2007). Self-poisoning decreased in England between 2000 and 2007 (Bergen *et al*, 2010). Older adults have a high suicide rate, with 1.5% taking their own life within 1 year of a non-fatal self-poisoning (Murphy *et al*, 2012).

Just 0.6% of paracetamol overdose cases attending emergency departments result in acute liver failure, but overdose can be a portent of further self-harm in young people, with 17.7% of adolescents self-harming a second time withn 1 year of first attendance at hospital with self-poisoning (Hawton *et al*, 2012a), and 27.3% repeating self-harm after follow-up by up to 7 years (Hawton *et al*, 2012b).

It is generally accepted that there is a lifetime risk of suicide of about 15% in those prescribed antidepressants, but only 5% of these use the drug they are prescribed which represents less than 1% of all depressed patients (Henry, 1992). Certified deaths from fatal poisoning (accidents, suicides and open verdicts) in England and Wales have declined steadily over the years (from 3952 in 1979 to 2565 in 2004). There was also a small annual reduction in suicides (all causes) in males and in females over this period. In 2004, self-poisoning accounted for 25% of suicides and open verdicts in males ($n=862$) and 45% in females ($n=540$).

The common clinical consequences of overdose are diverse and usually non-specific:

- diarrhoea
- hallucinations
- dizziness
- abdominal pain
- ataxia

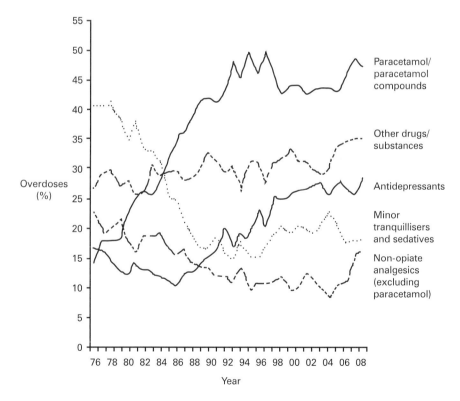

Fig. 19.1 Substances used in deliberate self-poisoning by patients presenting to John Radcliffe Hospital, Oxford in 1976–2009. Reproduced with permission from Hawton *et al* (2011a).

- seizures
- vomiting
- drowsiness
- confusion
- visual problems
- internal bleeding
- abnormal pupil size
- sweating
- hyperacusis or tinnitus
- severe headache
- hyperthermia
- arrhythmias
- hyper/hypotension
- tachycardia
- seizures
- sleepiness
- coma.

History

Where overdose is suspected, a tactful and sympathetic approach is essential. Core assessment is focused on several key questions:

- Which drug or drugs were taken?
- How much was taken?
- When was it taken?
- What are the symptoms and onset times?
- What other factors are involved (e.g. vomiting)?

It is best to err on the side of caution, particularly when the patient is confused, intoxicated or hostile. History from family or friends can be invaluable but has to be carefully evaluated, as views from relatives can be over-optimistic or otherwise flawed (Goulding, 1993). Poly-drug ingestion can cause complex interactions that are impossible to predict and difficult to manage. Paracetamol and salicylate levels should always be checked, as polydrug ingestion is common in overdose cases. Possible and toxic paracetamol levels should be assessed 4–6 h post-ingestion when the time of overdose is known, or immediately when this time is unknown or serial overdose suggested.

Immediate management and examination

Keep calm and recruit help, for example to keep the telephone line open. Priority is determined by clinical assessment. An emergency ambulance should be called in urgent cases, such as when breathing distress, severe dysrhythmia, loss of consciousness or prolonged seizures are seen. Overall, the most important aspects of a critically ill patient who has self-poisoned are maintenance of the patient's airway, ventilation and circulation (Worthley, 2002).

- In cases of cardiac arrest, perform cardiopulmonary resuscitation (CPR).
- In cases of status epilepticus, where support is not imminent, seizure has been protracted or signs are critical (e.g. cyanosis), the use of benzodiazepines might be justified (e.g. intravenous lorazepam 2 mg/min, repeated if necessary; intramuscular diazepam is limited in effect). Avoid non-GABA (gamma-aminobutyric acid) mediated anticonvulsants (e.g. phenytoin) that might potentiate calcium-channel-mediated dysrhythmias with overdosed drugs. Check glucose levels if possible.
- In cases of respiratory distress, keep the patient quiet and calm, avoiding unnecessary exertion. Be prepared to initiate mouth-to-mouth ventilation if the patient becomes apnoeic. Do not try and intubate unless competent as, if incorrectly performed, it can cause laryngeal spasm/vomiting.
- Do not induce vomiting, and avoid giving ipecac.
- Do not give milk or anything similar. It can have unhelpful effects on toxin absorption and might buffer the benefits of subsequent treatments (e.g. activated charcoal).
- Avoid activated charcoal unless advised to use it by a senior specialist or poisons unit. It is unhelpful after ingestion of bleach, acids or similar substances, as it will obscure emergency endoscopy. Seek advice from the regional poisons unit.
- Stay with your patient while awaiting transport. Mobilise a CPR trolley.
- Use the time to get a supplementary history (if possible), check glucose levels, do a baseline echocardiogram (ECG), prepare a succinct written referral summarising the case for emergency department colleagues (including any known critical times).
- Heroics on psychiatric wards should be avoided. There is very little that cannot await safe transfer to the general hospital.

Physical examination

Appearance

Assess the patient's level of consciousness. Look for cuts, abrasions, ligature marks, injection sites, bruising, abscesses, twitching/fasciculation, hallucinations, cyanosis, vomiting, haematemesis and haemoptysis.

Observations

Observations should include weight (noted from records, if available), temperature, blood pressure, pulse rate and respiratory rate. Temperature is an under-used marker of toxicity and core temperature and should be recorded frequently, if this is feasible. Anticholinergic and sympathomimetic substances increase heart rate, blood pressure and temperature. Conversely, organophosphates, opiates, barbiturates, beta-blockers, benzodiazepines, alcohol, and clonidine can cause hypothermia, bradycardia, and respiratory depression. Overdose-related flushing of the skin might indicate an allergic reaction, anticholinergic poisoning or a disulfiram-alcohol reaction. The possibility of alcohol withdrawal should not be forgotten.

Sweating could be a sign of hypoglycaemia, serotonin syndrome, neuroleptic malignant syndrome or poisoning (e.g. organophosphate, salicylate, paracetamol, cocaine or thyroxine). Alcohol withdrawal should be considered as a possibility. Jaundice might indicate delayed presentation after paracetamol poisoning or other hepatotoxic agents such as arsenic or carbon tetrachloride. Nasal mucosa erosion might signal chronic cocaine use. Anticoagulant overdose can present petechiae (small, multiple skin haemorrhages), but exclude meningoccaemia (meningitis, associated with a similar skin sign). Characteristic breath odours can indicate the ingestion of alcohol, diabetic acidosis, turpentine or other distillates, or organophosphorous compounds.

Cardiovascular system

Many drugs have cardiotoxic potential, especially in overdose. QTc interval prolongation might occur with antipsychotic or methadone overdose, with a resulting risk of ventricular fibrillation. Prolonged QRS complex after tricyclic-antidepressant overdose can also result in cardiac arrest. An urgent ECG and cardiology opinion should be sought where drugs that can compromise cardiac function are implicated. Drug and toxin causes of cardiac arrhythmia include:

- tricyclic antidepressants
- phenothiazines
- carbon monoxide
- clonidine
- chloral hydrate
- cocaine
- ethanol
- phenol
- digitalis
- calcium channel blockers
- beta-blockers
- arsenic
- quinine.

Central nervous system

Look for signs of confusion, psychosis, seizure (e.g. bitten tongue, incontinence), nystagmus, pupil size, retinal haemorrhage, reflexes. Seizures can occur after the ingestion of some poisons, such as the slug killer metaldehyde, or be caused by withdrawal from alcohol or other drugs (e.g. anticonvulsants). The possibility of a space-occupying lesion should be considered.

Ocular findings

Anticholinergic and sympathomimetic drugs typically cause mydriasis. In comparison with anticholinergic overdose, the pupils remain somewhat light-responsive in cocaine intoxication. Horizontal nystagmus is common in alcohol intoxication, but also has other causes, including toxicity caused by lithium, carbamazepine and various solvents.

Respiratory system

Airway obstruction, cyanosis and respiratory rate and pattern should be quickly assessed. Auscultation of the lungs can signal pulmonary oedema secondary to tricyclic-antidepressant or opiate overdose, or indicate aspiration. Wheezing can occur in organophosphorus poisoning and some allergic reactions. The pattern of breathing can give clues: Cheyne–Stokes, apneustic or ataxic breathing can all be indicative of a structural lesion necessitating imaging, and rapid deep breathing could indicate metabolic acidosis caused by salicylate, methanol or ethylene glycol. Diligence for respiratory arrest is essential, especially after opiate or barbiturate poisoning.

Gastrointestinal tract

Weighing the patient is important when practical, allowing accurate assessment of toxin load and calculation of the antidote dose. Consider mouth mucosa ulceration, bleeding or oedema, abdominal tenderness, increased or decreased bowel sounds (the latter being more common after overdose). Acute abdominal symptoms and signs must be excluded, especially after trauma. Diarrhoea and vomiting are characteristic of poisoning by lithium, theophylline, organophosphorus compounds, mushrooms and heavy metals such as mercury. Hypovolaemia should be treated with normal saline and intravenous anti-emetics might be indicated, but avoid metoclopramide if extrapyramidal side-effects are evident after drug overdose.

Management of coma

Coma, or unarousable unconsciousness, is common after acute overdose. It can be caused by systemic brain toxicity, brain stem lesions (unusually) or certain metabolic states. Other causes include head trauma, anoxia, meningitis, cardiovascular accident and hypothermia. Note that poisoned patients might seem brain dead with fixed, dilated pupils, coma and absent cold calorific response, yet recover fully on removal of the assaulting drug.

Repeated examination is critical. Priority should be given to ensuring a clear airway, with the patient being completely intubated as soon as is feasible. An intravenous drip of normal saline should be started. Indicated investigations include:

- paracetamol and salicylate
- full blood count
- urea and electrolytes
- glucose
- liver enzymes
- clotting factors (prothrombin time – baseline)
- urine pH
- blood gases
- toxicology (e.g. lithium, anticonvulsants).

Supra-tentorial mass must be excluded and magnetic resonance imaging of the head is indicated whenever there is disproportionate or unexpected impaired consciousness, or relevant history or signs. Look for evidence of coning: changes in respiratory pattern, disconjugate gaze or lateralising signs.

Capacity

If the patient refuses to accept transport, offer a blood sample or receive treatment, consider seeking legal advice. Document important points and times meticulously. An unconscious patient can usually be transported and treated under common law, if urgency and best interest dictates this course of action. Capacity will be an issue in cases where a patient who has overdosed is declining appropriate treatment. Seek advice from a senior colleague if possible. It might be difficult to conclude that capacity is sufficient to refuse life-saving treatment, even in a case of apparent suicide. The level of capacity necessary for a patient to make such decisions will increase with the gravity of the consequences of the decision. Furthermore, there is a 'very heavy burden on those advocating a course which would lead inevitably to the cessation of a human life' (Jones, 2008). This might reasonably be taken to include acts of omission. Legal guidance should be sought where possible and time allows, but where urgent treatment is imperative to save a life, this should not be delayed if capacity is in question. A solicitor will be on call at all times for hospital trusts. If capacity is questioned and treatment is not an immediate life-saving imperative, direction from the courts must be sought.

Key questions in assessing capacity are:

- Can the patient understand information given?
- Can they believe it?

- Can they retain pertinent information?
- Can they weigh this information and make a decision?

It is important to remember that the decision they make need not be rational or sensible. Remember that capacity might fluctuate over time, requiring reassessment and review.

It is a common misperception that only a psychiatrist can assess capacity. In fact, all doctors can assess capacity and indeed are required to do so. Crucial treatment should not be delayed in a critical situation to wait for the attendance of a psychiatrist. Another misperception is that the Mental Health Act 2007 authorises treatment for physical conditions. This is not the case. Although the Mental Health Act may be invoked to treat a depressive illness, it cannot be used to sanction treatment with acetylcysteine following a paracetamol overdose. Medical treatment must be undertaken either with consent, which might be indicated by cooperation in practice, or by relying on doctrine of necessity or best interest where the patient lacks capacity. Having said this, the Act is increasingly being expanded by case law to include physical treatments that might bear on mental state. However, urgent treatment should not be delayed by waiting for a Mental Health Act assessment.

General treatment principles

Get clear and direct notification of poison levels and blood results. Do not rely on second-hand messages in busy departments or psychiatry units from staff who may be unfamiliar with the nomenclature or clinical or operational issues that might cause miscommunication. Gastric lavage is not used routinely and can complicate management, leading to longer intensive care unit stay and admission times.

Activated charcoal use is limited to within 2 h of ingestion or, in less common circumstances, where the drug ingested delays gastric emptying/motility. Drugs with slow absorption, such as *Amanita* mushrooms and monoamine oxidase inhibitors (MAOIs), are the exception rather than the rule. Enteric-coated or sustained-release tablets can cause unpredictable delays in peak serum levels or multiphasic fluctuation. Activated charcoal is not given when the ingested agent is non-toxic or is not absorbed by charcoal. Toxins and drugs not absorbed by activated charcoal include alcohol, hydrocarbons, organophosphates, carbamates, acids, potassium, alkali, iron and lithium.

Patients who are intoxicated or otherwise confused, have physical complications (e.g. arrhythmias) or show acute signs of poisoning warrant continued medical monitoring (Hillard & Zitek, 2004). As a rule, patients who are asymptomatic after 6 h of observation, have normal paracetamol/salicylate levels and have an unremarkable physical examination are deemed fit for psychiatric assessment.

Specific drugs and substances used to self-poison

Paracetamol

Paracetamol (acetaminophen) is the most frequently used analgesic. Some 3500 million 500 mg tablets were bought in the UK in 2000 (Sheen *et al*, 2002). Its pain relieving and antipyretic properties were first noted in the 19th century after its synthesis in Germany. The onset of analgesic effect begins 10–11 min after ingestion. Remarkably, parecetamol's hepatotoxicity was not described until 1966. It is now the most frequently overdosed drug in the UK, USA, Australia and New Zealand. In the UK, mortality due to paracetamol self-poisoning has reduced by 47% since retail restrictions (e.g. pack size) were introduced, but paracetamol still caused 90–155 deaths annually between 2000 and 2008 (Hawton *et al*, 2011b). Some 15–20 liver transplants result from paracetamol poisoning annually in the UK.

Peak serum paracetamol concentrations occur within 1–2 h with standard tablet formulations and within 30 min with liquid preparations. Overall, 20% of the ingested dose undergoes first-pass metabolism in the gut wall. Further elimination occurs by hepatic metabolism. The half-life of paracetamol at recommended, prescribed doses is 1.5–3 h. About 90% is metabolised to sulphate and glucuronide conjugates that are excreted in the urine. The rest is metabolised via cytochrome P450 enzymes, resulting in the highly reactive intermediary compound *N*-acetyl-*p*-benzoquinone imine (NAPQI). In normal conditions, NAPQI is quickly bound by intracellular glutathione and eliminated in the urine as mercapturic compounds. It is the depletion of glutathione by overdose that causes critical hepatotoxic levels of NAPQI.

The resulting mortality starts from day 2 and peaks at day 4. Possible preventative measures include making paracetamol prescription only and adding methionine to paracetamol (a glutathione donor). The introduction of blister packs in the UK in 1998 decreased fatalities from paracetamol overdose by 22% and referrals for liver transplant after paracetamol-induced poisoning by 30% (Hawton *et al*, 2004). To determine when to use acetylcysteine, refer to the *British National Formulary* nomogram in Fig. 19.2 (Joint Formulary Committee, 2011).

Factors that increase the toxicity of paracetamol include the following (Young & Mazure, 1998):

- chronic alcohol use
- HIV positivity
- use of certain enzyme-inducing drugs (e.g. phenytoin, rifampicin, carbamazepine, St John's wort)
- hepatic incapacity (e.g. viral hepatitis)
- glutathione depletion
- anorexia
- bulimia

- malnutrition
- cachexia
- cystic fibrosis
- combinations of these (e.g. carbamazepine and anorexia).

The accepted toxic dose of paracetamol is 150 mg/kg, but half this amount can be toxic in susceptible individuals compromised by depleted hepatic glutathione stores or induction of P450 microenzymes (Greene *et al*, 2005). *N*-acetylcysteine (NAC) is virtually 100% effective if given within 8 h of initial ingestion, but its efficacy when given later is less certain. It seems to be safe in pregnancy. The prothrombin time is a sensitive index of liver damage: 50% of patients with a prothrombin time of ≥36 s at 36 h will develop acute hepatic failure; a falling prothrombin time indicates recovery (Dargan & Jones, 2002). The onset of abdominal pain and other symptoms and signs frequently occur after the safe treatment window post-ingestion. Acute renal failure with oliguria, metabolic acidosis and encephalopathy can also occur.

After 24 h, plasma paracetamol concentration cannot be used to determine the extent of toxicity and other clinical considerations then inform management and prognosis:

- vomiting
- right-upper-quadrant tenderness
- dose ingested >150 mg per 24 h (75 mg per 24 h if high risk)
- international normalized ratio, liver function tests, creatinine, venous bicarbonate trends.

If there is significant serum paracetamol and the timing of ingestion has not been ascertained accurately, NAC treatment should be commenced

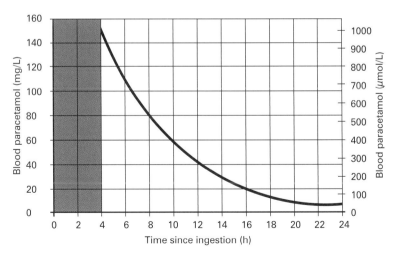

Fig 19.2 Simple nomogram for paracetamol poisoning (Joint National Formulary, 2011; reproduced with permission from All Wales Therapeutics and Toxicology Centre).

and alanine aminotransaminase level determined. If at the end of repeated infusion the alanine aminotransaminase level normalises or is decreasing, NAC may be discontinued. If further history subsequently becomes available and the serum paracetamol level can be accurately plotted on the nomogram, this should be done and NAC discontinued if appropriate (Daly *et al*, 2008).

Prognosis is not necessarily dismal. In 306 paracetamol self-poisonings, 6.9% were hepatotoxic, though not severely so. All made a good recovery. Predictably, poor prognosis correlates to higher drug intake and length of time to presentation (Sheen *et al*, 2002).

Non-steroidal anti-inflammatory drugs

Ibuprofen is the most frequently overdosed non-steroidal anti-inflammatory drug. It has a rapid absorption rate of 80% in 30–120 min. Elimination is by urinary excretion: 90% as metabolites. The half-life is about 2 h, so a single 400 mg dose is normally undetectable in serum at 12 h. Symptoms arise in 47% of adults who have taken an overdose, but severe consequences are relatively rare (Hall *et al*, 1986). Generally confined to the first 6 h after ingestion, symptoms are mainly gastrointestinal, and include vomiting, abdominal pain and diarrhoea. Mild sedation is common. Apnoea, seizures and coma have been reported, but are rare.

Salicylates (aspirin)

Salicylates were more frequently overdosed 30 years ago than they are now, but are still commonly used in self-poisoning. Symptoms of salicylate poisoning are dose-dependent (Box 19.1).

Serum levels peak 12–18 h after overdose but this is unpredictable, especially when enteric-coated tablets have been taken. Blood salicylate, electrolyte and glucose levels need monitoring every 4 h until the salicylate blood level decreases. Activated charcoal can be given if blood salicylate levels are above 125 mg/kg and gastric lavage considered if levels are more than 500 mg/kg within 1 h of ingestion.

Urine alkalinisation speeds up the excretion of salicylates. Urine pH should be checked every 30 min to ensure that a value of 7.5–8.5 is achieved. If metabolic acidosis is severe, with a pH of less than 7.3, sodium bicarbonate can be given with carefully titrated potassium chloride under close medical supervision. Where very high levels of salicylates are present (>800 mg/L in adults or >700 mg/L in children and the elderly), haemodialysis is usually indicated to remove the drug and correct electrolyte levels (Greene *et al*, 2005).

Benzodiazepines

Benzodiazepines comprise the most widely prescribed drug group in the world. Prescribed as hypnotic, anxiolytic and anticonvulsant agents, their

---

Box 19.1   Symptoms of salicylate poisoning are dose-dependent

Mild (> 150 mg/kg)

- Nausea
- Vomiting
- Tinnitus
- Deafness

Moderate (> 250 mg/kg)

- Agitation
- Sweating
- Vasodilation
- Hypoglycaemia
- Petechial/subconjunctival haemorrhage

Severe (> 500 mg/kg)

- Metabolic acidosis
- Seizures
- Renal failure
- Cardiovascular collapse
- Pulmonar oedema (rare)
- Coma

Greene *et al* (2005)

---

use has decreased because of dependency concerns. Prevalence (defined as benzodiazepine use at some time in the previous year) reduced from 11.2% in 1982 to 3.3% in 1986; most of this decrease was caused by curtailment of their use as anxiolytics (Ashton, 1997). Benzodiazepines are commonly used to self-poison, although their popularity for this purpose has declined. Overdose is more likely to be repeated if the index overdose included a benzodiazepine (Hawton & van Heeringen, 2000).

At least historically, the suicide rate in women taking a benzodiazepine at the time of the index overdose is increased 10-fold over 10 years, compared with those who are not (Allgulander & Nasman, 1991). The cause of this association is unclear. It might be that benzodiazepines were prescribed inappropriately instead of antidepressants, or that this group was more distressed than those who were not taking benzodiazepines. Benzodiazepines might provoke suicide attempts. Alprazolam disinhibits individuals, leading to impulsive acts, and this could indicate that a class effect of benzodiazepines is predisposition to overdose (O'Sullivan *et al*, 1994; Bond *et al*, 1995; Cowdry & Gardner, 1996; Hawton & van Heeringen, 2000).

The main effect of benzodiazepine toxicity is depression of the central nervous system, including respiratory drive. Complications and effects are exacerbated by the ingestion of other depressant drugs, including alcohol, when risk of aspiration of vomit is significant. Benzodiazepines taken alone, however, are unlikely to result in a Glasgow Coma Scale score of less than ten

(Teasdale & Jennett, 1974). Common features of benzodiazepine overdose are drowsiness, mid-sized or dilated pupils, dysarthria, hypotension (with large doses), ataxia, and respiratory depression (again, with large doses).

Treatment of overdose is supportive when a benzodiazepine is taken alone. Tolerance can be compromised in the elderly and where there is a concurrent ailment like chronic obstructive pulmonary disease. Activated charcoal can be considered for very large overdoses presenting within 1 h of ingestion (Greene *et al*, 2005). The use of the benzodiazepine antagonist flumazenil is not recommended, as benzodiazepine-dependent individuals are at risk of withdrawal complications including seizures. Furthermore, flumazenil can exacerbate complications when other drugs have been taken (e.g. the development of arrhythmias caused by tricyclics). Flumazenil use is limited to the uncommon circumstance where a benzodiazepine alone has caused severe respiratory depression without facility to intubate and ventilate. In these rare cases only, cautious incremental administration of flumazenil is an option. It has been described as 'an antidote in search of an overdose' (Goldfrank, 1997).

Antidepressants

In the period 1993–2004, the poisoning death rate per million prescriptions was about 10 times higher for tricyclic antidepressants than for selective serotonin reuptake inhibitors (SSRIs) in England and Wales. Despite increased SSRI prescription, there has been only a slight decrease (10%) in the annual number of antidepressant-related poisoning deaths, in line with the similar reduction in suicides (all methods) over this period and increase in prescriptions for the less-toxic SSRIs.

Citalopram seems to have higher overdose toxicity than other SSRIs. Of the non-SSRIs, the toxicity of venlafaxine, although lower than that of tricyclic antidepressants, seems to be higher than that of SSRIs; serotonin syndrome, seizures, rhabdomyolysis, renal failure and hepatic failure have all been reported (Flanagan, 2008). There are fewer data on other antidepressants, but management is predominantly conservative, with supportive monitoring for cardiac effects or seizures. Prophylactic benzodiazepine cover might be indicated to prevent seizures. Where widened QRS time occurs, cardiac conduction stabilisation with intravenous bicarbonate might be necessary and expert cardiologist advice should be sought.

Tricyclic antidepressants

In total, 33.1 million prescriptions for tricyclic antidepressants were made in 1998–2000 in England and Wales. In the same period, there were 12 deaths per million tricyclic prescriptions, compared with two per million for SSRIs (Cheeta *et al*, 2004). Tricyclic antidepressants are toxic in overdose, most seriously causing cardiovascular complications such as ventricular dysrhythmias. The tricyclic antidepressants amitriptyline and dosulepin (formerly known as dothiepin) were frequently prescribed before the advent of SSRIs. They were among the most toxic tricyclics. The least toxic is lofep-ramine, by a factor of up to 21; this low toxicity is attributed to its intrinsic membrane-stabilising properties (Cheeta *et al*, 2004).

Symptoms of tricyclic toxicity include dilated pupils, confusion, hallucinations and arrhythmias. The cardiotoxicity of this class is mediated by ion-channel-induced dysfunction in the myocardium. Myocardial infarc-tion and *torsade de pointes* (TdP) have been described. Fatal arrhythmias and death usually occur within 24 h of ingestion (Thanacoody & Thomas, 2005).

Treatment is by activated charcoal, and is most efficient when given within 1–2 h of ingestion. Intravenous fluid and sodium bicarbonate may be administered to counter metabolic acidosis, hypotension and destabilisation of the myocardium. Expert management on an intensive care unit can involve giving anti-arrhythmia drugs and anti-seizure benzodiazepines.

SSRIs and modern atypical antidepressants

Since their introduction in the early 1990s, SSRIs have become the most frequently prescribed class of antidepressant. As they are safer than tricyclics, it is unlikely that overdoses of less than 500 mg will cause untoward symptoms (25 fluoxetine capsules or equivalent). Symptoms of overdose include blurred vision, sinus tachycardia, drowsiness, nausea and vomiting. Toxic levels of up to 1390 ng/mL have been managed by supportive care only (Borys *et al*, 1992). Until 2004, fatal overdoses with SSRIs occured in combination with other drugs in 93% of cases, and with tricyclics in 25% of this number (the largest subgroup; Cheeta *et al*, 2004).

Ingestion of higher doses can lead to seizures (Braitberg & Curry, 1995), which can be managed with benzodiazepines, or serotonin syndrome (Stork, 2002). Serotonin syndrome is characterised by changes in mental state, autonomic instability and neuromuscular dysfunction. Very high doses of SSRIs can result in coma. Diagnosis is clinical, as laboratory findings are non-specific. Activated charcoal is indicated when presentation occurs within 1 h of taking ten or more tablets. Treatment is otherwise supportive, with agitation managed with benzodiazepines, cardiac monitoring and cooling measures if the patient is pyrexial (Greene *et al*, 2005).

Venlafaxine, a serotonin–noradrenaline reuptake inhibitor (SNRI), has a half-life of 4 h or less and a maximum serum concentration that is reached 1–2 h after ingestion. However, its active metabolite *O*-demethylvenlafaxine has a half-life of 10 h and monitoring for 2 days after overdose is recommended (White *et al*, 1997). Activated charcoal, given promptly enough, can be useful. Ipecac is contraindicated where there is a risk of seizure (Stork, 2002). Venlafaxine has a similar overdose symptom profile to that of SSRIs, but is associated with more severe cardiovascular toxicity, including hypertension and cardiac conduction problems, urinary retention and seizures (White *et al*, 1997). Some very rare side-effects (e.g. thrombocytopaenia, blood dyscrasias) are idiosyncratic reactions, and are not dose related. Venlafaxine might differ somewhat from other members of the SNRI class in relation to the frequency of hypertension-related reactions.

Coma is less likely with venlafaxine or SSRI overdose than with tricyclic-antidepressant overdose, but serotonin toxicity is more common and can be fatal. Death usually results from QRS prolongation and ventricular dysrhythmia (Daniels, 1998; Stork, 2002). Interaction with MAOIs can predispose the patient to serotonin syndrome (White *et al*, 1997). MAOIs are not commonly prescribed and are infrequently seen in overdose, but it is important to be aware of it when they are, as MOAIs have implications for other drugs ingested, including opiates. Mirtazapine has a low epileptogenic potential and seems to be substantially benign in overdose, mainly causing self-limiting somnolence (Montgomery, 1995).

Antipsychotics

Sudden death has been reported with antipsychotic use since the early 1960s. Poisoning deaths involving antipsychotics are far fewer than those involving antidepressants (713 and 5602 deaths, respectively, in England and Wales in 1993–2004). Following the restriction of thioridazine in 2000, thioridazine-related fatal poisonings fell to zero by 2002. An increase in deaths associated with atypical antipsychotics, including clozapine and olanzapine, counters this. Antipsychotic-related poisoning deaths were higher in 2004 than at any time since 1993 (Flanagan, 2008).

Interest has centred on the QTc interval (pathological prolongation of the time between Q and T waves on the ECG, corrected for heart rate) and TdP, a subsequent polymorphic ventricular arrhythmia that can progress to ventricular fibrillation and sudden death. The QTc interval represents the time between the onset of electrical depolarisation (contraction) of the ventricles and the end of repolarisation. Prolongation of the QTc interval increases any potential a drug has to cause TdP. In individual patients, an absolute QTc interval of >500 ms or an increase of 60 ms from baseline is regarded as raising the risk of TdP. However, TdP can occur with lower QTc values. Concern about a relationship between QTc prolongation, TdP and sudden death applies to a wide range of drugs and has led to the withdrawal or restricted labelling of some. The degree of QTc prolongation is probably dose dependent in an individual and varies between antipsychotics, reflecting their differing capacity to derange ion-flux in the myocardium and its coordinating cardiac conduction bundles (Haddad & Anderson, 2002).

Toxic doses of atypical antipsychotics are variable; some patients die while taking therapeutic doses and others survive massive overdoses with supportive measures only. For example, overdoses of quetiapine of

9.6 g (Hustey, 1999) and even up to 20 g have been successfully treated in an intensive care setting (Dev & Raniwalla, 2000). However, second-generation antipsychotics might be more hazardous than first-generation antipsychotics (Ciranni *et al*, 2009). Toxicity is increased with the ingestion of certain other agents, particularly drugs competing with cytochrome-P450-mediated metabolic pathways.

Arrhythmia is more likely to occur if drug-induced QTc prolongation coexists with other risk factors (Haddad & Anderson, 2002):

- presence of congenital long QT syndromes
- heart failure
- bradycardia
- electrolyte imbalance
- overdose of another QTc prolonging drug
- female gender
- restraint
- old age
- hepatic or renal impairment
- slow metaboliser status
- stimulant drugs.

A study of 29 deaths concluded that olanzapine toxicity in overdose is variable and ill-defined. The symptoms in olanzapine overdose include somnolence, mydriasis, blurred vision, respiratory depression, hypotension and extrapyramidal and anticholinergic effects. Metabolism of olanzapine varies as much as 20-fold between individuals. The probable adverse effects on mortality from overdose, of higher rates of cardiovascular disease and sudden death in people with schizophrenia was highlighted (Chue & Singer, 2003). Similarly, the major effects in one study of risperidone overdose included lethargy, spasm/dystonia, hypotension, tachycardia and dysrhythmia (Acri & Henretig, 1993).

Although deaths due to atypical antipsychotics are often related to cardiovascular factors, pulmonary, neurological, endocrine and gastro-intestinal complications have also caused fatalities (Trenton *et al*, 2003).

Lithium

Lithium salts have been used for at least 150 years to treat gout and other ailments. Use declined in the 19th century because of toxicity concerns. In the 20th century, lithium salts were used to treat affective disorder; safety was facilitated by monitoring serum levels. Lithium is now an established treatment for severe depression and bipolar disorder, reducing suicidal action by seven-fold in the latter (Tondo *et al*, 1997; Hawton & van Heeringen, 2000).

Lithium is absorbed from the upper gastrointestinal tract over about 8 h, with peak serum levels occurring 1–2 h after oral administration. Lithium is also available in sustained-release preparations; serum levels peak 4–5 h after ingestion, but can continue to rise for 3–4 days. Lithium has a half-life of 12–27 h after a single dose, but this can increase to 58 h in elderly individuals or patients taking lithium chronically. Lithium is distributed in total body water and does not bind to serum proteins. Tissue distribution is complex. The concentration in cerebrospinal fluid is only 40% of serum level because of transport out of the cerebrospinal fluid by brain capillary endothelium and arachnoid membranes.

Sequential monitoring of lithium levels is necessary after overdose because its rate of elimination is variable and unpredictable. Gastric lavage can be considered within 1 h of ingestion. All that is usually necessary is to increase fluids to increase urine production, but diuretics should be avoided.

Patients with acute lithium toxicity might have only mild symptoms and signs, despite elevated levels, and need conservative management only. Patients developing toxicity while on chronic maintenance therapy, on the other hand, are more likely to have significant symptoms. Severe symptoms and serum lithium levels above the therapeutic range can require haemodialysis (Gadallah *et al*, 1988). Significant symptoms include weakness, tremor, drowsiness, vomiting, headache, confusion, diarrhoea, dysarthria, ataxia, renal failure, seizures and coma. Persistent neurological side-effects are not common but can be serious after acute toxicity or during maintenance therapy, when toxicity is more insidious. Irreversible neurologic complications generally result in persistent cerebellar signs, especially ataxia and dysarthria (Kores & Lader, 1997).

Opiates

There are approximately 300 deaths from opiate overdose per year in the UK, often involving heroin, morphine, codeine or methadone. These overdoses are usually accidental and death by respiratory depression prior to arrival at hospital accounts for most fatalities. Overdose in opiate users may be associated with confusion and or chaotic lifestyle. A check for the presence of paracetamol will be indicated in most cases (Greene *et al*, 2005).

Symptoms and signs of opiate poisoning include reduced consciousness, respiration-rate depression and pin-point pupils. Naloxone is usually used to reverse the effects of opiate overdose and is best given intravenously for a quick onset of action. Optimum administration is an intravenous infusion, typically 1200–2000 µg in 10 mL of normal saline. This can be slowly injected or dripped, allowing titration against clinical improvement. However, in an emergency, it can also be administered intramuscularly, intranasally or via an endotracheal tube. After a large overdose, up to 10 mg of naloxone may be needed (administered in increments). The half-life of naloxone is short (30–100 min), compared with some of the opiates. For example, methadone has a half-life as long as 24 h in some patients. This can necessitate repeated administration of naloxone and vigilant observation to prevent deterioration over time after an initial response to naloxone.

Pesticides

Poisoning by pesticides is a major cause of morbidity and mortality worldwide. Suicide by this means is especially common in rural India and other Asian communities, where it seems to be culturally sanctioned and adequate treatment facilities are often inaccessible. Pesticides are typically complex compounds without specific antidotes that can cause various symptoms that remit with supportive management in the majority of cases. Some insecticides, such as pyrethroid compounds, are relatively benign. Two of the more harmful pesticides often taken in suicide acts are the organophosphorous insecticides, for instance dimethoate and the contact herbicide paraquat. The latter has been banned in the EU since 2007.

However, organophosphorous insecticides are extremely toxic compounds that can poison through contact and inhalation as well as ingestion. They are potent anticholinesterase inhibitors and rapidly cause autonomic nervous system acetylcholine dysregulation and collapse. Urgent treatment with intravenous atropine 3 mg is indicated, to be repeated as necessary until atropinisation is achieved. In cases of severe poisoning, this might require upwards of 100 mg of atropine.

Paraquat poisoning has a poor prognosis and, although cases with ingestion of minute amounts can have a reasonable outlook with supportive measures, just a few mL can be fatal. Large doses usually cause death in 2 or 3 days due to respiratory failure. Oropharyngeal ulceration is an ominous sign indicating poor outlook. Intermediate levels of poisoning typically lead to death after 2–3 weeks by pulmonary fibrosis. Review of the literature on paraquat belies the complex toxicity of this compound and the sophistication of the measures employed to improve prognosis. Fuller's earth and activated charcoal are advocated as an initial measure, but gastric lavage is contraindicated. Urgent transfer to a suitable emergency facility and liaison with the regional poisons unit is imperative.

Summary

Deliberate self-poisoning is common. The role of the psychiatrist is to expedite referral and coordinate transfer to a suitable treatment centre as necessary. Active prioritisation, monitoring and maintenance of basic life support while achieving this is imperative.

References

Acri AA, Henretig FM (1993) Effects of risperidone in overdose. *American Journal of Emergency Medicine*, **16**: 498–501.

Allgulander C, Nasman P (1991) Regular hypnotic drug treatment in a sample of 32,679 Swedes: associations with somatic and mental health, inpatient psychiatric diagnoses and suicide, derived with automated record-linkage. *Psychosomatic Medicine*, **51**: 708–712.

Ashton H (1997) *Cambridge Handbook of Psychology and Medicine.* Cambridge University Press.

Bergen H, Hawton K, Waters K, *et al* (2010) Epidemiology and trends in non-fatal self-harm in three centres in England, 2000 to 2007. *British Journal of Psychiatry*, **197**: 493–498.

Bond AJ, Curran HV, Bruce MS, *et al* (1995) Behavioural aggression in panic disorder after 8 weeks' treatment with alprazolam. *Journal of Affective Disorders*, **35**: 117–123.

Borys DJ, Setzer SC, Ling LJ, *et al* (1992) Acute fluoxetine overdose: a report of 234 cases. *American Journal of Emergency Medicine*, **10**: 115–120.

Braitberg G, Curry SC (1995) Seizure after isolated fluoxetine overdose. *Annals of Emergency Medicine*, **26**: 234–237.

Cheeta S, Shifano F, Oyefeso A, *et al* (2004) Antidepressant-related deaths and antidepressant prescriptions in England and Wales, 1998–2000. *British Journal of Psychiatry*, **184**: 41–47.

Chue P, Singer P (2003) A review of olanzapine toxicity and fatality in overdose. *Journal of Psychiatry and Neuroscience*, **28**: 253–261.

Ciranni MA, Kearnay TE, Olson KR (2009) Comparing acute toxicity of first- and second-generation antipsychotic drugs: a 10-year, retrospective cohort study. *Journal of Clinical Psychiatry*, **70**: 122–129.

Cowdry RW, Gardner DL (1996) Alprazolam, carbamazapine, trifluoperazine and tranylcypromine. *Advances in Psychiatric Treatment*, **3**: 66–71.

Daly FS, Fountain JS, Murray L, *et al* (2008) Guidelines for the management of paracetamol poisoning in Australia and New Zealand – explanation and elaboration. *The Medical Journal of Australia*, **188**: 296–302.

Daniels RJ (1998) Serotonin syndrome due to venlafaxine overdose. *Journal of Accident and Emergency Medicine*, **15**: 333–337.

Dargan PI, Jones AL (2002) Acetaminophen poisoning – an update for the intensivist. *Critical Care*, **6**: 108–110.

Dev V, Raniwalla J (2000) Quetiapine: a review of its safety in the management of schizophrenia. *Drug Safety*, **23**: 295–307.

Flanagan RJ (2008) Fatal toxicity of drugs used in psychiatry. *Human Psychopharmacology*, **23** (Suppl 1): 43–51.

Gadallah MF, Feinstein EL, Massry SG (1988) Lithium intoxication: clinical course and therapeutic considerations. *Mineral and Electrolyte Metabolism*, **14**: 146–149.

Goldfrank LR (1997) Flumazenil: a pharmacological antidote with limited medical toxicology utility, or … an antidote in searth of an overdose. *Academic Emergency Medicine*, **4**: 935–936.

Goulding R (1993) The fatal paracetamol dosage – how low can you go? *Medicine, Science, and the Law*, **33**: 274.

Greene SL, Dargan PI, Jones AL (2005) Acute poisoning: understanding 90% of cases in a nutshell. *Postgraduate Medical Journal*, **81**: 204–216.

Haddad PM, Anderson IM (2002) Antipsychotic-related QTc prolongation, torsades de points and sudden death. *Drugs*, **62**: 1649–1671.

Hall AH, Smolinske SC, Conrad FL, *et al* (1986) Ibuprofen overdose: 126 cases. *Annals of Emergency Medicine*, **15: 1308–1313.**

Hawton K, van Heeringen K (eds) (2000) *The International Handbook of Suicide and Attempted Suicide.* Wiley.

Hawton K, Fagg J, Simkin S, *et al* (1997) Trends in deliberate self-harm in Oxford, 1985–1995. Implications for clinical services and the prevention of suicide. *British Journal of Psychiatry*, **171**: 556–560.

Hawton K, Simkin S, Deeks J, *et al* (2004) UK legislation on analgesic packs: before and after study of long-term effect on poisonings. *BMJ*, **329**: 1076.

Hawton K, Bergen H, Casey D, *et al* (2007) Self-harm in England: a tale of three cities. Multicentre study of self-harm. *Social Psychiatry and Psychiatric Epidemiology*, **42**: 513–521.

Hawton K, Casey D, Bale E, *et al* (2011a) *Deliberate Self-Harm in Oxford 2009.* Centre for Suicide Research, University of Oxford.

Hawton K, Bergen H, Simkin S, *et al* (2011b) Impact of different pack sizes of paracetamol in the UK and Ireland on intentional overdoses: a comparative study. *BMC Public Health*, **11**: 460.

Hawton K, Bergen H, Kaput N, *et al* (2012a) Repetition of self-harm and suicide following self-harm in children and adolescents: findings from the Multicentre Study of Self-harm in England. *Journal of Child Psychology and Psychiatry and Allied Disciplines*, **53**: 1212–1219.

Hawton K, Bergen H, Waters K, *et al* (2012b) Epidemiology and nature of self-harm in children and adolescents: findings from the Multicentre Study of Self-harm in England. *European Child and Adolescent Psychiatry*, **21**: 369–377.

Henry JA (1992) The safety of antidepressants. *British Journal of Psychiatry*, **160: 439–441.**

Hillard R, Zitek B (2004) *Emergency Psychiatry*. McGraw–Hill.

Hustey FM (1999) Acute quetiapine poisoning. *Journal of Emergency Medicine*, **17: 995–997.**

Joint Formulary Committee (2011) *British National Formulary (61st edn)*. BMJ Group and Pharmaceutical Press.

Jones R (2008) *Mental Capacity Act (3rd edn)*. Sweet & Maxwell.

Kores B, Lader ML (1997) Irreversible lithium neurotoxicity – an overview. *Clinical Neuropharmacology*, **20**: 283–299.

Montgomery SA (1995) Safety of mirtazapine: a review. *International Clinical Psychopharmacology*, **10** (Suppl 4): 37–45.

Murphy E, Kapur N, Webb R, *et al* (2012) Multicentre cohort study of older adults who have harmed themselves: risk factors for repetition and suicide. *British Journal of Psychiatry*, **200**: 399–404.

O'Sullivan GH, Noshirvani H, Basoglu M (1994) Safety and side-effects of alprazolam: controlled study in agoraphobia with panic disorder. *British Journal of Psychiatry*, **165**: 79–86.

Sheen CL, Dillon JF, Bateman DN, *et al* (2002) Paracetamol toxicity: epidemiology, prevention and cost to the health-care system. *QJM*, **95**: 609–619.

Stork C (2002) Serotonin reuptake inhibitors and atypical antidepressants. In *Goldfrank's Toxicologic Emergencies* (eds LS Nelson, NA Lewin, MA Howland, *et al*). McGraw–Hill.

Teasdale G, Jennett B (1974) Assessment of coma and impaired consciousness. A practical scale. *The Lancet*, **13**: 81–84.

Thanacoody HK, Thomas SH (2005) Tricyclic antidepressant poisoning: cardiovascular toxicity. *Toxicological Reviews*, **24**: 205–214.

Tondo L, Jamison JR, Baldessarini RJ (1997) Effect of lithium maintenance on suicidal behavior in major mood disorders. *Annals of the New York Academy of Sciences*, **836**: 339–351.

Trenton A, Currier G, Zwerner F (2003) Fatalities associated with therapeutic use and overdose of atypical antipsychotics. *CNS Drugs*, **17**: 307–324.

White CM, Gailey TA, Levin GM, *et al* (1997) Seizure resulting from a venlafaxine overdose. *Annals of Pharmacotherapy*, **31**: 178–180.

Worthley LI (2002) Clinical toxicology: Part II. Diagnosis and management of uncommon poisonings. *Critical Care and Resuscitation*, **4**: 216–230.

Young CR, Mazure CM (1998) Fulminant hepatic failure from acetaminophen in an anorexic patient treated with carbamazepine. *Journal of Clinical Psychiatry*, **59**: 622.

Index

Compiled by Linda English